# *Understanding*
# *ıman Anatomy*
# *and Physiology*

## Eldra Pearl Solomon

*Adjunct Biology Professor*
*Hillsborough Community College*
*Tampa, Florida*

## Gloria A. Phillips

*Formerly Chairperson, Allied Health Program*
*Hillsborough Community College*
*Tampa, Florida*

**1987   W.B. Saunders Company**

*Philadelphia / London / Toronto*
*Sydney / Tokyo / Hong Kong*

W. B. Saunders Company:   West Washington Square
Philadelphia, PA 19105

**Library of Congress Cataloging-in-Publication Data**

Solomon, Eldra Pearl.
  Understanding human anatomy and physiology.

  Includes index.
  1. Human physiology.   2. Anatomy, Human.
I. Phillips, Gloria A.   II. Title.   [DNLM: 1. Anatomy.
2. Physiology.   QS 4 S689u]
QP34.5.S694   1987       612       86-17759
ISBN 0-7216-1994-0

A number of the illustrations, tables, and focus boxes in this text are reproduced by courtesy of Saunders College Publishing from
  Davis, W.P., and Solomon, E.P.: The World of Biology. 3rd ed., 1986;
  Solomon, E.P., and Davis, W.P.: Human Anatomy and Physiology. 1983;
  Villee, C.A., Solomon, E.P., and Davis, W.P.: Biology. 1985.

*Editor:*  Michael Brown

*Developmental Editor:*  Frances P. Mues

*Designer:*  Saunders Staff

*Production Manager:*  Bob Butler

*Manuscript Editor:*  Terry Russell

*Illustrators:*  Philip Ashley, Glenn Edelmayer, and Karen Giacomucci

*Illustration Coordinator:*  Peg Shaw

*Page Layout Artist:*  Meg Jolly

Understanding Human Anatomy and Physiology                    ISBN 0-7216-1994-0

Last digit is the print number:     9     8     7     6     5     4     3     2     1

This book is dedicated to the memory of my colleague, coauthor, and friend,

## Dr. Gloria A. Phillips

Gloria was one of the most remarkable human beings I have ever known. She was a nurse, mental health counselor, teacher, author, college administrator, and developer of innovative programs. Most important, she was a friend par excellence. Her warmth and caring touched my life and the lives of countless others in a profound and lasting way.

Gloria and I first spoke of writing this book in 1979 when we team-taught a course in human anatomy and physiology for Human Services students. However, both of us were involved in other projects and it was not until 1985 that we began the task in earnest. Gloria coauthored this book during her last year of life—between a dozen hospitalizations. At a time when most mortals would not have dragged themselves out of bed my courageous coauthor learned to use a word processor and developed manuscript. Gloria remains an inspiration to me. I miss her very much.

# Preface

That body which allows us to think, to see, hear, and feel, to run and play, to create, to experience the planet we inhabit is a marvel of biological engineering. One of our main goals in writing this book is to transmit to the student some of our own excitement about the intricate design and function of the human body.

*Understanding Human Anatomy and Physiology* is designed to meet the needs of students pursuing careers in nursing and the allied health fields. Because the structures of the body are so exquisitely adapted to carry out specific functions, we believe that students can best understand and appreciate anatomy and physiology when they are presented together. For this reason, we have thoroughly integrated anatomy and physiology. We have used a systems, rather than a regional, approach, which further facilitates our focus on the relationship between structure and function.

No assumptions have been made about the student's background in chemistry, physics, or even basic biology. Principles of these disciplines are introduced as necessary for an understanding of the concepts presented.

From our own teaching experience we have found that students learn most effectively and pleasurably when they can immediately apply or relate what they are learning to familiar issues or experiences. Accordingly, as we discuss the workings of the world within, we continuously relate them to the more familiar external world. For example, when discussing pigment cells and melanin we immediately relate their function to tanning and sunburn. When discussing insulin, we describe the metabolic effects of diabetes. The chapter on immune mechanisms considers allergy, organ transplantation, and AIDS. Paragraphs dealing with clinical material are highlighted so that it can be easily identified if the instructer chooses to omit this type of material.

## ORGANIZATION

We have organized the book into seven parts, or units. As indicated in the Table of Contents, each part consists of chapters that focus on a particular aspect of body function. Because instructors may want to vary the sequence of topics covered, or even omit certain chapters, each chapter is self-contained. This permits maximum flexibility in course organization.

## LEARNING AIDS

In developing this book, a great deal of thought and effort have been devoted to the learning process. The following features will help the student master the principles of anatomy and physiology.

**Readability.** Students will find the writing style clear and enjoyable. The reading level is appropriate, and new technical terms are set in boldface. A pronunciation guide is provided immediately following the introduction of each new term that may prove difficult to pronounce correctly. New terms are carefully defined.

**Chapter Outline.** An outline of topics at the beginning of each chapter shows the student how the material is organized and divides the chapter into manageable sections.

**Learning Objectives** at the beginning of each chapter indicate just what the student must be able to do to demonstrate mastery of the material in the chapter.

Numerous **Tables,** many of them illustrated, organize and summarize material throughout the text.

**Focus Boxes** present clinical applications or case studies, or other enrichment material.

**Illustrations** have been carefully designed to support the material in the text. Medical art rendered by qualified medical illustrators helps the student accurately visualize anatomic detail presented in the text. Diagrams, such as the teeter-totters used to illustrate homeostatic mechanisms, aid in understanding concepts presented. Full color is used throughout the book, increasing the teaching value of the illustrations and adding visual appeal. In addition, many anatomic photographs, photomicrographs, radiographs, and CT scans have been included.

A **Summary** in outline form at the end of each chapter helps the student review the main concepts presented in the chapter. An objective **Post-test** at the end of each chapter encourages the student to evaluate mastery of the material. Answers to post-test questions are given in Appendix C at the end of the book. **Review Questions** provide the student with the opportunity to further check understanding of concepts, to apply them, and to synthesize some of the material presented.

The combined Index-Glossary includes definitions for important terms used in the book.

Appendix A presents common prefixes, suffixes, and word roots.

Metric system information and equivalents are given in Appendix B.

# Acknowledgments

Many people—colleagues, editors, friends, family members—contributed to the development of this book. Special thanks to Al Brod, M.D., who carefully reviewed clinically oriented portions of the manuscript and offered valuable input. I appreciate Dr. Richard Schmidt's expertise in reviewing the medical illustrations. I thank Professor Sherry Kersey for her suggestions and Nell Gillis for casting her skilled editorial eye through the manuscript. I am grateful to my friends Dr. Ann Landsman, Larry Pasman, Drs. James and Connie Messina for their support and encouragement during Gloria Phillip's illness and after her untimely death. I also thank Gloria's family, especially Randy Phillips and Aggie Dollar.

I want to thank Phala Pesano for doing the bulk of the word processing and for helping us put the Index-Glossary together. I am grateful to Amy Solomon for jumping in whenever additional word processing help was needed, and to Mical Solomon for keeping the computer systems going. Belicia Efros willingly lent a helping hand whenever asked.

The editorial staff at W. B. Saunders was wonderful. Our acquisitions editor, Michael Brown, helped us design the project and was there throughout to solve expertly every problem that emerged. Our talented and dedicated developmental editor, Fran Mues, offered many valuable suggestions for improving the manuscript. In the Production Department, we especially thank Wynette Kommer, Pat Morrison, Philip Ashley, and copy editor Terry Russell.

We appreciate the input of the following reviewers.

Marilyn Boyer, RN, BSN
Erwin Vocational-Technical Center
Tampa, Florida

Gene H. Campbell, BSN, MEd
Opelika Vocational School
Opelika, Alabama

Eva Kasten, MS
Bergen Pines County Hospital
Paramus, New Jersey

Mary E. Schwalb, RN, BSNEd
Rochester General Hospital
Rochester, New York

Jean Stutes Broussard, BSN
Southwest Louisiana Vocational-
   Technical Institute
Crowley, Louisiana

Jan Harris, EdD, MS, MSEd, BSEd
Central Oklahoma AUTS
Drumright, Oklahoma

Aileen L. Rowand, RN, BSNEd, MEd
Decatur Vocational Center
Decatur, Illinois

Lorraine Soda, RN, BS Health
   Education
Essex County Technical Career Center
Newark, New Jersey

ELDRA PEARL SOLOMON

# Contents

# I

# ORGANIZATION OF THE BODY

# Introducing the Human Body

LEARNING OBJECTIVES

**After you study this chapter you should be able to**
1. Define anatomy and physiology and give examples of their subdisciplines, as given in this chapter.
2. List in sequence the levels of biological organization in the human body, beginning with the chemical level.
3. List the functions of the 10 principal body systems.
4. Define metabolism and homeostasis and give examples of these processes.
5. Describe the anatomical position.
6. Define and use properly the principal directional terms used in human anatomy.
7. Identify on diagrams sagittal, transverse, and frontal sections of the body or its structures such as blood vessels or the brain.
8. Define and locate the principal regions and cavities of the human body.

No machine known, not even the most sophisticated computer, begins to rival the complexity of the human body. How each of its millions of parts are constructed, and how they work together in the living, functioning body, is the fascinating subject matter of this book.

This book can be considered an owner's manual for the human body. It is an introduction to **anatomy** (uh-**nat'**-uh-me), the science of body structure, and to **physiology** (fiz-ee-**ol'**-uh-jee), the study of body function. The anatomy and physiology of the body are intricately interrelated. Each structure is marvelously adapted for carrying out its specific function. The muscular walls of the heart, for example, are especially constructed for pumping blood from its hollow chambers. Blood is forced into large blood vessels with elastic walls that permit the vessels to expand as they fill with blood and then snap back to normal size. Between the chambers of the heart, flaplike valves prevent the blood from flowing backward.

As you proceed with your study of the human body look for the relationships between the structure and function of the body parts you are studying. Try to understand how the size, shape, and structure of each part is related to the job it must perform.

Anatomy and physiology are broad fields with many subdisciplines. **Gross anatomy**, for example, deals with organs and structures of the body that can be studied by dissection, whereas microscopic anatomy, the study of tissue, is known as **histology**. The study of the structure of individual cells is called **cytology**. **Embryology** is the study of the development of the organism before birth, and **pathology** is the study of disease processes. In our study of the human body we will deal with all these subdisciplines, and many others.

Medical science is an applied form of anatomy and physiology that uses the findings of anatomists and physiologists to maintain health and to treat disease. Some career applications are briefly described in the Focus on Some Careers in the Health Sciences.

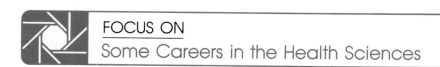

## FOCUS ON
## Some Careers in the Health Sciences

| | |
|---|---|
| **Nursing** | Registered nurses (RN) or licensed practical nurses (LPN) assist physicians in the examination and care of patients. |
| **Radiologic technology** | Radiologic technologists assist physicians with diagnostic radiologic procedures, including routine x-ray, computerized tomography (CT), magnetic resonance imaging (MRI), and angiographic procedures (visualizing blood vessels). |
| **Radiation therapy technology** | Radiation therapy technologists assist physicians with the management, control, and care of patients receiving radiation therapy treatment. |
| **Nuclear medicine technology** | Nuclear medicine technologists assist in the preparation and examination of patients when radioactive substances are used, such as in nuclear scanning. |
| **Emergency medical technology** | Emergency medical technicians with ambulance training perform basic life support measures at the scene of accidents. Paramedics are further trained in advanced life support. |
| **Human services technology** | Human services technicians serve as paraprofessionals in community agencies dealing in human services/mental health. Under professional supervision they perform such services as counseling and case management. |
| **Occupational therapy** | Occupational therapists work with patients debilitated by accidents, stroke, or other diseases. The therapist's job is to teach patients how to manage everyday tasks within their physical limitations. |
| **Physical therapy** | Physical therapists work with patients debilitated by accidents, stroke, or other diseases. They teach patients exercises to maintain muscle tone and strengthen muscles. |
| **Respiratory therapy** | The respiratory therapist administers treatments for respiratory tract disorders as prescribed by the patient's physician. |

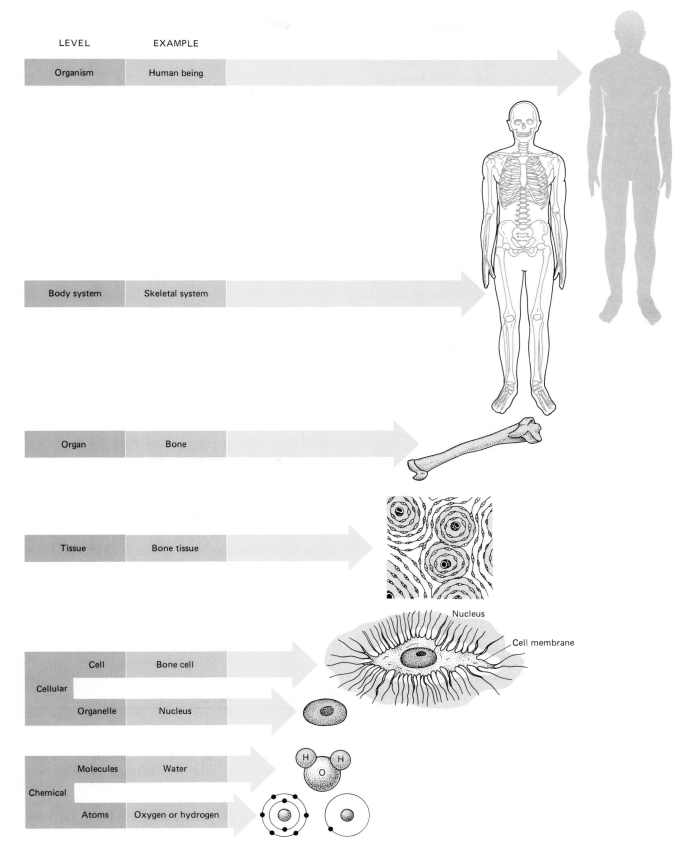

LEVEL

EXAMPLE

Organism — Human being

Body system — Skeletal system

Organ — Bone

Tissue — Bone tissue

Cell — Bone cell

Cellular

Organelle — Nucleus

Nucleus

Cell membrane

Molecules — Water

Chemical

Atoms — Oxygen or hydrogen

H    H

O

**Figure 1–1.** Levels of structural organization in the human body. Note the hierarchy from simple to complex.

## THE ORGANIZATION OF THE BODY

One of the most striking features of the body is its exquisite organization. The simplest level of structural organization is the **chemical level**, consisting of atoms and molecules. **Atoms** are the basic units of all matter. An atom is the smallest amount of a chemical element (pure chemical substance such as iron or calcium) that retains the characteristic properties of that element. Atoms can combine chemically to form **molecules**. For example, two atoms of hydrogen combine with one atom of oxygen to produce a molecule of water.

In our hierarchy of organization, the next most complex level is the **cellular level** (Fig. 1–1). In living organisms atoms and molecules associate in specific ways to form cells, the basic building blocks of the body. The human body is composed of about 100 trillion cells of many distinct types, such as blood cells and muscle cells. Although cells vary in size and shape according to their functions, most are so small that they are visible only with a microscope. Each cell consists of specialized cell parts called **organelles**. One organelle, the **nucleus**, serves as the information and control center of the cell. Several other kinds of organelles scattered throughout the cell perform specific functions such as manufacturing needed substances or breaking down fuel molecules to provide energy.

A **tissue** is a group of closely associated cells specialized to perform particular functions. The four main types of tissue in the body are muscle tissue, nervous tissue, connective tissue, and epithelial tissue. Tissues will be discussed in Chapter 3.

Various types of tissue are organized into functional structures called **organs**, such as the brain, stomach, or heart. Although the heart consists mainly of a type of muscle tissue called cardiac muscle, it is covered by epithelial tissue and also contains connective and nervous tissue.

A coordinated group of tissues and organs makes up a **body system**, or organ system. The circulatory system, for example, consists of the heart, blood vessels, blood, lymph structures, and several other organs. Working together with great precision and complexity the body systems make up the living **organism (or′-guh-nizm)**—that is, you yourself.

## THE BODY SYSTEMS

A body system consists of a group of tissues and organs that work together to perform specific func-tions. Each system contributes to the dynamic, carefully balanced state of the body. Table 1–1 summarizes and Figure 1–2 illustrates the 10 systems of the human body.

## METABOLISM

All the chemical processes that occur within the body are collectively referred to as its **metabolism (meh-tab′-oh-lizm)**. Metabolic processes are essential to digestion, growth and repair of the body, and conversion of food energy into forms useful to the body. Other metabolic processes maintain the routine operations of the nerves, muscles, and other body parts.

## HOMEOSTASIS

Metabolic activities take place continuously and must be precisely regulated to maintain a constant internal environment, or **steady state**. The steady state of the body must be preserved even in the face of changing conditions in the external environment. Temperature within the body must be maintained within narrow limits and an appropriate concentration of nutrients, oxygen and other gases, and various chemicals must be present at all times.

The term **homeostasis (home-ee-oh-stay′-sis)** refers to the body's automatic tendency to maintain its steady states. The control systems that maintain a constant, appropriate internal environment are called **homeostatic mechanisms** (Fig. 1–3). Any stimulus that disrupts homeostasis is a **stressor**. When homeostatic mechanisms are unable to compensate for the resulting stress and restore the steady state, the stress may lead to a malfunction, which can cause disease or even death.

## PLAN OF THE BODY

The body consists of right and left halves that are mirror images, that is, it exhibits **bilateral symmetry**. Two other important features are the **cranium (kray′-nee-um)**, or brain case, and the **vertebral column**, or backbone, structures that characterize us as vertebrates. Humans are also mammals and so have hair, mammary (milk) glands, and four limbs, each with five digits bearing nails.

TABLE 1–1
**The Body Systems**

| System | Components | Functions | Homeostatic ability |
|---|---|---|---|
| *Integumentary* | Skin, hair, nails, sweat glands | Covers and protects body | Sweat glands help control body temperature; as barrier, skin helps maintain steady state |
| *Skeletal* | Bones, cartilage, ligaments | Supports body, protects; muscles attach to bones; provides calcium storage | Helps maintain constant calcium level in blood |
| *Muscular* | Skeletal muscle, cardiac muscle, smooth muscle | Moves parts of skeleton, locomotion; pumps blood; aids movement of internal materials | Ensures such vital functions as nutrition through body movements; smooth muscle maintains blood pressure; cardiac muscle circulates the blood |
| *Nervous* | Nerves and sense organs, brain and spinal cord | Receives stimuli from external and internal environment, conducts impulses, integrates activities of other systems | Principal regulatory system |
| *Endocrine* | Pituitary, adrenal, thyroid, and other ductless glands | Regulates body chemistry and many body functions | Together with nervous system, regulates metabolic activities and blood levels of various substances |
| *Circulatory* | Heart, blood vessels, blood; lymph and lymph structures | Transports materials from one part of body to another; defends body against disease | Transports oxygen, nutrients, hormones; removes wastes; maintains water and ionic balance of tissues |
| *Respiratory* | Lungs and air passageways | Exchanges of gases between blood and external environment | Maintains adequate blood oxygen content; eliminates carbon dioxide |
| *Digestive* | Mouth, esophagus, stomach, intestines, liver, pancreas | Ingests and digests foods, absorbs them into blood | Maintains adequate supplies of fuel molecules and building materials |
| *Urinary* | Kidney, bladder, and associated ducts | Excretes metabolic wastes; removes substances present in excess from blood | Regulates blood chemistry in conjunction with endocrine system |
| *Reproductive* | Testes, ovaries, and associated structures | Reproduction; provides for continuation of species | Passes on genetic endowment of individual; maintains secondary sex characteristics |

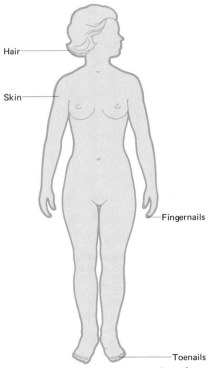

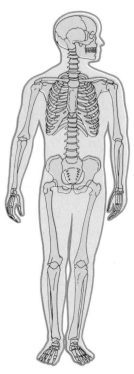

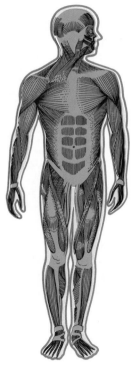

Hair

Skin

Fingernails

Toenails

(1) The integumentary system consists of the skin and the structures derived from it. This system protects the body, helps to regulate body temperature, and receives stimuli such as pressure, pain, and temperature.

(2) The skeletal system consists of bones and cartilage. This system helps to support and protect the body.

(3) The muscular system consists of the large skeletal muscles that enable us to move, as well as the cardiac muscle of the heart and the smooth muscle of the internal organs.

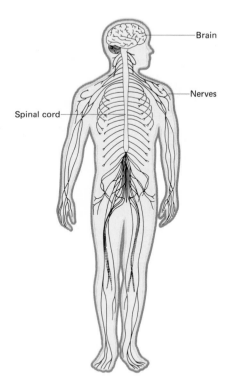

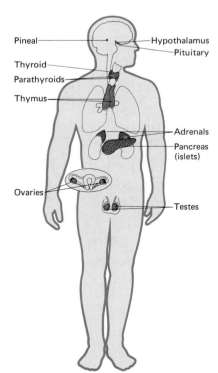

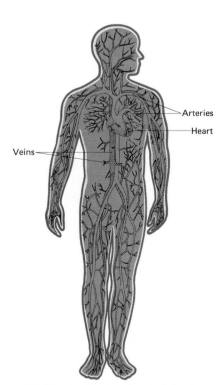

Brain

Nerves

Spinal cord

Pineal

Hypothalamus

Pituitary

Thyroid

Parathyroids

Thymus

Adrenals

Pancreas (islets)

Ovaries

Testes

Arteries

Heart

Veins

(4) The nervous system consists of the brain, spinal cord, sense organs, and nerves. The nervous system is the principal regulatory system.

(5) The endocrine system consists of the ductless glands that release hormones. It works with the nervous system in regulating metabolic activities.

(6a) The circulatory system includes the heart and blood vessels. This system serves as the transportation system of the body.

*Figure 1–2.* *The principal systems of the human body.*

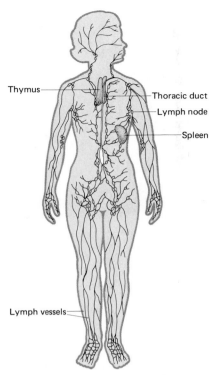

Thymus

Thoracic duct

Lymph node

Spleen

Lymph vessels

(*6b*) The lymphatic system is a subsystem of the circulatory system; it returns excess tissue fluid to the blood and defends the body against disease.

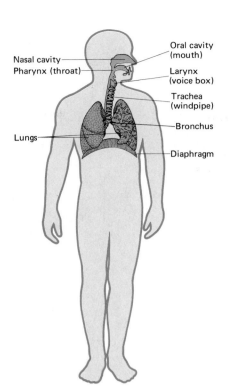

Nasal cavity
Pharynx (throat)

Oral cavity (mouth)

Larynx (voice box)

Trachea (windpipe)

Bronchus

Lungs

Diaphragm

(*7*) The respiratory system consists of the lungs and air passageways. This system supplies oxygen to the blood and rids the body of carbon dioxide.

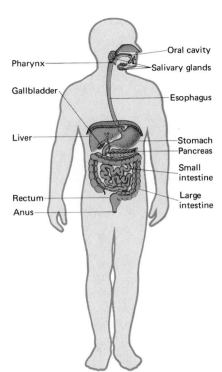

Pharynx

Oral cavity

Salivary glands

Gallbladder

Esophagus

Liver

Stomach
Pancreas

Small intestine

Rectum

Large intestine

Anus

(*8*) The digestive system consists of the digestive tract and glands that secrete digestive juices into the digestive tract. This system mechanically and chemically breaks down food and eliminates wastes.

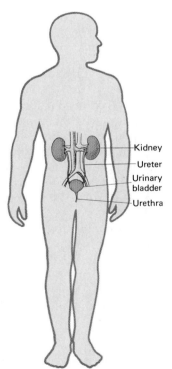

Kidney

Ureter

Urinary bladder

Urethra

(*9*) The urinary system is the main excretory system. The kidneys remove wastes and excess materials from the blood and produce urine. This system helps regulate blood chemistry.

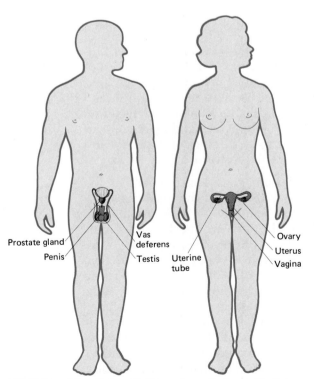

Prostate gland

Penis

Vas deferens

Testis

Uterine tube

Ovary

Uterus

Vagina

(*10*) Male and female reproductive systems. Each reproductive system consists of gonads and associated structures. The reproductive system maintains sexual characteristics and perpetuates the species.

*Figure 1–2* Continued

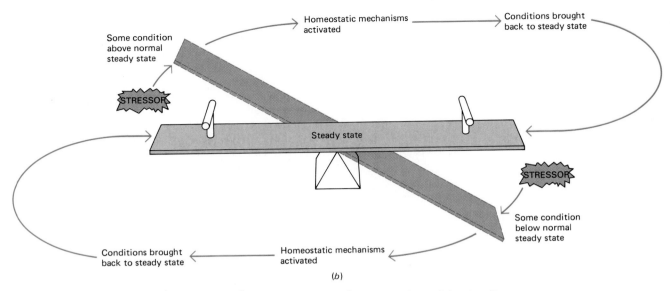

**Figure 1–3.** *Homeostasis: the process of maintaining steady states. Stressful stimuli, called stressors, disrupt homeostasis. In the body, any deviation from the steady state is regarded as stress. Stress activates an appropriate homeostatic mechanism that brings conditions back toward the steady state.*

## The General Directions

To identify the structures of the body it is useful to learn some basic terms and directions. Directional terms in human anatomy are relative, somewhat like directional terms in geography. Thus one could say that New York City is north of Washington, D.C., but south of Boston or that Chicago is west of Philadelphia but east of San Francisco. Bear this in mind as you learn the anatomical directional terms. These terms are applied to the body when it is in the **anatomical position**, which means that the body is standing erect, eyes looking forward, arms at the sides of the body, and palms and toes directed forward (Fig. 1–4).

1. **Superior/inferior**. The "North Pole" of the human body is the top of the head, its superior point. Its "South Pole" is represented by the soles of the feet, its most inferior part (Fig. 1–4). Thus the heart is superior to the stomach because it is closer to the head. The heart is inferior to the brain. The stomach is inferior to the heart. The terms **cephalic** (seh-fal′-ik) and **cranial** are sometimes used instead of the word superior. In human anatomy, the term **caudal** (toward the tail) is sometimes used instead of the word inferior.
2. **Anterior/posterior**. The front (belly) surface of the body is anterior, or **ventral**. The stomach is anterior to the vertebral column (backbone). The back surface of the body is posterior, or **dorsal**. The vertebral column is posterior to the stomach.
3. **Medial/lateral**. The body axis is an imaginary line extending from the center of the top of the head to the groin. This main superior-inferior body axis is medial, going right through the midline of the body. A structure is said to be medial if it is closer to the midline of the body than to another structure. The naval is medial to the hip bone. A structure is lateral if it is toward one side of the body. Thus the hip bone is lateral to the navel.
4. **Proximal/distal**. When a structure is closer to the body midline or point of attachment to the trunk, it is described as proximal. This term is used especially in locating limb structures. Thus the wrist is proximal to the fingers. Distal means farther from the midline or point of attachment to the trunk. The fingers are distal to the wrist.
5. **Superficial/deep**. Structures located toward the surface of the body are superficial. Blood vessels in the skin are superficial to those lying beneath in the muscle. Structures located farther inward (away from the body surface) are deep. Blood vessels in the muscle are deep to those in the skin.

## Body Planes and Sections

In anatomic study as well as in clinical practice it is often helpful to visualize internal structures by cutting the body into sections, or slices. Such

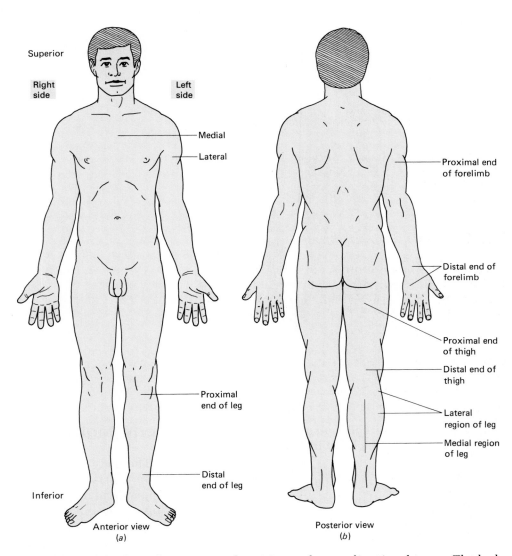

**Figure 1–4.** *The body in the anatomical position and some directional terms. The body is erect, eyes forward, arms at the sides, and palms and toes directed forward. (a) Anterior view. (b) Posterior view.*

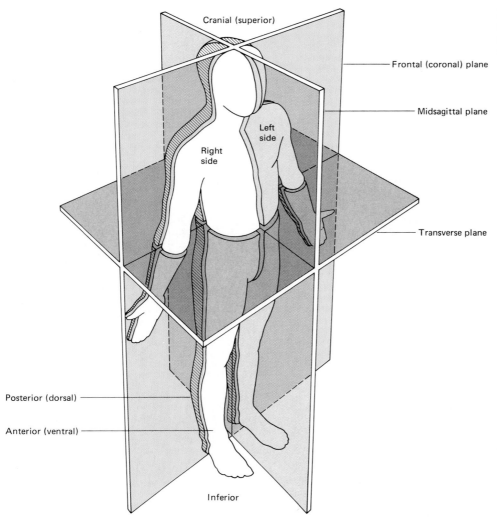

*Figure 1–5. Planes of section. The body or its parts may be cut in sagittal, transverse, or frontal sections.*

cuts are made along body planes, imaginary flat surfaces that divide the body into parts (Fig. 1–5).

1. **Sagittal** (**sadj'**-i-tul). A sagittal plane divides the body into right and left parts. A midsagittal (or median) plane passes through the body axis and divides the body into two (almost) mirror-image halves.
2. **Transverse.** A plane at right angles to the body axis is a transverse or **cross section**. It divides the body into superior and inferior parts.
3. **Frontal** (or **coronal**). A plane that divides the body into anterior and posterior parts is a frontal section.

In many diagnostic procedures bits of tissues or organs are removed from the body and sliced (sectioned) so that they can be examined by a pathologist for signs of disease. Many of the illustrations in this book depict blood vessels or other structures that have been cut in various planes.

## Body Regions

The body may be subdivided into an **axial** portion, consisting of head, neck, and trunk, and an **appendicular** (ap-pen-**dik'**-u-lar) portion, consisting of the limbs. The trunk, or **torso**, consists of the thorax, abdomen, and pelvis (Fig. 1–6).

Some of the terms used to indicate specific body regions or structures follow.

| Term | Region of the Body Referred To |
|---|---|
| Abdominal | Portion of trunk below the diaphragm |
| Arm | Technically, the part of the upper extremity between the shoulder and the elbow, as distinguished from the forearm (popularly, the term arm refers to the entire upper extremity) |

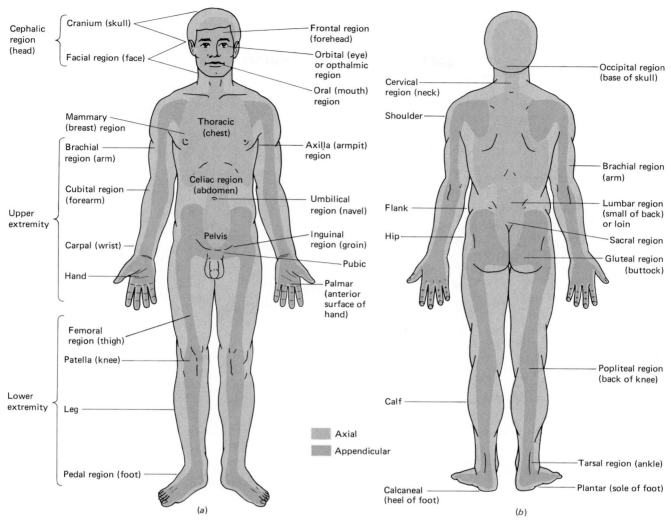

**Figure 1–6.** *Some specific regions of the body. (a) Anterior view. (b) Posterior view.*

| | | | |
|---|---|---|---|
| Axillary (**ak′**-sih-lar″-ee) | Armpit area | Costal (**kos′**-tal) | Ribs |
| Brachial (**bray′**-kee-al) | Arm | Cranial | Skull |
| Buccal (**buk′**-al) | Inner surfaces of the cheeks | Cubital | Elbow or forearm |
| Carpal (**kar′**-pal) | Wrist | Cutaneous (ku-**tay′**-nee-us) | Skin |
| Celiac (**see′**-lee-ak) | Abdomen | Femoral (**fem′**-or-al) | Thigh; the part of the lower extremity between the hip and the knee |
| Cephalic | Head | Forearm | Upper extremity between the elbow and the wrist |
| Cervical | Neck region | Frontal | Forehead |

Gluteal
(**gloo'**-tee-al)
— Buttock

Groin — Depressed region between the abdomen and the thigh

Inguinal
(**ing'**-gwih-nal)
— Groin

Leg — Lower extremity, especially the part from the knee to the foot

Lumbar — Loin; the region of the lower back and side, between the lowest rib and the pelvis

Mammary — Breasts

Occipital
(ok-**sip'**-ih-tal)
— Back of the head

Ophthalmic
(of-**thal'**-mik)
— Eyes

Oral — Mouth

Palmar — Palm

Pectoral
(**pek'**-tow-ral)
— Chest

Pedal — Foot

Pelvic — Pelvis; the bony ring that girdles the lower portion of the trunk

Perineal
(per"-ih-**nee'**-al)
— Region between the anus and the pubic arch; includes the region of the external reproductive structures

Plantar — Sole of the foot

Popliteal
(pop-**lit'**-ee-al)
— Area behind the knee

Tarsal — Ankle

Thoracic
(thow-**ras'**-ik)
— Chest; the part of the trunk below the neck and above the diaphragm

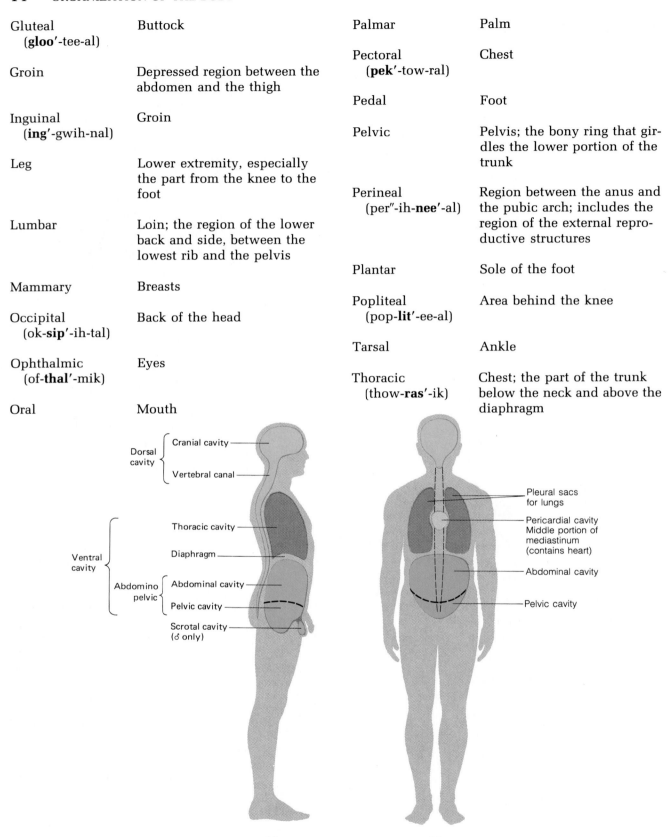

(a)    (b)

**Figure 1–7.** Principal cavities of the human body. (a) Lateral view of the body showing dorsal and ventral cavities and some of their subdivisions. (b) Anterior view, showing subdivisions of the ventral cavity.

## Body Cavities

The spaces within the body, called **body cavities**, contain the internal organs, or **viscera** (vis'-ur-uh). The two principal body cavities are the **dorsal cavity** and the **ventral cavity** (Fig. 1–7). The bony dorsal cavity, located near the dorsal (posterior) body surface, may be subdivided into the **cranial cavity**, which holds the brain, and the **vertebral** or **spinal canal**, which contains the spinal cord. The ventral cavity, located near the ventral (anterior) body surface, is subdivided in turn into the **thoracic**, or chest, **cavity** and the **abdominopelvic** (ab-dom"-ih-no-**pel**'-vik) **cavity**.

Thoracic and abdominopelvic cavities are separated by a broad muscle, the **diaphragm** (die'-uh-fram), which forms the floor of the thoracic cavity. Divisions of the thoracic cavity are the **pleural sacs**, each containing a lung, and the **mediastinum** (me"-dee-as-tie'-num) between them. Within the mediastinum lie the heart, thymus gland, and parts of the esophagus and trachea. The heart is

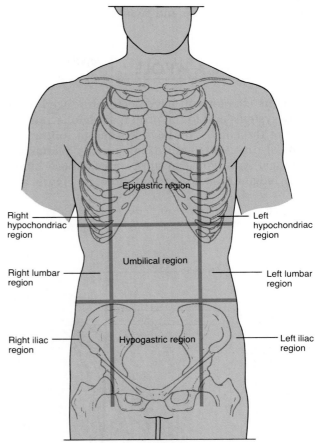

Right hypochondriac region

Left hypochondriac region

Epigastric region

Right lumbar region

Umbilical region

Left lumbar region

Right iliac region

Hypogastric region

Left iliac region

*Figure 1–9.* The abdominopelvic cavity can be divided into nine regions using two transverse and two sagittal planes. These regions can be used clinically to locate internal organs.

surrounded by yet another cavity, the **pericardial** (per"-ee-**kar**'-dee-al) **cavity**.

The upper portion of the abdominopelvic cavity is the **abdominal cavity**, which contains the stomach, small intestine, much of the large intestine, liver, pancreas, spleen, kidneys, and ureters. Although not separated by any kind of wall, the lower portion of the abdominopelvic cavity is the **pelvic cavity**, which holds the urinary bladder, part of the large intestine, and in the female, the reproductive organs. In males, the pelvic cavity has a small outpocket called the **scrotal cavity**, which contains the testes.

To simplify the task of identifying structures or locating pain, health professionals sometimes divide the abdominopelvic cavity into four quadrants: right upper or superior; right lower or inferior; left lower or inferior; and left upper or superior (Fig. 1–8). These quadrants are established by a midsagittal and a transverse plane that pass through the umbilicus. Another system divides the abdominopelvic cavity into nine regions

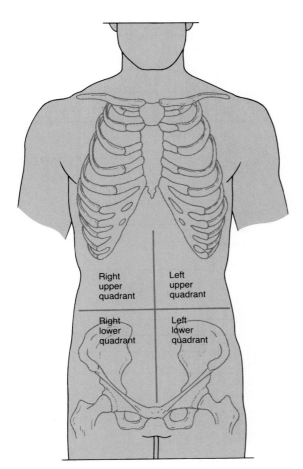

Right upper quadrant

Left upper quadrant

Right lower quadrant

Left lower quadrant

*Figure 1–8.* The abdominopelvic cavity can be divided into four quadrants by drawing imaginary transverse and sagittal lines through the umbilicus (navel).

using two transverse and two sagittal planes (Fig. 1–9).

## THE BODY AS A WHOLE

In this chapter you have been introduced to the body systems and to the principal regions and cavities of the body. You have learned to follow anatomical directions and visualize body planes and sections. Now you can apply all of these bits of knowledge to the body as a whole. In Figure 1–10 all the parts have been put back together so that you can study them in relation to one another and to the body as an integrated, functioning organism. In Figure 1–11 some of the more superficial anterior structures have been removed so that you can see the structures that lie beneath them.

Anterior structures have been progressively removed in Figures 1–11 through 1–13 so that you can study the relationships of the deeper organs. Figure 1–14 is a dorsal view. A different perspective is provided in Figure 1–15; the transverse sections through the head, mediastinum, and abdo-

*Text continued on page 22*

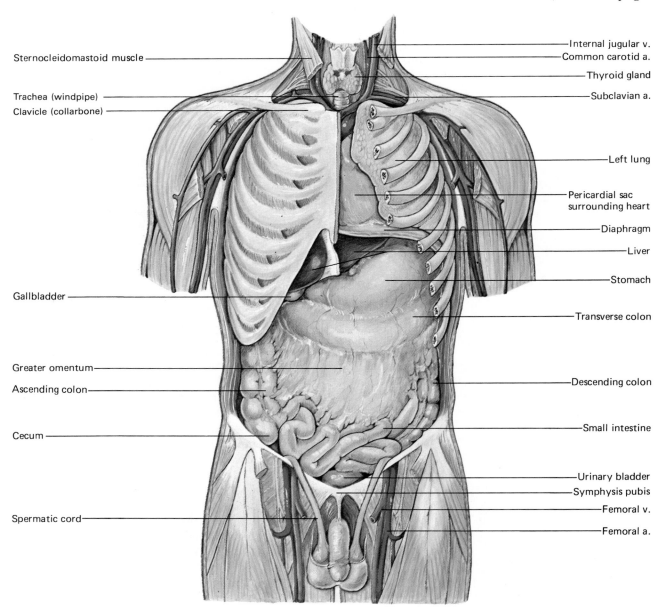

Sternocleidomastoid muscle

Trachea (windpipe)

Clavicle (collarbone)

Gallbladder

Greater omentum

Ascending colon

Cecum

Spermatic cord

Internal jugular v.

Common carotid a.

Thyroid gland

Subclavian a.

Left lung

Pericardial sac surrounding heart

Diaphragm

Liver

Stomach

Transverse colon

Descending colon

Small intestine

Urinary bladder

Symphysis pubis

Femoral v.

Femoral a.

**Figure 1–10.** *Anterior view of the body with skin and muscles removed. Note that much of the abdominal viscera is covered by the greater omentum, a fatty membrane that hangs down from the stomach. (a., Artery; v., vein.) Many of the structures shown here and in Figures 1–11 through 1–15 will be discussed in later chapters.*

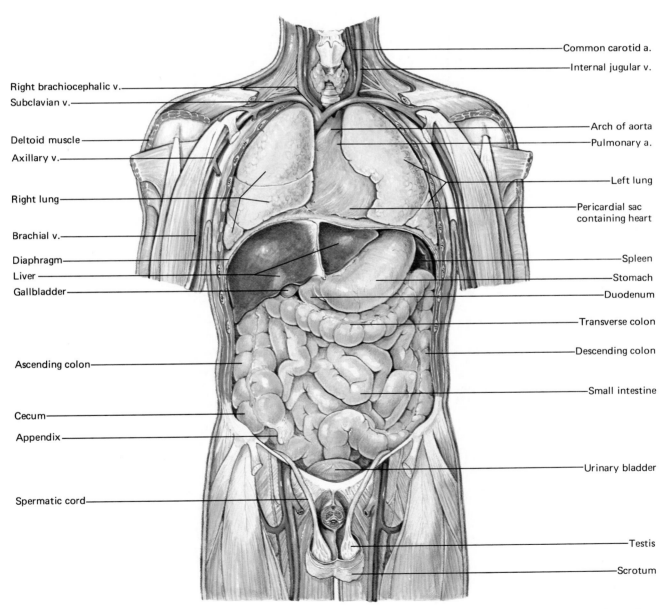

Common carotid a.

Internal jugular v.

Right brachiocephalic v.

Subclavian v.

Deltoid muscle

Axillary v.

Right lung

Brachial v.

Diaphragm

Liver

Gallbladder

Ascending colon

Cecum

Appendix

Spermatic cord

Arch of aorta

Pulmonary a.

Left lung

Pericardial sac containing heart

Spleen

Stomach

Duodenum

Transverse colon

Descending colon

Small intestine

Urinary bladder

Testis

Scrotum

**Figure 1–11.** Anterior view of the body. The rib cage and greater omentum have been removed to show the locations of the underlying viscera.

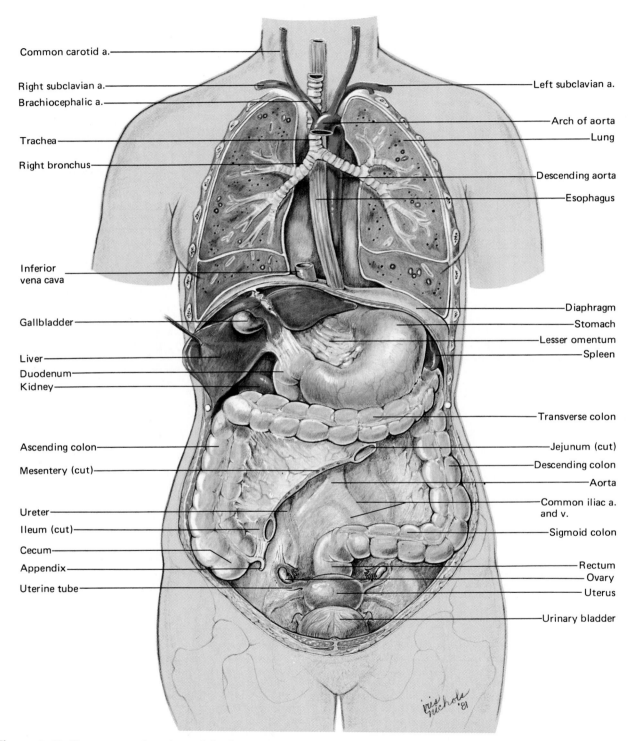

**Figure 1–12.** Deeper anterior view of the body. The lungs have been sectioned and the heart and small intestine have been removed.

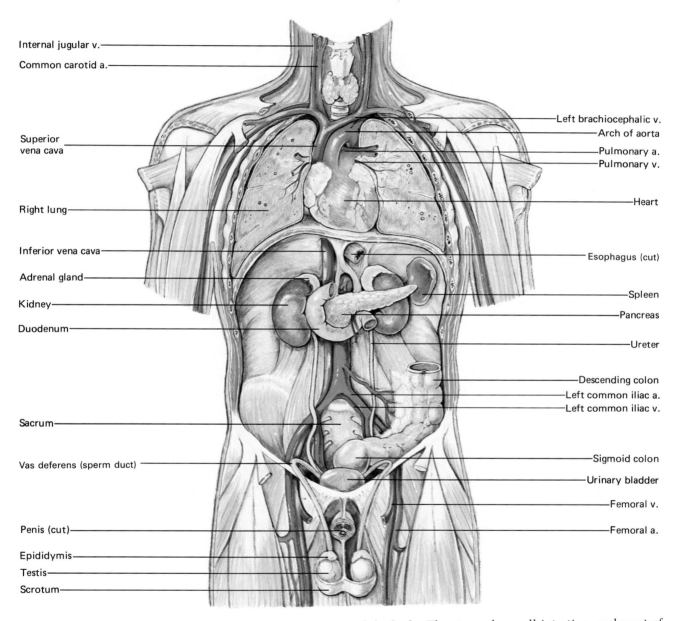

Internal jugular v.
Common carotid a.
Superior vena cava
Right lung
Inferior vena cava
Adrenal gland
Kidney
Duodenum
Sacrum
Vas deferens (sperm duct)
Penis (cut)
Epididymis
Testis
Scrotum

Left brachiocephalic v.
Arch of aorta
Pulmonary a.
Pulmonary v.
Heart
Esophagus (cut)
Spleen
Pancreas
Ureter
Descending colon
Left common iliac a.
Left common iliac v.
Sigmoid colon
Urinary bladder
Femoral v.
Femoral a.

***Figure 1–13.*** *Deep anterior view of the body. The stomach, small intestine, and most of the large intestine have been removed. The kidneys, pancreas, and other deep structures are visible.*

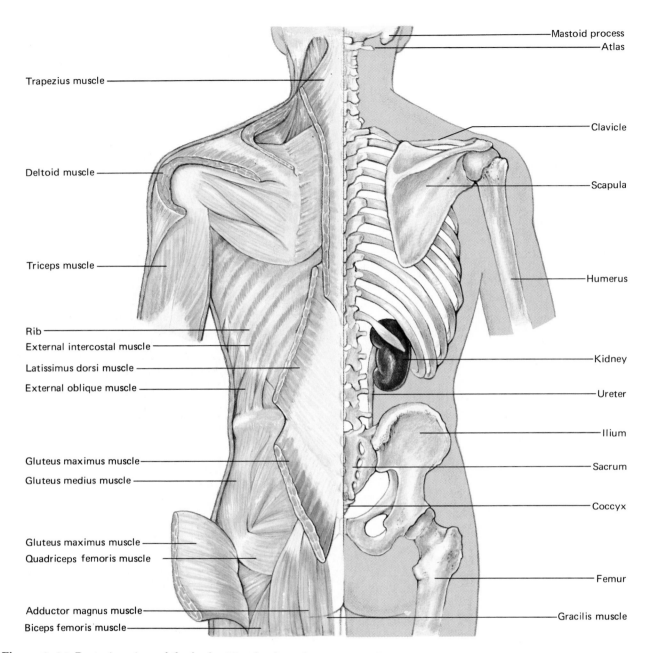

Trapezius muscle

Deltoid muscle

Triceps muscle

Rib
External intercostal muscle
Latissimus dorsi muscle
External oblique muscle

Gluteus maximus muscle
Gluteus medius muscle

Gluteus maximus muscle
Quadriceps femoris muscle

Adductor magnus muscle
Biceps femoris muscle

Mastoid process
Atlas

Clavicle

Scapula

Humerus

Kidney

Ureter

Ilium

Sacrum

Coccyx

Femur

Gracilis muscle

**Figure 1–14.** *Posterior view of the body. Muscles have been removed to show the skeletal structures and position of the kidneys.*

**Figure 1–15.** *A series of CT scans through various regions of the body. The level of the scan is indicated on the figure of the body. The color spectrum bar indicates the gradient of structure density as represented by color. The most dense structures, such as bone, appear white in the CT scans. The least dense structures appear orange. (CT scans courtesy of Professor Jon H. Ehringer.)*

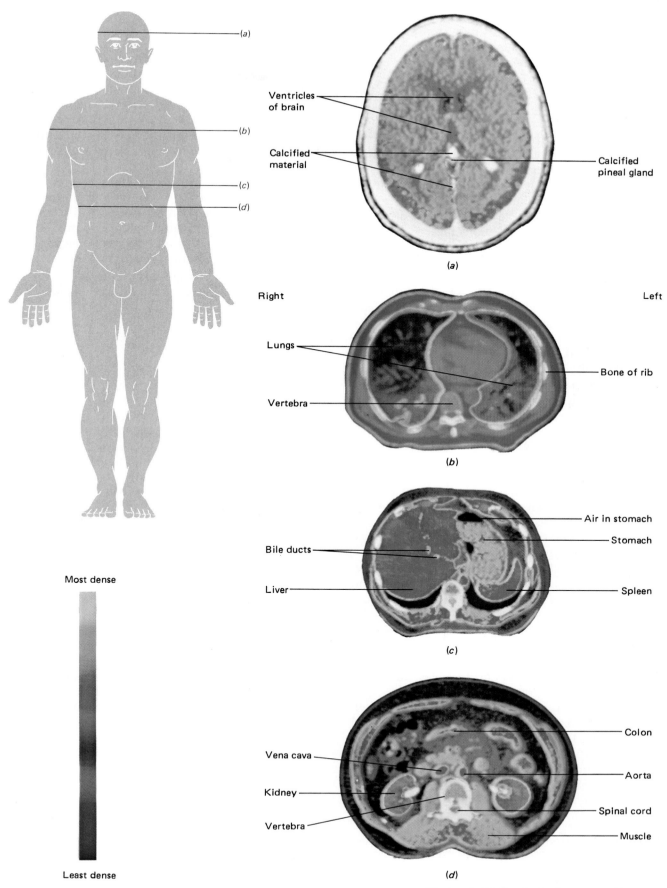

Most dense

Least dense

Ventricles
of brain

Calcified
material

Calcified
pineal gland

(a)

Right                                                              Left

Lungs

Bone of rib

Vertebra

(b)

Air in stomach

Stomach

Bile ducts

Liver

Spleen

(c)

Colon

Vena cava

Aorta

Kidney

Spinal cord

Vertebra

Muscle

(d)

***Figure 1–15.*** See legend on opposite page

men provide the opportunity to study the relationships between anterior and posterior structures within each of these body regions.

## SUMMARY

I. Anatomy is the science of body structure; physiology is the study of function, or how the body works.

II. We can identify several levels of organization within the human body.
   A. The chemical level of organization includes atoms and molecules.
   B. Atoms and molecules associate to form cellular organelles and cells.
   C. Cells associate to form tissues, which are specialized to perform specific functions.
   D. Tissues may be organized to form organs such as the brain or heart.
   E. Tissues and organs may function together to make up a body system.
   F. Ten body systems work together to make up the human organism.

III. The body can be divided into 10 different body systems that operate to maintain its integrity.
   A. The integumentary system (1) provides a protective covering for the body and helps regulate body temperature.
   B. The skeletal (2) and muscular (3) systems work together as a mechanical system to permit effective movement.
   C. The nervous (4) and endocrine (5) systems regulate the activities of the body.
   D. The circulatory system (6) transports nutrients and oxygen to all body cells and carries waste from the cells to the excretory organs. The cardiovascular and lymphatic systems are part of the circulatory system.
   E. The respiratory system (7) delivers oxygen to the blood and removes carbon dioxide from the body.
   F. The digestive system (8) breaks down food so that nutrients can be absorbed into the blood.
   G. Waste disposal and regulation of blood composition are the functions of the urinary system (9).
   H. The reproductive system (10) of the male

produces and delivers sperm; the reproductive system of the female produces ova (eggs) and incubates the developing offspring. Both systems secrete hormones that establish and maintain sexuality.

IV. Metabolism includes all of the chemical processes that take place within the body. Homeostasis is the body's automatic tendency to maintain a constant internal environment, or steady state.

V. Anatomical directional terms are applied to the body when it is in the anatomical position. In this position the body is standing erect, eyes looking forward, arms at the sides, and palms and toes directed forward. The principal directional terms are

| Term | Orientation |
|---|---|
| Superior (cephalic) | Upward; toward the head |
| Inferior | Downward; toward the feet |
| Anterior (ventral) | Belly surface; toward the front of the body |
| Posterior (dorsal) | Back surface; toward the back of the body |
| Medial | Toward the midline |
| Lateral | Toward the side |
| Proximal | Toward the midline or points of attachment to the trunk |
| Distal | Away from the midline or point of attachment to the trunk |
| Superficial | Toward the body surface |
| Deep | Within the body |

VI. The body or its organs may be cut along imaginary planes to produce different types of sections.
   A. A sagittal plane divides the body into right and left parts.
   B. A transverse (or cross) plane divides the body into superior and inferior parts.
   C. A frontal (or coronal) plane divides the body into anterior and posterior parts.

VII. The body may be divided into axial and appendicular regions. Terms such as abdominal, pectoral, and lumbar are used to refer to specific body regions or structures.

VIII. Two principal body cavities are the dorsal cavity and the ventral cavity.
   A. The dorsal cavity includes the cranial cavity and the vertebral canal.
   B. The ventral cavity is subdivided into the thoracic and abdominopelvic cavities.

## POST TEST

1. The science of body structure is _____; the study of body function is _____.

2. Atoms combine chemically to form _____.
3. The basic building blocks of the body are called _____.
4. Various types of tissues may be organized to form _____.
5. The system that includes the pituitary and thyroid glands is the _____ system.
6. The automatic tendency of the body to maintain a constant internal environment is called _____.

*Select the most appropriate answer from Column B for each item in Column A. You may use an answer once, more than once, or not at all.*

| **Column A** | **Column B** |
|---|---|
| 7. _____ The body's principal regulatory system | a. endocrine system |
| 8. _____ Includes the skin | b. integumentary system |
| 9. _____ Functions to support and protect the body | c. circulatory system |
| 10. _____ Transportation system | d. nervous system |
| 11. _____ Maintains adequate blood oxygen content | e. respiratory system |
| 12. _____ Its organs are the ductless glands that secrete hormones | f. skeletal system |

| **Column A** | **Column B** |
|---|---|
| 13. _____ Heart in relation to lung | a. superficial |
| 14. _____ Wrist in relation to elbow | b. medial |
| 15. _____ Knee in relation to ankle | c. lateral |
| 16. _____ Skin in relation to muscle | d. deep |
| 17. _____ Stomach in relation to vertebral column | e. proximal |
| | f. distal |
| | g. anterior |
| | h. posterior |

18. A plane that divides the body into right and left parts is a _____ _____ section.
19. A cut at right angles to the body is a _____ section.
20. The head, neck, and trunk make up the _____ portion of the body, whereas the limbs make up the _____ portion.
21. The internal organs within the body cavities are referred to as _____ _____.

*Select the most appropriate answer from Column B for each item in Column A.*

| **Column A** | **Column B** |
|---|---|
| 22. _____ Head | a. cervical |
| 23. _____ Skull | b. cephalic |
| 24. _____ Skin | c. cranial |
| 25. _____ Chest | d. cutaneous |
| 26. _____ Neck | e. pectoral |
| 27. _____ Armpit | f. axillary |

28. Thoracic and abdominopelvic cavities are separated by the _____.

## REVIEW QUESTIONS

1. Describe the position of each of the following using anatomical terms: (a) navel (b) ear (c) great toe (d) elbow (e) vertebral column (backbone).
2. Define homeostasis and give an example.

3. List in sequence the levels of organization within the human organism, from atom to organism.
4. List the body systems, give their functions, and tell how each is homeostatic.
5. Define anatomical position. Why might this definition be useful?
6. Identify the body cavities and name an organ or structure found in each.
7. Define each of the following: (a) cephalic (b) cervical (c) cranial (d) abdominal (e) sagittal (f) proximal (g) distal (h) bilateral symmetry.

# 2

# The Chemistry of Life

LEARNING OBJECTIVES

**After you study this chapter you should be able to**
1. Describe the basic structure of an atom, locating protons, neutrons, and electrons.
2. Identify the biologically significant elements listed in Table 2–1 by their chemical symbols and summarize the main functions of each in the body.
3. Interpret simple chemical formulas and equations.
4. Define chemical bond and distinguish between covalent and ionic bonds.
5. Contrast acids and bases and use the pH scale in describing the acidity or alkalinity of a solution.
6. Distinguish between inorganic and organic compounds.
7. Compare the major groups of organic compounds—carbohydrates, lipids, proteins, and nucleic acids—with respect to their functions.

TABLE 2-1
**Elements That Make Up the Human Body**

| Name | Chemical Symbol | Approximate Composition of Human Body by Mass (%) | Importance or Function |
|------|-----------------|---------------------------------------------------|------------------------|
| Oxygen | O | 65 | Required for cellular respiration; present in most organic compounds; component of water |
| Carbon | C | 18 | Forms backbone of organic molecules; can form 4 bonds with other atoms |
| Hydrogen | H | 10 | Present in most organic compounds; component of water |
| Nitrogen | N | 3 | Component of all proteins and nucleic acids |
| Calcium | Ca | 1.5 | Structural component of bones and teeth; important in muscle contraction, conduction of nerve impulses, and blood clotting |
| Phosphorus | P | 1 | Component of nucleic acids; structural component of bone; important in energy transfer |
| Potassium | K | 0.4 | Principal positive ion (cation) within cells; important in nerve function; affects muscle contraction |
| Sulfur | S | 0.3 | Component of most proteins |
| Sodium | Na | 0.2 | Principal positive ion in interstitial (tissue) fluid; important in fluid balance; essential for conduction of nerve impulses |
| Magnesium | Mg | 0.1 | Needed in blood and body tissues; part of many important enzymes |
| Chlorine | Cl | 0.1 | Principal negative ion (anion) of interstitial fluid; important in fluid balance |
| Iron | Fe | Trace amount | Component of hemoglobin and myoglobin; component of certain enzymes |
| Iodine | I | Trace amount | Component of thyroid hormones |

Other elements, found in very small amounts in the body (the trace elements), include manganese (Mn), copper (Cu), zinc (Zn), cobalt (Co), fluorine (F), molybdenum (Mo), selenium (Se), and a few others.

The body is composed of an array of atoms and molecules, and life processes depend on the specific organization and interaction of these chemical units. To understand anatomy and physiology (for example, digestion and assimilation of food, muscle contraction, how breathing is regulated, production of urine by the kidneys), we must have some knowledge of the basic principles of chemistry. The branch of chemistry that focuses on life processes is called *biochemistry* (life chemistry).

## CHEMICAL ELEMENTS

All matter, living and nonliving alike, is composed of chemical **elements**, substances that cannot be broken down into simpler substances by chemical reactions. Chemists have identified 92 naturally occurring elements, ranging from hydrogen, the lightest, to uranium, the heaviest.

About 98% of an organism's mass is composed of only six elements—oxygen, carbon, hydrogen, nitrogen, calcium, and phosphorus. Approximately 14 other elements are consistently present in living things but in smaller quantities. Some of these, such as iodine and copper, are known as **trace elements** because they are present in such

minute amounts. Table 2-1 lists the elements that make up a living organism and explains why each is important.

Instead of writing out the name of each element, chemists use a system of abbreviations called **chemical symbols**, usually the first one or two letters of the English or Latin name of the element. For example, O is the symbol for oxygen, C for carbon, Cl for chlorine, N for nitrogen, and Na for sodium (its Latin name is natrium). Chemical symbols for the elements found in living organisms are given in Table 2-1.

## THE ATOM

Imagine a bit of gold being divided into smaller and smaller pieces. The smallest possible particle of gold that could be obtained would be an atom of gold. An **atom** is the smallest unit of an element that retains the characteristic chemical properties of that element. No matter what physical state matter may assume—solid, liquid, or gas—its basic building blocks are atoms. Atoms are almost unimaginably small. If they could be lined up end to end, it would take more than 100 million atoms to measure an inch!

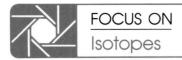

## FOCUS ON
## Isotopes

Atoms of the same element containing the same number of protons but different numbers of neutrons have different mass numbers and are called **isotopes**. The three isotopes of hydrogen, contain zero, one, and two neutrons, respectively. Elements usually occur in nature as a mixture of isotopes.

All isotopes of a given element have essentially the same chemical characteristics. Some isotopes with excess neutrons are unstable and tend to break down, or decay, to a more stable isotope (usually of a different element). Such isotopes are termed **radioisotopes** because they emit high-energy radiation when they decay.

Radioisotopes have been extremely valuable research tools in biology and are useful in medicine for both diagnosis and treatment. Despite the difference in the number of neutrons, the body treats all isotopes of a given element the same chemically.

The reactions of a chemical—a fat, a hormone, a drug—can be followed in the body by tagging the substance with a radioisotope, such as carbon-14 or tritium. For example, the active component in marijuana (tetrahydrocannabinol) has been tagged and administered intravenously. By measuring the amount of radioactivity in the blood and urine at successive intervals, experimenters have determined that this compound remains in the blood for more than 3 days and products of the metabolism of this substance can be detected in the urine for more than 8 days. Because radiation from radioisotopes can interfere with cell division, such isotopes have been used in the treatment of cancer (a disease characterized by rapidly dividing cells). Radioisotopes are also used to test thyroid gland function, measure the rate of red blood cell production, and study many other aspects of body chemistry.

## Atomic Structure

An atom is composed of smaller components called **subatomic particles**. For our purpose we need consider only three types—protons, neutrons, and electrons. **Protons** have a positive electrical charge; **neutrons** are uncharged particles with about the same mass as protons. Protons and neutrons make up almost all of the mass of an atom and are concentrated in the **atomic nucleus**. **Electrons** have a negative electrical charge and an extremely small mass (only about 1/1800 of the mass of a proton). The electrons spin about in the space surrounding the atomic nucleus (Fig. 2–1).

Each kind of element has a fixed number of protons in the atomic nucleus. This number, known as the **atomic number** of the element, determines the chemical identity of the atom. The total number of protons plus neutrons in the nucleus is termed the **mass number**. The common form of oxygen atom, with eight protons and eight neutrons in its nucleus, has an atomic number of 8 and a mass number of 16. (See Focus on Isotopes.)

## Energy Levels

Knowing the locations of electrons enables chemists to predict how atoms combine with one another to form chemical compounds such as salts or sugars. An atom may have several **energy levels**, or **electron shells**, where electrons are located. The lowest energy level is the one closest to the nucleus. Only two electrons can occupy this energy level. The second energy level can accomodate a maximum of eight electrons. Although the third and outer shells can each contain more than eight electrons, they are most stable when only eight are present. We may consider the first energy level to be complete when it contains two electrons and every other energy level to be complete when it contains eight electrons.

The atomic structures of some elements important in biological systems—hydrogen, carbon, oxygen, nitrogen, sodium, and chlorine—are shown in Figure 2–2. Although the simple diagrams of atoms shown in Figure 2–2 are helpful in understanding atomic structure, they are oversimplified.

*Figure 2–1. Two ways of representing an atom. (a) Model of a carbon atom. Although this type of model is not an accurate way to show the location of electrons, it is commonly used because of its simplicity and convenience. (b) An electron cloud. Dots represent the probability of the electron's being in a particular location at any given moment.*

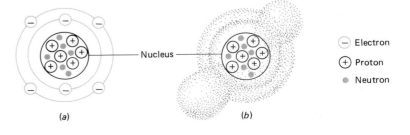

Nucleus

⊖ Electron
⊕ Proton
● Neutron

(a)　　　(b)

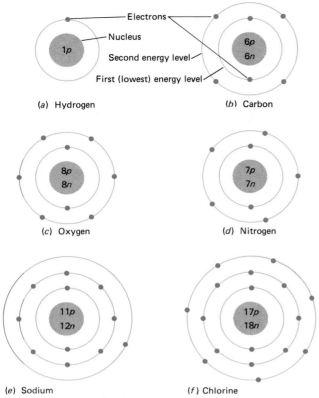

**Figure 2–2.** *Models of some biologically important atoms. (a) Hydrogen. (b) Carbon. (c) Oxygen. (d) Nitrogen. (e) Sodium. (f) Chlorine. Each circle represents an energy level, or electron shell. Dots on the circles represent electrons. (p, Proton; n, neutron.)*

Within energy levels, electrons occur in characteristic regions of space known as **orbitals**. There may be several orbitals within a given energy level, but each orbital can contain at most two electrons.

Electrons are thought to whirl around the nucleus, now close to it, now farther away. Orbitals represent the places where electrons are most probably found. In fact, one way of illustrating an atom is to show its occupied orbitals as electron clouds. The density of the shaded areas represents the likelihood that an electron is present at a given time (Fig. 2–1).

## CHEMICAL COMPOUNDS

Two or more atoms may combine chemically to form a **molecule**. When two atoms of oxygen combine chemically, a molecule of oxygen is formed. Different kinds of atoms can combine, forming **chemical compounds**. A chemical compound is a substance that comprises two or more different elements combined in a fixed ratio. Water is a chemical compound consisting of two atoms of

hydrogen chemically combined with one atom of oxygen.

## What Are Formulas?

A **chemical formula** is a shorthand method for describing the chemical composition of a molecule. Chemical symbols are used to indicate the types of atoms in the molecule and subscript numbers are used to indicate the number of each type of atom present. The chemical formula for molecular oxygen, $O_2$, tells us that this molecule consists of two atoms of oxygen. The chemical formula for water, $H_2O$, indicates that each molecule consists of two atoms of hydrogen and one atom of oxygen. (Note that when a single atom of one type is present, it is not necessary to write 1; we do *not* write $H_2O_1$.) Another type of formula is the **structural formula**, which shows not only the types and numbers of atoms in a molecule but also their arrangement.

## Chemical Equations

When we discuss body processes such as oxygen transport or digestion of food we will describe chemical reactions. Such reactions can be described on paper by means of *chemical equations*. The chemical equation describing the reaction between methane (natural gas) and oxygen provides a simple example.

$$CH_4 \quad + \; 2\,O_2 \quad \rightarrow \; CO_2 \quad + \; 2\,H_2O$$

Methane    Oxygen    Carbon    Water
                              dioxide

The **reactants** (the substances that participate in the reaction) are written on the left side of the equation and the **products** (the substances formed by the reaction) are written on the right side. The arrow means "yields" and indicates the direction in which the reaction tends to proceed. The number preceding a chemical symbol or formula indicates the number of atoms or molecules reacting. Thus $2\,O_2$ means two molecules of oxygen and $2\,H_2O$ means two molecules of water. The absence of a number indicates that only one atom or molecule is present.

In some cases the reaction will proceed in the reverse direction as well as forward. At **equilibrium** a certain amount of the product continuously breaks up to form the reactants and the rate of the forward reaction equals the rate of the reverse action. Reversible reactions are indicated by double arrows:

$$N_2 \quad + \ 3 \ H_2 \quad \rightleftarrows 2 \ NH_3$$

Nitrogen    Hydrogen    Ammonia

## HOW ATOMS COMBINE: CHEMICAL BONDS

The chemical properties of an element are determined primarily by the number of **valence (vay'-lunce) electrons**, the electrons in the *outermost* energy level. When the outer shell of an atom contains fewer than eight electrons, the atom tends to lose or gain electrons to achieve eight in the outer shell (zero or two in the case of the lightest elements). A **chemical bond** is the attractive force that holds two atoms together. Each bond represents a certain amount of potential chemical energy. Two important types of chemical bonds are covalent bonds and ionic bonds.

## Covalent Bonds

**Covalent bonds** involve the sharing of electrons between atoms. A simple example of a covalent bond is the one joining two hydrogen atoms in a molecule of hydrogen gas, $H_2$ (Fig. 2–3).

The carbon atom has four electrons in its outer energy level. When one carbon and four hydrogen atoms share electrons a molecule of methane ($CH_4$) is formed

$$\begin{array}{c} H \\ | \\ H - C - H \\ | \\ H \end{array}$$

Each bond (represented by a line) represents one electron pair shared between two atoms.

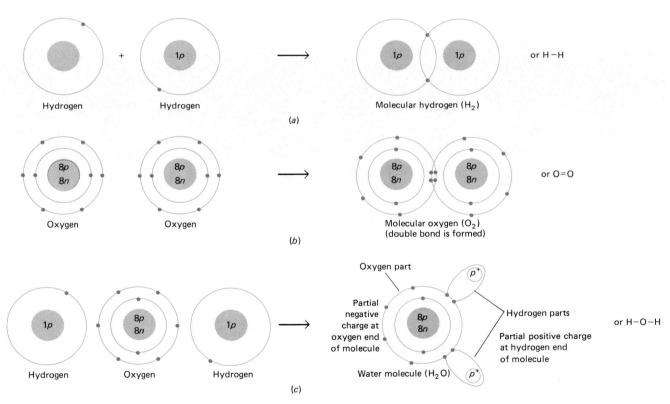

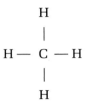

***Figure 2–3.*** *Formation of covalent compounds. (a) Two hydrogen atoms achieve stability by sharing electrons, thereby forming a molecule of hydrogen. The structural formula shown on the right is a simpler way of representing molecular hydrogen. The straight line between the hydrogen atoms represents a single covalent bond. (b) Two oxygen atoms share two pairs of electrons to form molecular oxygen. Note the double bond. (c) When two hydrogen atoms share electrons with an oxygen atom, the result is a molecule of water. Note that the electrons tend to stay closer to the nucleus of the oxygen atom than to the hydrogen nuclei. This results in a partial negative charge on the oxygen portion of the molecule and in a partial positive charge at the hydrogen end of the molecule. The water molecule as a whole is electrically neutral.*

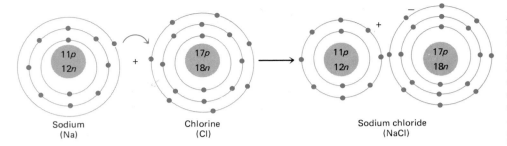

Sodium
(Na)

Chlorine
(Cl)

Sodium chloride
(NaCl)

*Figure 2–4. Formation of an ionic compound. Sodium donates its single valence electron to chlorine, which has seven electrons in its outer energy level. With this additional electron chlorine completes its outer energy level. The two atoms are now electrically charged ions. They are attracted to one another by their unlike electric charges, forming sodium chloride. The force of attraction holding these ions together is called an ionic bond.*

## Ionic Bonds

Atoms with one, two, or three electrons in the outer shell tend to *donate* electrons to other atoms. In doing so they become positively charged because of the excess of protons in the nucleus (Fig. 2–4). When an atom becomes electrically charged, it is called an **ion** (**eye′**-on). Positively charged ions are known as **cations**.

Atoms with five, six, or seven electrons in their outer shell tend to *gain* electrons from other atoms and become negatively charged **anions** (for example, $Cl^-$, chloride ion). Charged particles, anions and cations, play many important roles in biological systems, such as the transmission of impulses by nerves and the contraction of muscles (Fig. 2-5).

An **ionic bond** forms when one atom donates an electron to another. Each atom becomes electrically charged as a result of this exchange, and because of these opposite charges the atoms are attracted to one another. Thus, an ionic bond is the force of electrical attraction between two oppositely charged ions. When held together by ionic bonds, oppositely charged ions form an **ionic compound**. Sodium chloride, table salt, is a good example of an ionic compound.

When an ionic compound such as an acid, base, or salt is dissolved in water, its component ions separate. Because these charged particles can conduct an electrical current, they are called **electrolytes**. Substances, such as sugars, that do not ion-

ize in water do not conduct an electrical current and are termed **nonelectrolytes**.

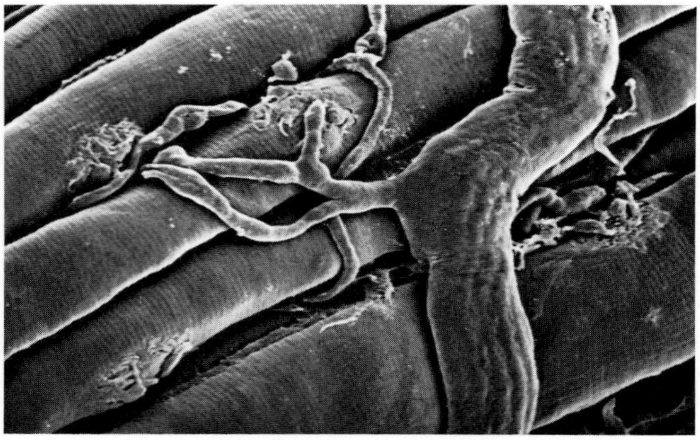

## ACIDS, BASES, AND pH

An **acid** is a compound that dissociates in solution to produce hydrogen ions and some type of anion. An acid is a proton, or $H^+$, donor. Acids have a sour taste. Perhaps the most familiar acid in the body is the hydrochloric acid (HCl) of the stomach. Another acid that plays an important role in body chemistry is carbonic acid ($H_2CO_3$).

The strength of an acid depends upon the degree to which it dissociates in water, producing $H^+$ ions. Thus, HCl is a strong acid because most of its molecules dissociate.

$$\text{HCl} \xrightleftharpoons{\text{in } H_2O} H^+ + Cl^-$$

Hydrochloric acid    Hydrogen ion    Chloride ion

Carbonic acid, on the other hand, is a weak acid because it scarcely dissociates. This compound is well tolerated in the body and occurs normally in the blood.

$$H_2CO_3 \xrightleftharpoons{\text{in } H_2O} H^+ + HCO^{3-}$$

Carbonic acid    Hydrogen ion    Bicarbonate ion

*Figure 2–5. Sodium, potassium, and chlorine ions are among the ions essential in the conduction of a nerve impulse. This scanning electron micrograph shows a nerve fiber communicating with several muscle cells (approximately ×900). The nerve fiber transmits impulses to the muscle cells, stimulating them to contract. The muscle cells are rich in calcium ions, which are essential for muscle contraction. (From Desaki, J.: Vascular autonomic plexuses and skeletal neuromuscular junctions: A scanning electron microscopic study. Biomedical Research Supplement, 139–143, 1981.)*

*Figure 2–6.* The pH scale. A solution with a pH of 7 is neutral because the concentrations of H⁺ and OH⁻ are equal. The lower the pH below 7, the more H⁺ ions are present, and the more acidic the solution is. As the pH increases above 7, the concentration of H⁺ ions decreases and the concentration of OH⁻ increases, making the solution more alkaline (basic).

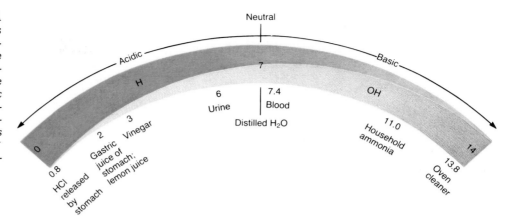

A **base** is defined as a proton acceptor. Most bases dissociate in water, yielding hydroxide ions (OH⁻) and a cation. Bases taste bitter and feel slippery. Sodium hydroxide (NaOH) is an example of a common base.

$$\text{NaOH} \rightleftharpoons \text{Na}^+ + \text{OH}^-$$

Sodium hydroxide → Sodium ion + Hydroxide ion

How can the acidity or alkalinity of a solution be determined? Although acids taste sour and bases are bitter, tasting is not a recommended method! Instead, solutions may be tested with litmus paper, an acid-base indicator found in basic chemistry sets. Litmus paper turns red when dipped in an acidic solution and blue when dipped in a basic solution.

A still more sophisticated method involves the use of a pH meter. This is an instrument that measures **pH**, the relative acidity or alkalinity of a solution, on a scale that ranges from 0 to 14. Seven, the pH of pure water, is neutral (Fig. 2–6). The higher the number above 7, the greater the alkalinity. Alkaline solutions contain more OH⁻ ions than H⁺ ions. A pH of less than 7 indicates an acidic solution, one that contains more H⁺ than OH⁻ ions. Each whole number on the scale represents a tenfold increase in the number of ions present. A pH of 5, for example, is ten times as acidic as a pH of 6—it represents a tenfold increase in hydrogen ion concentration. A pH of 4 represents another tenfold increase. Thus, a solution with a pH of 4 is 100 times more acidic than one with a pH of 6.

Many homeostatic mechanisms work to maintain appropriate pH levels. For example, the pH of blood is about 7.4 and must be maintained within narrow limits. Should the blood become too acidic, coma and death may result. A process known as buffering helps to maintain appropriate pH levels.

A **buffer** consists of a weak acid plus a salt of that acid. One of the most common buffering systems, and one that is important in human blood and tissues, involves the salt sodium bicarbonate (NaHCO₃) and carbonic acid (H₂CO₃). When excess hydrogen ions are present in blood or other body fluids, bicarbonate ions combine with them to form carbonic acid, a weak acid.

In this way a strong acid can be converted to a weak acid and a salt. Carbonic acid is unstable and breaks down, forming carbon dioxide and water. The carbon dioxide is excreted from the body by the lungs.

## INORGANIC COMPOUNDS

Chemical compounds can be divided into two broad groups—inorganic and organic. **Inorganic compounds** are relatively small, simple substances. Among the important groups of inorganic compounds are water, simple acids, bases, and salts. These substances are required in appropriate amounts for water balance, acid-base balance, and many cell activities such as transporting materials through cell membranes.

A **salt** is a compound that dissociates in water yielding a positive ion other than H⁺ and a negative ion other than OH⁻. Inorganic salts are a source of many important mineral ions such as so-

| Na⁺ | + | HCO³⁻ | + | H⁺ | + | Cl⁻ | → | H₂CO₃ | + | NaCl |
|---|---|---|---|---|---|---|---|---|---|---|
| Sodium ion | | Bicarbonate ion | | Hydrogen ion | | Chloride ion | | Carbonic acid | | Sodium chloride |

dium, chloride, calcium, and magnesium. Such ions are essential for fluid balance, acid-base balance, nerve and muscle function, blood clotting, bone formation, and many other aspects of body function.

## ORGANIC COMPOUNDS

**Organic compounds** are large, complex compounds containing carbon. They are the main structural components of the body and also serve as fuel molecules that provide energy for body processes. Organic compounds are the essential regulators of and participants in thousands of metabolic reactions. In all organic compounds the chain of atoms that makes up the principal axis of the molecule consists of carbon atoms. The most important groups of organic compounds in the body include carbohydrates, lipids, proteins, and nucleic acids.

### Carbohydrates

Carbohydrates are familiar to us as sugars and starches. These compounds are used by the body as fuel molecules. Glucose is a simple sugar, or **monosaccharide** (mon-oh-**sak′**-uh-ride). **Disaccharides** (die-**sak′**-uh-rides) can be degraded into two simple sugars; table sugar (sucrose) is an example. A **polysaccharide** (pol-ee-**sak′**-uh-ride) is a large molecule consisting of repeating units of a simple sugar, usually glucose. In plants glucose is stored as the polysaccharide we know as starch. We store glucose as glycogen, another polysaccharide.

### Lipids

Among the biologically important groups of **lipids** (**lip′**-ids) are the neutral fats, phospholipids,

and steroids. **Neutral fats** are an economical form for energy storage because they yield more than twice as much energy per gram as do carbohydrates. They are stored in the body's fat tissues. **Phospholipids** are structural components of cell membranes. **Steroids** include cholesterol, bile salts, and several hormones including the male and female sex hormones.

### Proteins

**Proteins** are important structural components of cells and tissues. Some serve as **enzymes**, catalysts that regulate the thousands of different chemical reactions that take place in the body. Each type of cell has characteristic kinds and amounts of proteins that determine what the cell looks like and how it functions. A muscle cell contains special contractile proteins that are largely responsible for its appearance and its ability to contract. The protein hemoglobin, found in red blood cells, is responsible for the specialized function of oxygen transport.

Proteins are composed of molecular subunits called **amino acids**. There are about 20 types of amino acids found in proteins. Each protein may contain chains of hundreds of amino acids joined in a specific linear order (Fig. 2–7). The various types of proteins differ from one another in the number, types, and arrangement of amino acids they contain. Amino acids are joined by a type of covalent chemical bond called a *peptide bond*. Two amino acids linked chemically are referred to as a **dipeptide**. Several linked amino acids form a **polypeptide**.

### Nucleic Acids

**Nucleic** (new-**klee′**-ik) **acids**, like proteins, are large, complex molecules. There are two classes of nucleic acids: **DNA** (deoxyribonucleic acid) and

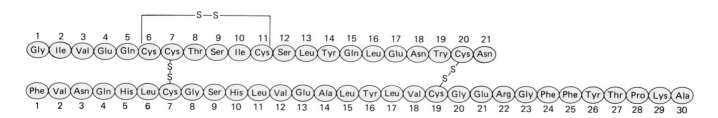

*Figure 2–7.* Protein structure. The structure of the two polypeptide chains that make up the small protein insulin. Each oval in the diagram represents an amino acid. The letters inside the ovals are symbols for the names of the amino acids.

RNA (ribonucleic acid). DNA is the chemical compound that makes up the genes, the hereditary material (see Fig. 22–1). DNA contains the instructions for making all of the proteins needed by the organism. The various kinds of RNA function in the process of manufacturing proteins.

## SUMMARY

I. The atom is the smallest unit of a chemical element that retains the characteristic properties of that element.
   A. A carbon atom is the smallest unit of carbon. A calcium atom is the smallest possible amount of calcium.
   B. An atom consists of subatomic particles, including electrons, protons, and neutrons.
II. A molecule consists of two or more atoms chemically bonded together. A chemical compound consists of two or more different elements combined in a fixed ratio.
   A. The composition of a molecule may be described by a chemical formula, such as $H_2O$.
   B. Chemical equations are used to describe the reactions that take place between atoms and molecules.
III. The atoms of a molecule are held together by forces of attraction between them called chemical bonds.

A. Covalent bonds are strong chemical bonds formed when atoms share electrons.
   B. An ionic bond is formed when one atom donates an electron to another, each atom thereby becoming charged and attracted to the other because of these electrical charges.
IV. Acids dissociate to form hydrogen ions; bases usually dissociate to form hydroxide ions.
   A. The stronger an acid, the lower its pH is. The stronger a base, the higher its pH is.
   B. Buffering, which requires a weak acid plus a salt of that acid, helps to maintain appropriate pH in an organism.
V. Inorganic compounds are simple substances such as water, salts, and certain acids and bases.
VI. Organic compounds are complex molecules that contain carbon; they are the main structural components of cells, serve as fuel for cells, and are important components of metabolic reactions.
   A. Carbohydrates include sugars and starches; they are used as fuel molecules.
   B. Lipids include the neutral fats, phospholipids, and steroids.
   C. Proteins, composed of molecular subunits called amino acids, are important structural components of cells and and some are enzymes.
   D. DNA and RNA are nucleic acids; DNA stores information that governs the structure and function of the organism.

## POST TEST

1. Negatively charged particles that whirl about the atomic nucleus are called _____.
2. The chemical formula for a compound containing one atom of calcium and two atoms of chlorine should be written as _____.
3. A(n) _____ bond is formed when one atom donates an electron to another.
4. Positively charged ions such as $Na^+$ are called _____.
5. The products are written on the _____ side of an equation.
6. Covalent bonds are formed when atoms share _____.
7. A(n) _____ is a compound that dissociates in solution to produce hydrogen ions and some type of anion.
8. A solution with a pH of 8 would be _____; one with a pH of 4 would be _____.
9. Buffers function to maintain appropriate _____.
10. Organic compounds are large, complex compounds that contain _____.

*Select the most appropriate answer from Column B for each item in Column A.*
*You may use an answer once, more than once, or not at all.*

| Column A | Column B |
|---|---|
| 11. _____ Simple sugar | a. protein |
| 12. _____ Glycogen is an example | b. monosaccharide |
| 13. _____ Cholesterol is an example | c. lipid |
| 14. _____ DNA is an example | d. nucleic acid |
| 15. _____ May serve as an enzyme | e. polysaccharide |
| | f. amino acid |

## REVIEW QUESTIONS

1. What is (a) an atom (b) a chemical compound (c) an electron (d) a covalent bond (e) an ion (f) an electrolyte?
2. How do organic compounds differ from inorganic compounds?
3. Characterize each of the following solutions: (a) solution with a pH of 9 (b) a solution with a pH of 6.
4. Why are each of the following biologically important: (a) carbon (b) proteins (c) steroids (d) glycogen?
5. To which class of organic compounds do each of the following belong: (a) glucose (b) DNA (c) steroids (d) enzymes (e) fats?

# 3

# Cells and Tissues

## LEARNING OBJECTIVES

**After you study this chapter you should be able to**
1. Explain why the cell is considered the basic unit of life and describe the general characteristics of cells.
2. Describe, locate, and list the functions of the principal organelles and label them on a diagram.
3. Explain how materials pass through cell membranes, distinguishing among passive and active processes.
4. Predict whether cells will swell or shrink under various osmotic conditions.
5. Describe the stages of a cell's life cycle and summarize the significance of mitosis with respect to maintaining a constant chromosome number.
6. Define the term tissue and give the functions of the principal types of tissue.
7. Compare epithelial tissue with connective tissue.
8. Compare the three types of muscle tissue.

Each of us began life as a single cell, the fertilized egg. That cell gave rise to the millions of cells that make up the complex tissues, organs, and systems of the body. In this chapter we will glimpse the fascinating workings of cells and tissues.

## THE CELL: BASIC UNIT OF LIFE

Cells are often referred to as building blocks of the body because the body is constructed of cells and substances produced by cells. Although it consists of many parts, the **cell** itself is considered the basic unit of life because it is the smallest part of the body, given the proper environment, that is capable of self-sufficient life. We might say that the cell is a complete metabolic unit, because it has all the basic equipment and chemical know-how needed for its own maintenance and growth. If their environmental needs are met, cells can be kept alive in laboratory glassware for many years. No cell part is capable of such survival.

Most cells are microscopic in size. A "typical" cell is about 10 micrometers (10 μm, or about 1/2500 inch) in diameter. (See Appendix B, The Metric System.) This means that if you could line

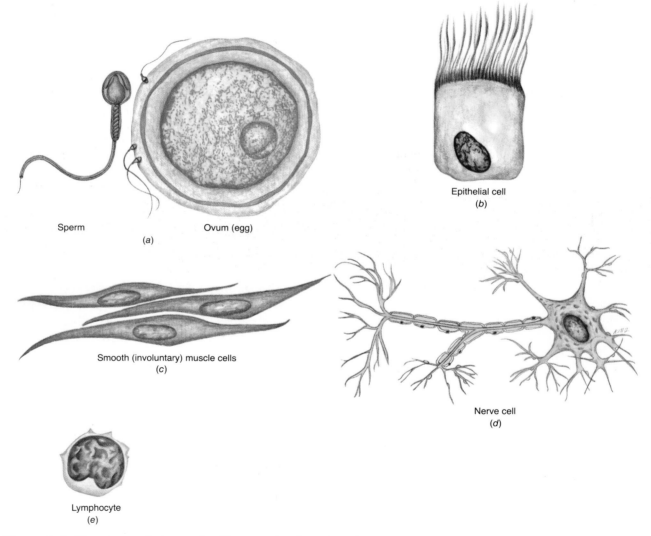

Sperm          Ovum (egg)
(a)

Epithelial cell
(b)

Smooth (involuntary) muscle cells
(c)

Nerve cell
(d)

Lymphocyte
(e)

*Figure 3–1.* *The size and shape of cells are related to their functions. (a) Ovum and sperm cells. Ova (egg cells) are among the largest cells in the body. Sperm cells are among the smallest. Note the long tail (flagellum) used by the sperm cell in locomotion. By whipping its flagellum, the sperm can move itself toward the ovum. (b) Epithelial cell. Epithelial cells join to form tissues that cover body surfaces and line body cavities. (c) Smooth muscle cells join to form the involuntary muscle tissues of the internal organs. For example, smooth muscle in the wall of the digestive tract moves food through the intestine. (d) A nerve cell (neuron) is specialized to transmit messages from one part of the body to another. (e) Lymphocyte, a type of white blood cell. This cell can move through the tissues of the body, destroying invading microorganisms.*

up about 2500 typical cells end to end, the resulting cellular parade would measure less than 3 cm (only about 1 inch). Even the egg cells, which are among the largest cells in the human body, are only about as large as a period on this page.

The size as well as the shape of a cell is related to the specific functions it must perform (Fig. 3–1). For instance, the lymphocyte, a type of white blood cell, has the ability to change its shape as it flows through the tissues of the body, destroying invading bacteria. Nerve cells have long extensions that permit them to transmit messages over great distances within the body. Sperm cells have long whiplike tails that are used for propulsion. Epithelial cells, which look like tiny building blocks, are specialized to cover body surfaces.

One of the biologist's most important tools for studying the internal structure of cells is the microscope. Most cell structures were first identified with an ordinary light microscope, which uses visible light as the source of illumination. (This is the kind of microscope used by students in most high school and college laboratories.) During the last three decades the development of the **electron microscope** has enabled researchers to study the fine detail (**ultrastructure**) of cells and their parts. Whereas the ordinary light microscope may magnify a structure about 1000 times, the electron microscope can magnify it 250,000 times or more. A photograph taken with an electron microscope is called an **electron micrograph**, or **EM** (Fig. 3–2).

## INSIDE THE CELL

Early biologists thought that the cell interior consisted of a homogeneous jelly that they called protoplasm. They recognized only a few structures, such as the nucleus, and with their limited tools they had no satisfactory means of exploring the inside of the cell in greater detail. With use of electron microscopes and other modern research tools, perception of the world within the cell has been vastly expanded. We now know that the cell is an amazingly complex structure with its own control center, internal transportation system, power plants, factories for making needed materials, packaging plants, and even a "self-destruct" system.

Today, the word protoplasm (if used at all) is used in a general way. Instead, the portion of the protoplasm outside the nucleus is called the **cytoplasm** (**sigh'**-toe-plazm) and the corresponding jellylike material within the nucleus is called nucleoplasm. Scattered throughout the cell are tiny structures called **organelles** (little organs), which perform jobs within the cell. Dissolved within the cytoplasm are a great variety of amino acids, simple sugars, and other substances used to manufacture larger molecules. Also present are thousands of different kinds of enzymes and structural proteins, as well as ions that maintain an appropriate biochemical environment.

Most of the organelles within the cell are enclosed by membranes that partition the cytoplasm into different compartments. The characteristics of the various cellular organelles are summarized in Table 3–1 and illustrated in Figures 3–2 and 3–3.

## The Cell Membrane

The **cell membrane**, or **plasma membrane**, is the thin, delicate membrane that surrounds every cell. The cell membrane protects the cell and regulates the passage of materials into and out of the cell.

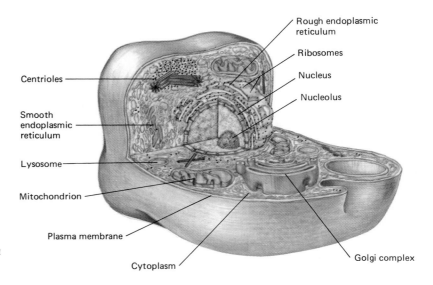

Centrioles

Smooth endoplasmic reticulum

Lysosome

Mitochondrion

Plasma membrane

Cytoplasm

Rough endoplasmic reticulum

Ribosomes

Nucleus

Nucleolus

Golgi complex

*Figure 3–2.* An artist's conception of a "typical" cell.

TABLE 3–1
**Cell Structures**

| Structure | Description | Function |
|---|---|---|
| Cell membrane | Lipid bilayer throughout which a variety of proteins are distributed in a mosaic pattern | Protection; regulates passage of materials into and out of cell; helps maintain cell shape; communicates with other cells |
| Endoplasmic reticulum (ER) | Network of internal membranes extending through cytoplasm; forms system of tubes and vesicles | Intracellular transport of materials |
| Smooth | Lacks ribosomes on outer surfaces | Produces steroids in certain cells; conduction of impulses in muscle cells |
| Rough | Ribosomes stud outer surfaces | Manufactures and transports proteins |
| Ribosomes | Nonmembranous granules composed of RNA and protein; some attached to ER | Manufacture protein |
| Golgi complex | Stacks of flattened membranous sacs | Packages secretions; manufactures lysosomes |
| Lysosomes | Membranous sacs containing digestive enzymes | Release enzymes to break down proteins and other materials, including ingested bacteria; play a role in cell death |
| Vesicles and vacuoles | Membranous sacs | Contain ingested materials or cellular secretions or wastes |
| Mitochondria | Sacs consisting of two membranes; inner membrane is folded to form cristae | Site of most of the reactions of cellular respiration; power plants of cell |
| Centrioles | Nonmembranous; a pair of hollow cylinders | Mitotic spindle forms between these structures during mitosis |
| Cilia | Nonmembranous; extend outside of cell | Movement of material outside the cell. Ciliated cells that line the respiratory tract beat to move mucus away from the lungs; not present in all cells |
| Flagella | Nonmembranous hollow tubes; extend outside of cell; longer than cilia | Found only in sperm cells |
| Nucleus | Large spherical structure surrounded by a double nuclear membrane; contains nucleolus and chromosomes | Control center of the cell; contains the chromosomes |
| Nucleolus | Nonmembranous; rounded granular body within nucleus; consists of RNA and protein | Assembles ribosomes; may have other functions |
| Chromosomes | Nonmembranous; long threadlike structures composed of DNA and proteins | Contain the genes (hereditary units) that govern the structure and activity of the cell |

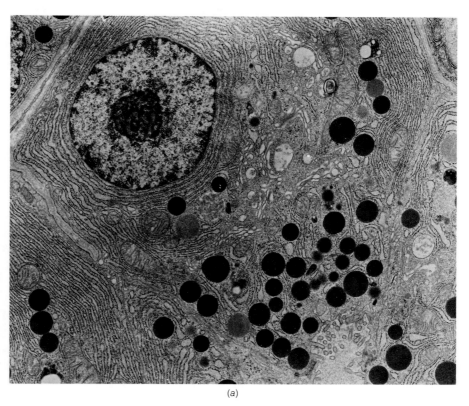

(a)

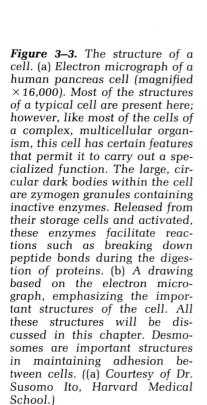

*Figure 3–3.* The structure of a cell. (a) Electron micrograph of a human pancreas cell (magnified ×16,000). Most of the structures of a typical cell are present here; however, like most of the cells of a complex, multicellular organism, this cell has certain features that permit it to carry out a specialized function. The large, circular dark bodies within the cell are zymogen granules containing inactive enzymes. Released from their storage cells and activated, these enzymes facilitate reactions such as breaking down peptide bonds during the digestion of proteins. (b) A drawing based on the electron micrograph, emphasizing the important structures of the cell. All these structures will be discussed in this chapter. Desmosomes are important structures in maintaining adhesion between cells. ((a) Courtesy of Dr. Susomo Ito, Harvard Medical School.)

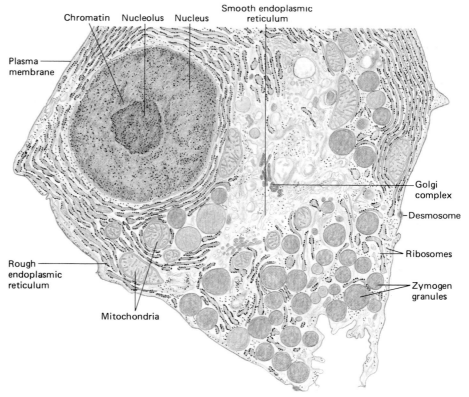

(b)

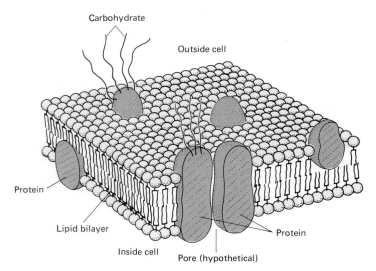

Carbohydrate

Outside cell

Protein

Lipid bilayer

Inside cell

Pore (hypothetical)

Protein

*Figure 3–4. An artist's conception of the cell membrane according to current theory.*

Because it is selectively permeable the cell membrane can allow certain materials to enter or leave the cell while preventing the passage of others. The cell membrane also communicates with other cells and organs. For example, certain proteins that project from the surface of the cell membrane act as receptors that receive chemical messages from endocrine glands or other types of cells.

The cell membrane consists of a rather fluid lipid bilayer (a double layer of lipid molecules) in which are embedded a variety of proteins distributed in a mosaic pattern (Fig. 3–4). Although the lipids of the membrane present a barrier to the passage of materials, the proteins permit selective transport of water-soluble substances. Some of the proteins are thought to form channels through the membrane that allow ions and small water-soluble molecules to enter and exit.

## Endoplasmic Reticulum and Ribosomes

The **endoplasmic reticulum** (**en'**-dow-plas-mik ret-**ik'**-yoo-lum) (**ER**) is a system of internal membranes that extends throughout the cytoplasm of many cells. Somewhat like a complex tunnel system, the ER provides passages through which materials can be transported from one part of the cell to another. Two types of ER can be distinguished, smooth and rough.

**Smooth ER** produces steroids in certain cells. In muscle cells it is involved in calcium storage and affects muscle contraction. The smooth ER of liver cells is thought to be specialized for detoxifying drugs. **Rough ER** has a granular appearance that results from the presence of organelles called **ribosomes** (**rye'**-bow-sowms) along its outer walls. Ri-

bosomes function as factories in which proteins are manufactured.

## The Golgi Complex

Looking somewhat like stacks of pancakes, the **Golgi** (**goal'**-jee) **complex** is composed of layers of platelike membranes. This organelle functions as a packaging plant. Within the Golgi complex a carbohydrate component may be added to a protein secretion. The secretion is then packaged within vesicles made from the Golgi complex membrane. These vesicles are released from the Golgi complex and move to the cell membrane. They release their contents outside the cell. Cells lining the digestive tract package and release digestive enzymes in this way. Not all cells secrete products but even in nonsecreting cells the Golgi complex is thought to package intracellular digestive enzymes in the form of lysosomes.

## Lysosomes

Small sacs of digestive enzymes called **lysosomes** (**lye'**-sow-sowms) are released from the Golgi complex and dispersed throughout the cytoplasm. When a white blood cell ingests bacteria or some other scavenger cell ingests debris or dead cells, this foreign matter is enclosed in a vacuole (little sac or vesicle) composed of part of the cell membrane. One or more of the cell's lysosomes then fuse with the vacuole containing the foreign matter. The lysosome pours its powerful digestive enzymes into the vacuole, destroying the material within it.

When a cell dies, lysosomes release their enzymes into the cytoplasm, where they break down the cell itself. This "self-destruct" system accounts for the rapid deterioration of many cells following death. Recent studies suggest that some forms of tissue damage and the aging process itself may be related to leaky lysosomes. Rheumatoid arthritis is thought to result in part from damage done to cartilage cells in the joints by enzymes that have been released from lysosomes. Cortisone-type drugs, which are used as antiinflammatory agents, stabilize lysosome membranes so that leakage of damaging enzymes is reduced.

## Mitochondria

Cells contain tiny power plants called **mitochondria** (my″-tow-**kon′**-dree-uh) in which most of the reactions of cellular respiration (fuel breakdown with release of energy) take place. A metabolically active cell such as a liver cell may contain more than 1000 mitochondria and a muscle cell even more. A typical mitochondrion is a sausage-shaped sac bounded by two membranes. Numerous folds of the inner membrane, called **cristae** (**kris′**-tee), project into the central space, or **matrix**, of the mitochondrion (Fig. 3–5). Just as shelves increase the storage surface of a closet, the cristae increase the available membrane surface within the mitochondrion. Some of the enzymes needed for cellular respiration are arranged along the cristae. Other enzymes are dissolved in the contents of the matrix.

## Cilia and Flagella

**Cilia** (**sil′**-ee-uh), tiny hairlike organelles projecting from the surfaces of many types of cells, help to move materials outside the cell. The cells lining the respiratory passages, for example, are equipped with cilia, which ceaselessly beat to propel a layer of mucus containing trapped dirt particles and other debris away from the lungs. Each human sperm cell is equipped with a whiplike tail, or **flagellum** (fla-**jel′**-um), that is used in locomotion.

## The Nucleus

The **nucleus** (**new′**-klee-us) is a large, spherical organelle that serves as the control center of the cell. Most cells have only one nucleus but some large cells (for example, skeletal muscle cells) are multinucleated. The nucleus is enclosed by a double membrane, the **nuclear membrane**, which is interrupted by pores that permit passage of materials into and out of the nucleus.

The **nucleoplasm** inside the nucleus is thicker and less fluid than the cytoplasm. In a cell that is not in the process of division, loosely coiled, fibrous material called **chromatin** can be seen as a darkly staining granular material scattered throughout the nucleoplasm (Fig. 3–2). When a cell prepares to divide, the chromatin fibers become more tightly coiled and condense to form discrete rod-shaped bodies, the **chromosomes**.

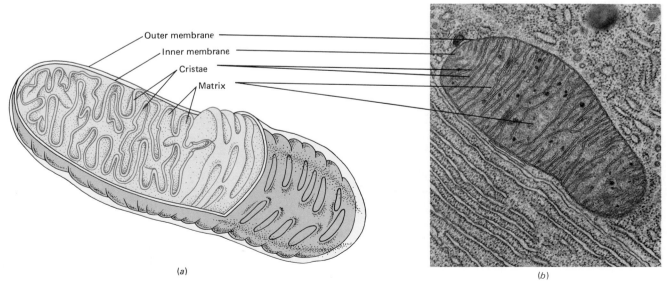

Outer membrane
Inner membrane
Cristae
Matrix

(a)

(b)

***Figure 3–5.*** *The mitochondrion. (a) Diagram of a mitochondrion cut open to show the cristae. (b) Electron micrograph of a typical mitochondrion showing the cristae and matrix (approximately ×80,000). Note the extensive rough ER at the lower left and some lysosomes at the upper right. (Courtesy of Dr. Keith R. Porter.)*

Each chromosome contains several hundred genes arranged in a specific linear order; the genes are composed of DNA. The chromosomes may be thought of as a chemical cookbook for the cell, with each gene being a recipe for a specific protein.

The **nucleolus** (little nucleus) is a specialized region within the nucleus. Studies indicate that the nucleolus may be a factory in which the RNA components of ribosomes are assembled. Ribosomes may also be stored there temporarily.

## MOVEMENT OF MATERIALS THROUGH CELL MEMBRANES

By regulating the passage of materials into and out of the cell, the cell membrane controls the composition of the cell. Materials may move passively by physical processes such as diffusion, osmosis, and filtration, or they can be moved actively by physiological processes such as active transport and phagocytosis. Such active physiological processes require the expenditure of energy by the cell.

### Diffusion

If we were to open a bottle of ammonia and place it on a front-row desk in a closed classroom, within a few moments students in the second row would begin to smell ammonia. Some time later the acrid odor would be evident in every part of the room. How does this happen? Molecules move out of the bottle and distribute themselves throughout the room. This is an example of **diffusion** (di-**few'**-shun), the movement of molecules or ions from a region of higher concentration to a region of lower concentration brought about by the energy of the molecules.

Molecules tend to move along a **concentration gradient**, that is from where they are more concentrated to where they are less concentrated (Fig. 3–6). Diffusion depends on the random movement of individual molecules, propelled by collision with other vibrating molecules or with the sides of the container. As diffusion occurs, each individual molecule moves in a straight line until it bumps into something—another molecule or the side of the container. Then it rebounds and moves in another direction. Molecules continue to move even when they have become uniformly distributed throughout a given space. However, as fast as some molecules move in one direction others move in the opposite direction, so that on the whole all the molecules remain uniformly distributed; an equilibrium exists.

Many substances are distributed throughout the cytoplasm by diffusion and this process is responsible for moving oxygen, carbon dioxide, water, and many other small ions and molecules into or out of the cell. However, diffusion through the cell membrane is limited both by molecular size and by the compatibility of substances with the lipid membrane.

### Osmosis

**Osmosis** (os-**mow'**-sis) is a special kind of diffusion—the diffusion of water molecules across a differentially permeable membrane from a region where water molecules are more concentrated to a region where they are less concentrated. Cell membranes selectively regulate the passage of most solutes (dissolved particles) but water is able to move rather freely into and out of the cell.

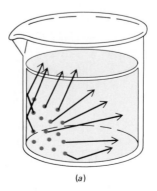  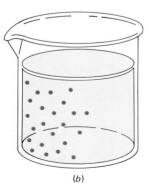  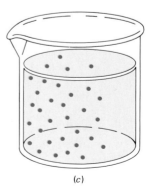  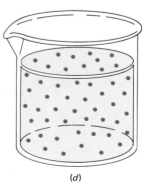

| | | | |
|---|---|---|---|
| (a) | (b) | (c) | (d) |

*Figure 3–6.* The process of diffusion. When a lump of sugar is dropped into a beaker of water, its molecules dissolve (a) and begin to diffuse (b) and (c). Eventually, diffusion results in an even distribution of sugar molecules throughout the water (d).

*Figure 3–7.* Osmosis and the living cell. (a) In an isotonic solution, the concentration of solutes (and thus water molecules) is the same in the solution as in the cell. The net movement of water molecules is zero. (b) A hypertonic solution has a greater solute concentration (thus a lower water concentration) than the cell and therefore exerts an osmotic pressure on the cell. This results in a net movement of water molecules out of the cell, causing the cell to dehydrate, shrink, and perhaps die. (c) A hypotonic solution has a lower solute (and thus a greater water) concentration than the cell. The cell contents thus exert an osmotic pressure on the solution, drawing water molecules inward. There is a net diffusion of water molecules into the cell, causing the cell to swell and perhaps even to burst. (Micrographs of human red blood cells courtesy of Dr. R.F. Baker, University of Southern California Medical School.)

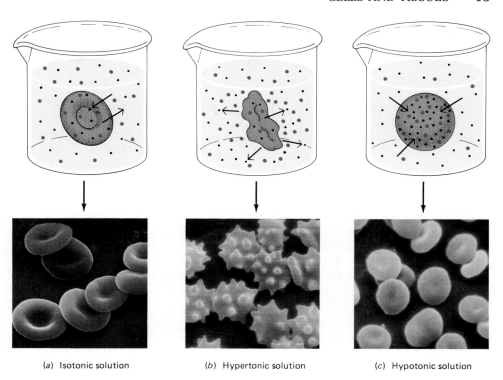

(a) Isotonic solution    (b) Hypertonic solution    (c) Hypotonic solution

When living cells are placed in a solution that has a solute concentration equal to that in the cells, the water molecule concentration is also equal and therefore water molecules move into and out of the cells at the same rate. The net movement of the water molecules is zero (Fig. 3–7). Such a solution is described as **isotonic** (eye″-so-**ton′**-ik) to the cells, that is, of equal solute concentration.

Cells may be placed in solutions that are of greater or lesser solute concentration relative to the solute concentration within the cytoplasm. If the solution is of greater solute concentration it is said to be **hypertonic** (hy-per-**ton′**-ik) (above strength) to that of the cell, whereas if it is of lesser concentration it is **hypotonic** (under strength) compared with the cell. Note that the terms hypertonic and hypotonic are relative to each other. A 5% solution is hypertonic to a 2% solution but is hypotonic to a 10% solution.

Suppose that we place some living cells in distilled water that contains 100% water molecules. If the total number of solute molecules in the cells amounted to 1% of the total molecules present, then water molecules would account for only 99% of the total. Like solute molecules, water molecules tend to move from a region where they are more concentrated to a region where they are less concentrated. Thus, water molecules diffuse inward across the cell membrane (Fig. 3–7). Although the solute molecules have a tendency to

diffuse in the opposite direction, the cell membrane prevents them from "leaking out" to any great extent. Instead, they may be thought of as being trapped within the cell and exerting an **osmotic pressure** on the less concentrated solution outside the membrane. So much water may enter the cell that it swells and bursts.

On the other hand, when cells are placed in a solution that is hypertonic to them, water tends to flow out of them. The cells may become dehydrated, shrink, and die. Can you explain this in terms of the relative concentrations of water molecules in the two solutions? Remember, as a solution contains more solute molecules it contains proportionately fewer water molecules, so that the solvent and solute concentrations are reciprocally related.

## Filtration

Substances may be forced through membranes by hydrostatic pressure, a process called **filtration**. Blood pressure forces some of the plasma (liquid portion) of the blood through the cells of the capillary wall in this way, forming tissue fluid. Ions and small molecules dissolved in the plasma leave the blood vessels with the plasma and become part of the tissue fluid. Filtration is also an important aspect of urine formation by the kidneys.

## Active Transport

A cell requires certain substances (potassium ions, for example) in greater concentration than they are present in the cell's surroundings. The potassium concentration is about 35 times greater inside the cell than outside. Other substances (for example, sodium ions) are more concentrated in the environment than could be tolerated inside the cell. Given the opportunity to do so, diffusion would quickly eliminate such differences in solute concentration and the cell would die. To maintain a steady state the cell must prevent diffusion from occurring in some cases or even reverse its direction. In **active transport** the cell moves materials from a region of lower concentration to a region of higher concentration. Working "uphill" this way against a concentration gradient requires energy. Expenditure of energy in active transport is an example of how even cells that appear to be resting are actually performing work just to remain alive.

## Phagocytosis

In diffusion and in active transport individual molecules and ions pass through the cell membrane. Larger quantities of material—particles of food, or even whole cells—must sometimes be transported into or out of the cell. Such cellular work requires the cell to expend energy. In **phagocytosis** ("cell eating"), the cell ingests large solid particles such as bacteria (Fig. 3–8). Folds of the cell membrane move outward and enclose the particle to be ingested forming a vacuole (little sac or vesicle) around it. The vacuole, still attached to the cell membrane, bulges into the cell interior. The membrane then tightens like a drawstring purse and fuses together, leaving the vacuole floating freely in the cytoplasm.

## HOW CELLS DIVIDE

Certain types of cells in the body divide almost continuously. As many as 10 million blood cells are produced in the body every second. Certain cells in the skin and in the intestinal lining also divide continuously, replacing cells that wear off. Other cells never divide at all after birth. For example, the highly specialized muscle and nerve cells are ordinarily unable to replace themselves. As they wear out or are destroyed, by disease or simply by aging, we are left with fewer and fewer.

## Mitosis

Before a cell physically divides to form two cells, it undergoes mitosis. In **mitosis** (my-**tow'**-sis) the chromosomes are precisely duplicated, and a complete set is distributed to each end of the parent cell. After the parent cell divides each new cell contains the identical number and types of chromosomes present in the parent cell. This means that when a fertilized egg divides to form two cells, each of the new cells receives a complete copy of all its genetic information. After hundreds of divisions every cell in the body (with the exception of the sex cells) contains a complete set of the original chromosomes contributed by the sperm and egg. (The sex cells undergo a special process called **meiosis** (my-o'-sis) which halves their number of chromosomes; see Chapter 22).

The life cycle of the cell may be divided into five phases: interphase, prophase, metaphase, anaphase, and telophase (Fig. 3–9). The cell spends most of its life in **interphase** (meaning between phases), the period between mitoses. During interphase the cell actively synthesizes new materials and grows, and just before mitosis begins, the chromosomes are duplicated.

During **prophase**, the first stage of mitosis, the chromatin fibers coil tightly, so that discrete chromosomes are visible under the light microscope. Although the chromosomes have already duplicated, the duplicated copies are still attached to one another by a special structure called the **centromere**. Thus, each chromosome consists of two identical **chromatids**.

During prophase the nuclear membrane dissolves. Two pairs of organelles known as centrioles function during mitosis. Each pair of centrioles migrates toward an opposite end, or pole, of the cell. Protein threads (microtubules) radiate out from the centrioles and form a structure resembling a spindle.

During **metaphase**, the second phase of mitosis, the chromosomes are aligned along the equator of the cell. The thickened chromosomes can be seen more clearly in metaphase than at any other time. They are sometimes photographed in this stage and studied clinically to determine whether chromosome abnormalities exist.

During **anaphase**, the chromatids of each chromosome separate at their centromeres and start to move away from one another. Once separated, each chromatid is considered an individual chromosome. The protein threads of the spindle begin to pull one set of chromosomes to one end of the cell and the other set to the opposite end.

With the arrival of a complete set of chromosomes at each end of the cell, **telophase** begins. Each chromosome now begins to uncoil and become threadlike chromatin again. The spindle disappears and a nucleus forms around each set of chromosomes.

## Two Cells From One

During telophase the cell constricts inward around its center and divides, forming two cells.

This division of the cytoplasm to form two cells is called **cytokinesis** (Fig. 3–10). Each new cell enters interphase and begins a new cell cycle.

The significance of mitosis is that all the genetic information contained within the chromosomes is precisely duplicated and distributed to each new cell. No genetic information is lost and no new information is added. Each of the two new cells has the potential to function exactly like the parent cell.

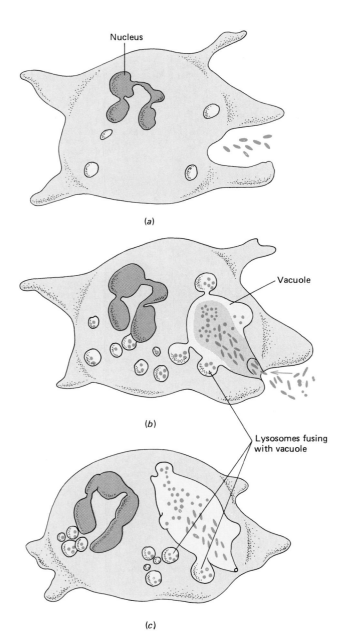

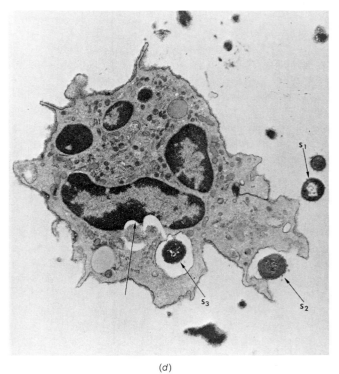

*(d)*

***Figure 3–8.*** *Phagocytosis. (a) The cell ingests large solid particles such as bacteria. Folds of the cell membrane surround the particle to be ingested, forming a small vacuole around it. (b) This vacuole then pinches off inside the cell. (c) Lysosomes may fuse with the vacuole and pour their potent digestive enzymes onto the ingested material. (d) A white blood cell in the presence of bacteria (approximately ×23,000). One bacterium ($S_1$) is free, one bacterium ($S_2$) is being phagocytized, and a third bacterium ($S_3$) has been phagocytized and is seen within a vacuole. Note that near the vacuole (see arrow) the white blood cell's own nucleus has been partly digested. (Phagocytosis, C.L. Sanders, Battelle Pacific Northwest Labs/BPS.)*

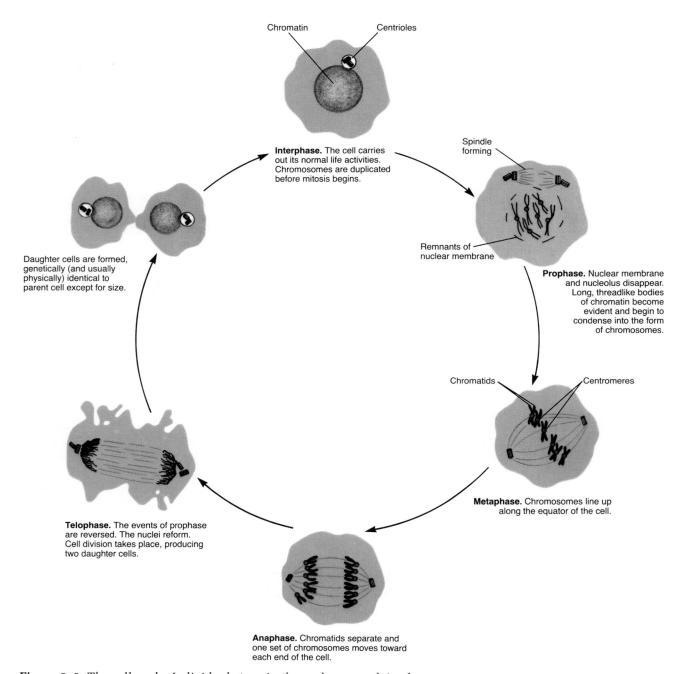

**Figure 3–9.** The cell cycle. Individual steps in the cycle are explained.

*Figure 3–10.* Cytokinesis in human cells grown in culture. These cells are stained with fluorescent dyes. Chromosomes are stained orange, and the microtubules yellow-green. (Jonathan G. Izant.)

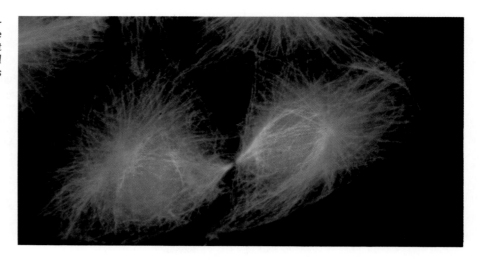

## TISSUES: THE FABRIC OF THE BODY

A **tissue** is a group of closely associated cells that work together to carry out a specific function or group of functions. The cells of a tissue produce the nonliving materials, called **intercellular substance**, that lie between the cells and are part of the tissue. If the body were composed only of cells it would be somewhat like a blob of jelly. The intercellular substances give the body its strength and help it to maintain its shape.

Four principal types of tissues make up the body.

1. **Epithelial tissue** protects the body by covering all of its free surfaces and lining its cavities. The outer layer of the skin consists of epithelial tissue. Some epithelial tissue is specialized to form glands.
2. **Connective tissue** supports and protects the organs of the body; it connects and holds parts of the body together. Bone and fat (adipose) tissue are examples of connective tissue.
3. **Muscle tissue** is specialized for moving the body and its parts.
4. **Nervous tissue** receives and transmits messages so that the various parts of the body can communicate with one another.

## Epithelial Tissue

Epithelial tissue, also called epithelium, serves several important functions.

1. **Protection.** The main job of epithelial tissue is protection. Epithelial tissue covers the body and lines all the body cavities, thus providing a protective shield for the underlying tissues.
2. **Absorption.** In some parts of the body epithelium is specialized to absorb certain materials. For example, epithelium lining the digestive tract absorbs molecules of digested food.
3. **Secretion.** In some epithelial tissues, certain cells are specialized to secrete specific substances. For example, goblet cells in the lining of the intestine secrete mucus, a slippery, protective substance. When large amounts of specialized secretions are needed, epithelium may be arranged to form complex glands.
4. **Excretion.** Epithelial cells lining the kidney tubules excrete certain materials.
5. **Surface transport.** In the respiratory passageways, epithelium transports mucus containing trapped particles. Such epithelial cells are equipped with cilia that beat in a coordinated manner so that a thin sheet of mucus containing trapped dirt particles is continuously moved away from the lungs.
6. **Sensory functions.** The taste buds in the mouth and olfactory (smelling) structures in the nose consist of epithelium specialized to receive sensory information.

Epithelial tissue consists of cells that fit tightly together (Table 3–2). Little intercellular substance is present. Epithelial tissue may be classified as (1) covering and lining epithelium and (2) glandular epithelium.

### Covering and Lining Epithelium

Epithelial tissue that covers body surfaces consists of tight-fitting cells that are firmly attached to one another, forming sheets of cells, or **membranes**. Epithelial membranes are all supported by

TABLE 3–2
**Epithelial Tissues**

| Tissue Name | Some Main Locations | Functions | Description and Comments |
|---|---|---|---|
| ***Simple Squamous Epithelium***<br>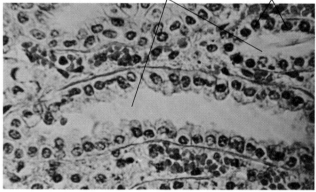<br>Nuclei<br>Approximately × 350 | Air sacs of lungs, lining of blood vessels (endothelium), lining of body cavities (mesothelium) | Passage of materials where little or no protection is needed | Like all epithelium, provided with a basement membrane secreted by the cells; cells are flat (often so flat that cytoplasm cannot be discerned) and arranged as a single layer; simplest of all epithelial tissues |
| ***Simple Cuboidal Epithelium***<br>Lumen of tubule   Nuclei of cuboidal epithelial cells<br>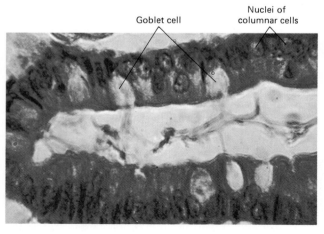<br>Approximately × 450 | Kidney tubules, gland ducts | Secretion and absorption | A single layer of cells that appears box-shaped in tissue sections |
| ***Simple Columnar Epithelium***<br>Goblet cell   Nuclei of columnar cells<br>Approximately × 450 | Lining of much of digestive tract; ciliated columnar epithelium lines upper part of respiratory tract | Secretion, especially mucus secretion; absorption, protection, movement of mucous layer | Single layer of columnar cells, often with nuclei basally located almost in a row; sometimes with enclosed secretory vacuoles (goblet cells), highly developed Golgi apparatus, and cilia |

TABLE 3–2
**Epithelial Tissues** *(continued)*

| Tissue Name | Some Main Locations | Functions | Description and Comments |
|---|---|---|---|
| *Stratified Squamous Epithelium* | Skin, mouth lining, vaginal lining | Protection only; little or no absorption or transport of materials; keratinized layer continuously sacrificed by friction and replaced from below | Several layers of cells, with only lower ones columnar and metabolically active; division of lower cells causes older ones to be pushed upward toward surface; not keratinized in moist membranes, but waterproofed with this substance in flattened dead upper layers of skin |

Approximately × 150

| | | | |
|---|---|---|---|
| *Pseudostratified Epithelium* | Some respiratory passages, ducts of many larger glands, some ducts of male reproductive system; sometimes ciliated | Secretion, protection, movement of mucus | Comparable in many ways to columnar epithelium, except that not all cells are same height; thus, though all cells contact the same basement membrane, the tissue appears stratified; nuclei not in line; may be ciliated or mucus-secreting |

Cilia        Goblet cell

Basement membrane

Approximately × 600

underlying connective tissue. The membrane is attached to the connective tissue beneath it by a **basement membrane,** a thin layer of nonliving material secreted by the cells. Epithelial membranes are nonvascular, that is, they lack blood vessels. The cells of an epithelial membrane are dependent on the connective tissue beneath for their blood supply.

Many epithelial membranes are subjected to continuous wear and tear. As outer cells are sloughed off they must be replaced by new ones from below. Such epithelial tissues have a rapid rate of mitosis so that new cells are continuously produced to take the place of those lost.

**Shapes of Cells.** We can identify three main shapes of epithelial cells.

1. **Squamous cells** are thin and flattened.
2. **Cuboidal cells** appear as small cubes when the tissue is cut at right angles to the surface.
3. **Columnar cells** look like tiny columns or cylinders when viewed from the side. The nu-

cleus may be seen toward the base of each cell. In cross section, or looking down at their top surface, these cells appear hexagonal in shape.

**Arrangement of Cells.** Epithelial tissue may be **simple**, that is, composed of one layer of cells, or **stratified**, composed of two or more layers. Simple epithelium is usually present in areas where materials must diffuse through the tissue or where substances are secreted, excreted, or absorbed. Stratified epithelial tissue is located in regions where protection is the main function. A third arrangement is **pseudostratified** epithelium, so called because its cells falsely appear to be layered.

Table 3–2 illustrates the types of epithelial tissue and indicates where they are found in the body. In stratified epithelium the shape of the cells at the free surface determines the name of the tissue.

### Glandular Epithelium

A **gland** consists of one or more epithelial cells that produce and discharge a particular product. Two main types of glands are endocrine and exocrine glands. **Endocrine glands** lack ducts (tubes through which the secretion is discharged) and release their products, chemical messengers called **hormones**, into the surrounding tissue fluid. The hormone usually diffuses into the blood, which transports it to its destination. The thyroid and adrenal glands are examples of endocrine glands.

**Exocrine glands**, in contrast, have **ducts**, also made of epithelial cells, which conduct the secretion to some body surface. For example, sweat passes from sweat glands through ducts to the surface of the skin and salivary gland ducts conduct saliva to the mouth. Exocrine glands may be unicellular (composed of one cell) like goblet cells (Fig. 3–11) but most are multicellular.

## Connective Tissue

The main function of connective tissue is to join together the other tissues of the body. Connective tissues also support the body and its structures and protect underlying organs. In addition, almost every organ in the body has a supporting framework of connective tissue. Some of the main types of connective tissue are (1) ordinary connective tissue, (2) adipose tissue, (3) cartilage, (4) bone, and (5) blood, lymph, and tissues that produce blood cells (see Table 3–3).

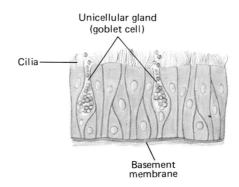

**Figure 3–11.** *A goblet cell is a unicellular gland that secretes mucus.*

Unlike the closely fitting cells of epithelial tissues, the cells of connective tissue are usually separated by large amounts of intercellular substance. The intercellular substance usually consists of threadlike, microscopic **fibers** scattered throughout an amorphous (without definite form) **matrix**. The matrix is usually a viscous, semifluid gel composed of polysaccharide and protein complexes and tissue fluid.

Three types of connective tissue fibers are collagen fibers, reticular fibers, and elastic fibers. **Collagen fibers**, the most numerous, are sometimes called white fibers because when they are present in great numbers the tissue containing them appears white. Collagen and the smaller **reticular fibers** contain the protein **collagen**, the most abundant protein in the body. Collagen is a tough substance and collagen fibers give great strength to structures in which they occur. (In fact, meat is tough because of its collagen content.) **Elastic fibers** can be stretched by a force and then can return to their original size and shape.

## Muscle Tissue

Muscle tissue is composed of cells specialized to contract. When muscle cells contract they become shorter and thicker, causing body parts attached to them to move. Because they are long and narrow, muscle cells are referred to as **fibers**. Muscle fibers are usually arranged in bundles or layers surrounded by connective tissue. Three types of muscle tissue are skeletal muscle, cardiac muscle, and smooth muscle (Table 3–4).

When we think of muscles we normally think of the voluntary muscles that enable us to walk, run, or move the body in some other way. Such movements are the job of the **skeletal muscles**, which are attached to the bones. Skeletal muscle fibers

TABLE 3–3
**Connective Tissues**

| Tissue Name | Some Main Locations | Functions | Description and Comments |
|---|---|---|---|
| ***Loose (Areolar) Connective Tissue*** Approximately × 200 | Every place where support must be combined with elasticity, e.g., subcutaneous layer | Support | Elastic and inelastic fibers produced by fibroblast cells embedded in a semifluid matrix and mixed with other kinds of cells |
| ***Dense Connective Tissue*** Approximately × 200 | Tendons, strong attachments between organs; dermis layer of skin | Support; transmission of mechanical forces | Bundles of interwoven collagen fibers interdigitated with rows of fibroblast cells |
| ***Elastic Connective Tissue*** Approximately × 300 | Structures that must both expand and return to their original size, such as lung tissue, large arteries | Confers elasticity | Branching elastic fibers interspersed with fibroblasts (cells that produce fibers) |
| ***Reticular Connective Tissue*** | Framework of liver, lymph nodes, spleen, thymus | Support | Consists of interlacing reticular fibers |

Approximately × 500 (From Bloom, W., and Fawcett, D.W.: A Textbook of Histology, 10th ed. Philadelphia, W.B. Saunders Co., 1975.)

*Table continued on the following page*

TABLE 3–3
**Connective Tissues (continued)**

| Tissue Name | Main Locations | Functions | Description and Comments |
|---|---|---|---|
| **Adipose Connective Tissue** Approximately × 150 | Subcutaneous layer; pads around certain internal organs | Food storage, insulation, support of such organs as breasts, kidneys | Fat cells are star-shaped at first; fat droplets accumulate until typical ring-shaped cells are produced |
| **Hyaline Cartilage** Chondrocytes — Lacuna — Intercellular substance Approximately × 300 | Forms ends of bones; synovial joint surfaces; respiratory tubes | Flexible support and reduction of friction in bearing surfaces | No visible fibers; cartilage cells (chondrocytes) are separated from one another by the gristly intercellular substance, and occupy little spaces (called lacunae) in it |
| **Bone** Lacunae — Haversian canal — Matrix Approximately × 150 | Bone tissue makes up bones of skeleton | Support, protection of internal organs, calcium reservoir; skeletal muscles attach to bones | Osteocytes (bone cells) located in small cavities called lacunae; in compact bone lacunae arranged in concentric circles about haversian canals |
| **Blood** Red blood cells — White blood cell Approximately × 1100 | Within heart and blood vessels of circulatory system | Transports oxygen, nutrients, wastes, and other materials | Consists of cells dispersed in fluid intercellular substance |

TABLE 3–4
**Types of Muscle Tissues**

|  | Skeletal | Smooth | Cardiac |
|---|---|---|---|
| *Location* | Attached to skeleton | Walls of stomach, intestines, etc. | Walls of heart |
| *Type of Control* | Voluntary | Involuntary | Involuntary |
| *Shape of Fibers* | Elongated, cylindrical, blunt ends | Elongated, spindle-shaped, pointed ends | Elongated, cylindrical fibers that branch and fuse |
| *Striations* | Present | Absent | Present |
| *Number of Nuclei per Fiber* | Many | One | One |
| *Speed of Contraction* | Most rapid | Slowest | Intermediate |
| *Ability to Remain Contracted* | Least | Greatest | Intermediate |

Nuclei    Cross striations

Nuclei

Nuclei

Intercalated disks

(a) Skeletal muscle fibers    (b) Smooth muscle fibers    (c) Cardiac muscle fibers

have a striped, or **striated**, appearance. Skeletal muscle fibers contract when stimulated by nerves.

**Cardiac muscle**, found in the walls of the heart, is considered involuntary because it is not generally regulated at will. Its striated muscle fibers are joined end to end and branch and rejoin to form complex networks.

**Smooth muscle** (also called visceral muscle) occurs in the walls of the digestive tract, uterus, blood vessels, and other internal organs. Its fibers are not striated, and its control is involuntary.

## Nervous Tissue

Nervous tissue consists of **neurons**, cells specialized for transmitting nerve impulses, and **glial cells**, cells that support and nourish the neurons. Typically, a neuron has a large cell body that contains the nucleus and from which two types of extensions project. Dendrites are specialized for receiving impulses, whereas the single axon conducts information away from the cell body (Fig. 3–12).

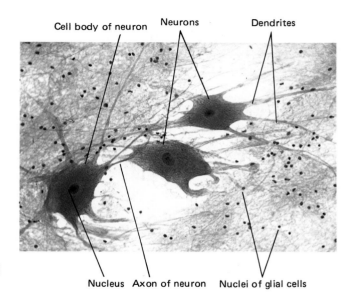

Cell body of neuron    Neurons    Dendrites

Nucleus    Axon of neuron    Nuclei of glial cells

*Figure 3–12. Nervous tissue consists of neurons and glial cells (approximately ×500).*

A **neoplasm** (new growth) is an abnormal mass of cells. Neoplasms, or **tumors**, can develop in many species of animals and plants. A benign ("kind") tumor tends to grow slowly and its cells stay together. Because benign tumors form discrete masses, often surrounded by connective tissue capsules, they can usually be removed surgically. Unless a benign neoplasm develops in a place where it interferes with the function of a vital organ, it is not lethal.

A malignant ("injurious") neoplasm, or **cancer**, usually grows much more rapidly than a benign tumor. Neoplasms that develop from connective tissues or muscle are referred to as **sarcomas** and those that originate in epithelial tissue are called **carcinomas**. Unlike the cells of benign tumors, cancer cells do not retain the typical structural features of the cells from which they originate.

Cancer is thought to be triggered when the DNA of a cell is mutated (altered) by radiation, certain chemicals or irritants, or viruses. When the mutated cell multiplies, all the cells derived from it bear the identical mutation. Should the mutation interfere with the cells' control mechanisms, the cells begin to behave abnormally. Two basic defects in behavior that characterize most cancer cells are rapid multiplication and abnormal relations with neighboring cells. Though normal cells respect one another's boundaries and form tissues in an orderly, organized manner, cancer cells grow helter-skelter upon one another and infiltrate normal tissues (see figure). Apparently they are no longer able to receive or respond to signals from surrounding cells.

Studies indicate that many neoplasms grow to only a few millimeters in diameter and then enter a dormant stage, which may last for months or even years. At some point, cells of the neoplasm release a chemical substance that stimulates nearby blood vessels to develop new capillaries that grow out toward the neoplasm and infiltrate it. Once a blood supply is ensured, the neoplasm grows rapidly and may become life-threatening.

Death from cancer is almost always caused by **metastasis**, which is a migration of cancer cells through blood or lymph channels to distant parts of the body. Once there, they multiply, forming new malignant neoplasms, which may interfere with normal function in the tissues being invaded. Cancer often spreads so rapidly and extensively that surgeons are unable to locate all the malignant masses.

Why some persons are more susceptible to cancer than others remains a mystery. Some researchers think that cancer cells form daily in everyone but that in most persons the immune system (the system that provides protection from disease organisms and other foreign invaders) is capable of destroying them. According to this theory cancer is a failure of the immune system. Another suggestion is that different persons have different levels of tolerance to environmental irritants. As many as 90% of cancer cases are thought to be triggered by environmental factors.

A cancer patient's survival depends upon early diagnosis and treatment with a combination of surgery, radiation therapy, and drugs that suppress mitosis (chemotherapy). Because cancer is actually an entire family of closely related diseases (there are more than 100 distinct varieties), it may be that there is no single cure. Most investigators agree, however, that a greater understanding of basic control mechanisms and communication systems of cells is necessary before effective cures can be developed.

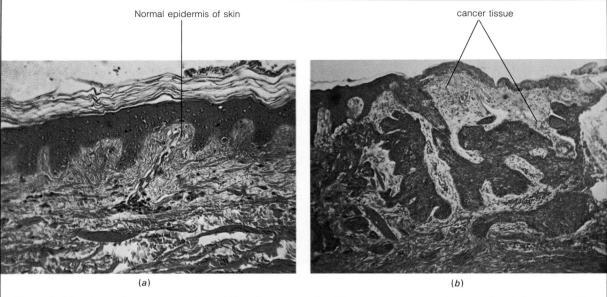

*Normal skin tissue (approximately ×200) (a) compared with cancerous tissue (approximately ×150) (b).*

# SUMMARY

I. The cell is considered the basic unit of life because it is the smallest self-sufficient unit in the body and because the body consists of cells and their products.

II. Most cells are bounded by a cell membrane and have a nucleus and other types of organelles dispersed within the cytoplasm.

   A. The cell membrane protects the cell and regulates the passage of materials into and out of the cell.

   B. The endoplasmic reticulum (ER) is a system of internal membranes that plays a role in the transport and storage of materials within the cell.

     1. The smooth ER lacks ribosomes; it produces steroids in certain types of cells.

     2. The rough ER is studded along its outer walls with ribosomes, granular organelles that manufacture proteins.

   C. The Golgi complex packages secretions for export from the cell and produces lysosomes.

   D. Lysosomes function in intracellular digestion and form the "self-destruct" system of the cell.

   E. Mitochondria, the power plants of the cell, are the sites of most of the reactions of cellular respiration, which yield energy for the cell.

   F. The nucleus, the control center of the cell, contains the chromosomes.

III. Materials move through the cell membrane passively by physical processes such as diffusion, osmosis, and filtration, or they can be actively transported by physiological processes such as active transport, phagocytosis, and pinocytosis. Passive processes do not require the expenditure of energy on the part of the cell; active processes do.

   A. Diffusion is the movement of molecules or ions from one region to another owing to their random molecular motion. Because of probability, the net movement of molecules in diffusion is from a region of greater concentration to a region of lower concentration.

   B. Osmosis is a kind of diffusion in which molecules of water diffuse through a selectively permeable membrane, resulting in a net movement from a region where the water molecules are more concentrated to a region where they are less concentrated.

   C. In filtration, substances are forced through a membrane by hydrostatic pressure.

   D. In active transport, cells expend energy to transport materials across membranes against their tendencies to diffuse.

   E. In phagocytosis, the cell ingests large solid particles by enclosing them in a vacuole pinched off from the cell membrane.

IV. The stages in the life cycle of a cell include interphase, prophase, metaphase, anaphase, and telophase. A cell reproduces itself by undergoing mitosis and then dividing to form two new cells.

V. A tissue is a group of closely associated cells that work together to perform a specific function or group of functions. Four main types of tissue are epithelial, connective, muscle, and nervous tissue.

VI. Epithelial tissue covers the body surfaces and lines its cavities; some epithelial tissue is specialized to form glands.

   A. The functions of epithelial tissue include protection, absorption, secretion, excretion, surface transport, and reception of sensory information.

   B. Epithelial cells may be squamous, cuboidal, or columnar in shape and epithelial tissue may be simple, stratified, or pseudostratified.

   C. Epithelial tissue that covers or lines body surfaces consists of epithelial membranes, sheets of cells that are firmly attached to one another.

   D. A gland consists of one or more epithelial cells specialized to produce and discharge a particular product. Endocrine glands lack ducts; exocrine glands discharge their secretions into ducts.

VII. Connective tissue joins other tissues of the body together, supports the body, and protects underlying organs.

   A. Some main types of connective tissue are ordinary connective tissue; adipose tissue; cartilage; bone; and blood, lymph, and tissues that produce blood cells.

   B. Cells of connective tissue are separated by large amounts of intercellular substance.

   C. Collagen fibers, reticular fibers, and elastic fibers are characteristic of connective tissue.

VIII. Muscle tissue is specialized to contract; the three types are skeletal, cardiac, and smooth.

IX. Nervous tissue is specialized to transmit neural impulses.

## POST TEST

*Select the most appropriate answer from Column B for each item in Column A.*
*You may use an answer once, more than once, or not at all.*

**Column A**

1. _____ Regulates passage of materials into the cell
2. _____ Network of internal membranes that extends throughout cytoplasm
3. _____ Site of cellular respiration
4. _____ Membranous sacs containing digestive enzymes
5. _____ Chromosomes located here
6. _____ Propels sperm
7. _____ Packages secretions
8. _____ Granules that manufacture protein

**Column B**

a. ribosomes
b. endoplasmic reticulum (ER)
c. mitochondria
d. cell membrane
e. nucleus
f. lysosomes
g. Golgi complex
h. flagellum

9. If a cell is placed in a hypertonic solution the net passage of water molecules will be from the _____ to the _____.
10. A cell engulfs a bacterium; this is an example of _____.
11. Active transport requires the expenditure of _____ by the cell.
12. A complete set of chromosomes is distributed to each end of the cell during _____.

*Select the most appropriate answer from Column B for each item in Column A.*
*You may use an answer once, more than once, or not at all.*

**Column A**

13. _____ Covers body surfaces
14. _____ Specialized to contract
15. _____ Contains collagen fibers
16. _____ Supports and protects
17. _____ Contains neurons and glial cells

**Column B**

a. muscle tissue
b. nervous tissue
c. connective tissue
d. epithelial tissue

18. Endocrine glands lack _____.

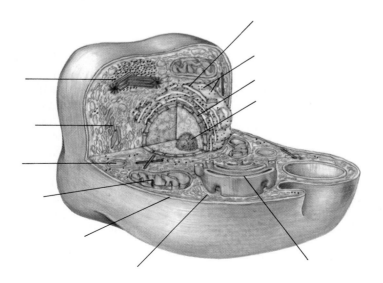

19. Bone and cartilage are examples of _____ tissue.
20. Chemical messengers released by endocrine glands are called _____.

Label the diagram of the cell. See Figure 3–2 for correct labeling.

## REVIEW QUESTIONS

1. What are the functions of the cell membrane? Describe its structure.
2. What is the function of the smooth endoplasmic reticulum? the rough ER?
3. Draw a diagram of a cell and label at least eight organelles. Give the function of each organelle you labeled.
4. Explain why the nucleus is considered the control center of the cell.
5. Compare diffusion with active transport.
6. If red blood cells are accidentally placed in a hypotonic solution, what happens to them? What would happen if red blood cells were placed in a hypertonic solution? an isotonic solution?
7. Why is mitosis important? What is cytokinesis?
8. What are some of the differences between epithelial and connective tissue?
9. The heart (like most organs) contains epithelial, connective, muscle, and nervous tissue. What function might each of these tissues perform in the heart?
10. What is the function of an epithelial membrane?

# The Skin

LEARNING OBJECTIVES

**After you study this chapter you should be able to**
1. List six functions of the skin and explain how each is important in homeostasis.
2. Compare the structure and function of the epidermis with that of the dermis.
3. Describe the subcutaneous layer.
4. Describe the origin and structure of hair.
5. Describe the functions of sebaceous glands and sweat glands.
6. Explain the function of melanin.
7. List the symptoms of inflammation and explain how inflammation is homeostatic.
8. Distinguish among first-, second-, and third-degree burns.
9. Identify the three types of skin cancer discussed in this chapter.

The skin with its glands, hair, nails, and other structures makes up the **integumentary** (in-teg"-u-**men'**-tar-y) **system**, the body's tough, outer protective covering. This is the body system with which you are most intimately acquainted for it is at least partly exposed to view. Perhaps for this reason a good deal of attention is lavished on it. It is scrubbed, creamed, and coated with cosmetics; its hair is cut, shaved, curled, and otherwise fashioned; and its nails are manicured.

The skin is also important in communication. You may shake hands or kiss, squeeze, stroke, or hit it. Involuntary changes in the skin reflect emotional states. For example, you may blush with embarrassment, blanch with fear or rage, redden with exertion, or sweat excessively when anxious. In addition, the appearance, coloration, temperature, and feel of the skin are important indicators of general health and of many disease states.

## FUNCTIONS OF THE SKIN

The skin is the outer boundary of the body—the part in direct contact with the external environment. The almost 6 square meters (20 or so square feet) of skin that cover the body are subjected to continuous wear and tear; to drying; to cold and heat; to toxic substances; and often to cuts, bruises, scrapes, and wounds. By performing the following functions, the skin also helps to preserve the balanced internal environment:

1. It serves as a protective barrier against mechanical and thermal injury. Located within the skin are sensory receptors for receiving stimuli of touch, pressure, heat, cold, and pain. These relay important information to the central nervous system when the body surface comes into contact with forces in the external world.

2. The skin is the body's first line of defense against disease organisms. Though many types of bacteria make their home on the body's surface, healthy skin prevents their entrance into the interior.

3. Skin also prevents the penetration of many kinds of harmful chemicals with which we may come into contact. Anyone who has suffered a bout with poison ivy knows, however, that some substances do manage to get through the skin. Absorption through the skin of some chemicals (for example, phenol) can cause damage to internal organs and absorption of biocides such as parathion can result in lethal poisoning. However, all in all

the skin does a remarkable job of keeping most foreign materials out of the body.

4. The skin prevents dehydration. The cells of the body are immersed in an internal sea, a carefully regulated, dilute salt solution essential to life. Yet, as terrestrial beings, humans move about in the relatively dry environment of air. The skin prevents excessive loss of fluid so that the cells do not dry out.

5. Humans are almost naked organisms. Their lack of an insulating fur coat is compensated for by a complex temperature-regulating system. Extensive capillary networks and sweat glands in the skin are an important part of the system.

6. Sweat glands also excrete excess water and some wastes (urea and uric acid) from the body.

7. Skin is also important as the site of vitamin D synthesis. Cholesterol compounds in the skin are converted to vitamin D when exposed to the ultraviolet rays of the sun.

## LAYERS OF THE SKIN

Skin consists of two main layers: an outer epidermis and an inner dermis. Beneath the skin is an underlying subcutaneous layer (Fig. 4–1).

### Epidermis

**Epidermis** (ep"-i-**der'**-mus) is composed of stratified squamous epithelium. Cells continuously proliferate from its deepest region, then mature as they are pushed toward the outer surface by newer cells beneath. Over most parts of the body the epidermis is only about as thick as a page of this book, yet it consists of four or five sublayers, or **strata** (**stray'**-ta).

The deepest portion of the epidermis is the **stratum basale** (ba-**say'**-lee). This is the reproductive layer of the epidermis. Its cells constantly divide by mitosis, providing a continuous supply of new cells for the upper strata.

As cells are pushed toward the body surface, they move into the outer horny layer of skin, the **stratum corneum** (**kor'**-nee-um). The nuclei and other organelles are destroyed by lysosomal enzymes and the cells die. **Keratin** (**ker'**-a-tin), the tough waterproofing protein of the epidermis, fills most of each cell. Stratum corneum consists of about 20 layers of dead cells in various stages of disintegration. As they are pushed outward these cells resemble dead scales. They are closely

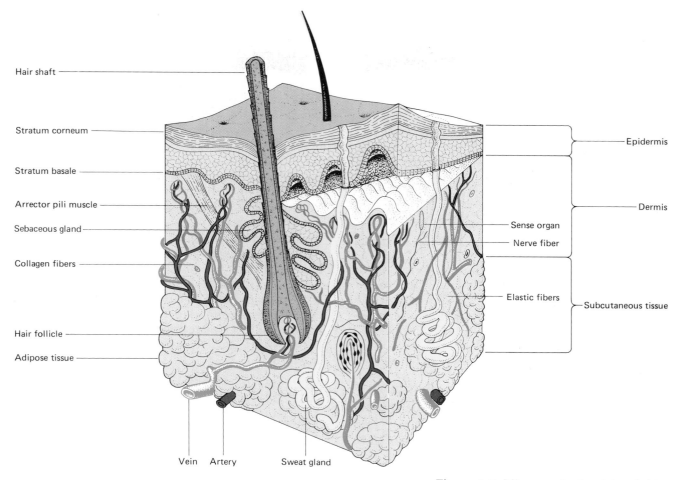

Hair shaft

Stratum corneum

Stratum basale

Arrector pili muscle

Sebaceous gland

Collagen fibers

Hair follicle

Adipose tissue

Vein   Artery   Sweat gland

Epidermis

Dermis

Sense organ

Nerve fiber

Elastic fibers

Subcutaneous tissue

***Figure 4–1.*** *Microscopic structure of skin.*

packed together and serve as a waterproof protective covering for the body.

It takes about 2 weeks for a basal cell to be pushed up into the stratum corneum, then another 2 weeks for the remains of that cell to slough off. Thousands of dead cells slough off the skin surface each day, only to be replaced by new ones from the deeper layers of the epidermis. In healthy individuals the cell population of the skin is carefully balanced.

## Dermis

The **dermis** (**der′**-mus) is the thick layer of skin beneath the epidermis (Fig. 4–1). Dermis is irregular dense connective tissue composed mainly of collagen fibers. The collagen is largely responsible for the mechanical strength of the skin. It also permits the skin to stretch and then contract again. The upper portion of the dermis has many small fingerlike projections called **papillae** (pah-**pill′**-ee), which project into the epidermal tissue. Exten-

sive networks of capillaries in the papillae deliver oxygen and nutrients to the cells of the epidermis and also function in temperature regulation.

Patterns of ridges and grooves visible on the skin of the soles and palms (including the fingertips) reflect the arrangement of the dermal papillae beneath. Unique to each individual, these patterns provide the fingerprints so useful to law enforcement officials, as well as serving as friction ridges.

Blood vessels and nerves, which are generally absent in epidermal tissue, are found throughout the dermis. Specialized skin structures such as hair follicles and glands are formed from cells of stratum basale that push down into the dermis and are located there. Cells of the dermis, as well as the deeper layers of the epidermis, are bathed by tissue fluid.

## Subcutaneous Layer

The **subcutaneous** (sub-koo-**tay′**-nee-us) **layer** beneath the dermis consists of loose connective tissue, usually including adipose tissue. The subcutaneous layer attaches the skin to underlying tissues, but because of its loose construction, the skin may be moved about over the muscle and bone beneath. This thick fatty layer helps to protect underlying organs from mechanical shock and also insulates the body, thus conserving heat. Fat stored within the adipose tissue can be mobilized and utilized for energy when adequate food is not available. Distribution of fat in the subcutaneous layer is largely responsible for the characteristic body contours of the female as compared with the male.

## SPECIALIZED STRUCTURES OF THE SKIN

During embryonic development thousands of small groups of epidermal cells from the stratum basale push down into the dermis. They multiply and differentiate to form hair follicles and glands.

### Hair

Hair serves a protective function and plays a role in sexual attraction. It is found on all skin surfaces except the palms and the soles. On the "less hairy" parts of the body the fine, downy hairs are hardly noticeable.

The part of the hair that we see is the **shaft**; the portion below the skin surface is the **root** (Figs. 4–1 and 4–2). The root together with its epithelial and connective tissue coverings is called the **hair follicle**. At the bottom of the follicle is a **papilla** (a little mound) of connective tissue containing capillaries that deliver nourishment to the cells of the follicle. Just above the papilla is a group of epithelial cells, derived from the stratum basale, which multiplies, giving rise to the cells of the hair.

Each hair consists of cells that proliferate, manufacture keratin as they move outward, and then die. The shaft of the hair consists of dead cells and their products. That is why hair can be cut without any sensation of pain. As long as the follicle remains intact, new hair will continue to grow. If the follicle is destroyed, as by electrolysis, no new hair can form.

Tiny bundles of smooth muscle are associated with hair follicles. These **arrector pili** muscles contract in response to cold or fear, making the hairs stand up straight. Skin around the hair shaft is pulled up into "gooseflesh."

### Glands

Like hair follicles, sebaceous glands and sweat glands also develop from epidermal cells that move down into the dermis.

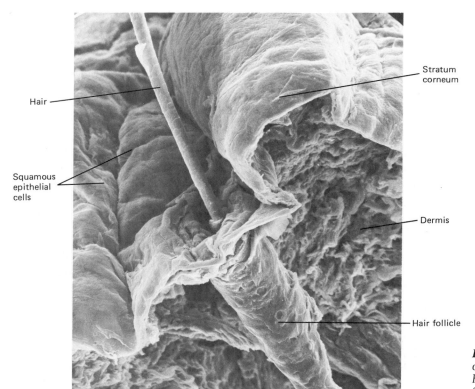

*Figure 4–2. Scanning electron micrograph of human skin showing hair follicle (approximately ×250). (Courtesy of Dr. Karen A. Holbrook.)*

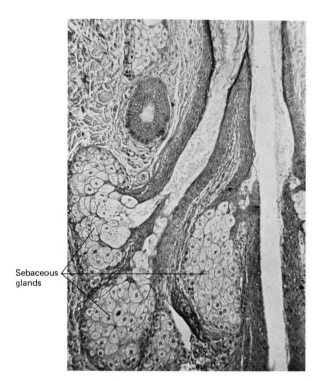

Sebaceous
glands

*Figure 4–3.* Hair follicle showing sebaceous glands
(×200).

## Sebaceous Glands

Two or more **sebaceous glands**, often called oil glands, are attached to each hair follicle by little ducts (Fig. 4–3). These glands are largest and most numerous on the face and scalp. Sebaceous glands secrete an oily substance called **sebum**, which functions to oil the hair, to lubricate the surface of the skin, and possibly to help retard water loss. It may also have some antibacterial and antifungal properties.

During childhood sebaceous glands are relatively inactive. At puberty they are activated by increased secretion of male hormone in both males and females. This stepped-up activity sometimes leads to the lesions (abnormal changes) characteristic of **acne**, a condition common during puberty.

Sometimes sebum accumulates in the duct of the sebaceous gland and hair follicle and obstructs it, forming a blackhead or whitehead (comedo). In a blackhead sebum and dead cells containing the dark pigment melanin block the duct. The black color is due to the melanin rather than to dirt.

Should the duct of a sebaceous gland rupture, allowing sebum, keratin, and perhaps bacteria to spill into the dermis, the skin becomes inflamed. The red papules (pimples) and pustules (lesions containing pus) characteristic of acne are formed in this way. Squeezing these lesions (as many persons do) causes an increase in the inflammation and may lead to scarring.

## Sweat Glands

Each **sweat gland** is a tiny coiled tube in the dermis or subcutaneous tissue, with a duct that extends up through the skin and opens onto the surface (Fig. 4–1). About 3 million sweat glands in the skin help regulate body temperature. They accomplish this by excreting sweat, which consists mainly of excess water with some salts and a trace of urea, a nitrogen waste product of metabolism. When profuse sweating occurs, the rate of salt reabsorption cannot keep up with the large amounts of sweat excreted, so that proportionately more salt is lost in the sweat. (This is why people engaged in strenuous exercise must replace salts lost in sweat.)

Small children lose heat more rapidly than adults because the skin surface accounts for a higher proportion of their bodies. With relatively more surface exposed, more heat is lost. It is also more difficult for an elderly person to maintain an appropriate body temperature than for a young adult. As people age, there is a decrease in the number of sweat glands making older individuals more prone to heat exhaustion.

Certain sweat glands found in association with hairs are concentrated in a few specific areas of the body such as the armpits and genital areas. These glands discharge into hair follicles. Their secretion is thick, sticky, and initially odorless. However, certain bacteria that inhabit the skin surface begin to decompose this secretion, causing it to become odorous. Deodorants kill these bacteria and replace the odor with a more perfumed scent; antiperspirants reduce moisture, thus inhibiting the growth of bacteria. Emotional stress or sexual stimulation promotes sweat gland secretion.

## Nails

**Nails** are a modification of the horny epidermal cells and consist mainly of a closely compressed, tough keratin. The nail bed beneath the **body** (the visible part) of the nail lacks a stratum corneum. Nails appear pink because of underlying capillaries. The actively growing area is the white crescent (lunula) at the base of the nail; growth is continuous at a rate of about 0.1 mm/day. Though continuously being worn down at their distal ends, nails are also deliberately trimmed. Lost nails are regenerated but the process requires several months.

## PIGMENTATION

Scattered throughout the basal layer of the epidermis are cells that produce pigment granules composed of a type of protein called **melanin** (**mel'**-ah-nin). Pigment cells have long projections of cytoplasm, which they use to transfer pigment granules to other epidermal cells. Cells that receive pigment carry it with them as they move into the stratum corneum, imparting a characteristic coloration to each person's skin. Pigment cells present in the lowest layer of hair follicle cells pass pigment granules on to hair cells, thereby giving color to hair as well as to skin.

Skin color is inherited. In dark-skinned individuals the pigment cells are more active and produce more and larger granules of melanin. Asiatic people have the yellowish pigment **carotene** in their skin, as well as melanin. The pinkish hue of light skin is due to the color of blood in the vessels of the dermis. An **albino** is a person of any race who has inherited the inability to produce pigment.

> Melanin is an important protective screen against the sun because it absorbs harmful ultraviolet rays. Exposure to the sun stimulates an increase in the amount of melanin produced and causes the skin to become darker. Thus suntan is a protective response.
>
> The tan so prized by sun worshippers is actually a sign that the skin has been exposed to too much ultraviolet radiation. When the melanin is not able to absorb all the ultraviolet rays the skin becomes inflamed, or sunburned. Excessive exposure to sun over a period of years, especially in fair-skinned individuals, eventually results in wrinkling of the skin and sometimes in skin cancer. Because dark-skinned people have more melanin, they suffer less sunburn, wrinkling, and skin cancer.

## THE SKIN IN STRESS

Though the skin is the outermost part of the body, providing protection from cuts, scratches, poisons, bacteria, and other insults, it also reflects inner turmoil. It flushes, pales, sweats, and bristles with the emotions; it scales, weeps, cracks, and swells with allergies. Pale skin may indicate anemia, yellowish skin may signal liver malfunction, and blue skin may indicate circulatory or respiratory disorder. In health and disease the skin mirrors much of one's physiology and experience.

## Inflammation and Repair of Wounds

Any bodily injury caused by physical means that disrupts the normal continuity of structures can be called a **wound**. When the skin (or any other tissue) is injured, it reacts homeostatically by attempting to protect itself against harmful agents and by repairing the wound. Mechanisms are activated to destroy bacteria that may have entered, dilute harmful chemicals, dispose of dead or injured cells, and even wall off the injured area. These reactions, collectively referred to as **inflammation**, are characterized by redness, swelling, heat, and pain. Inflammation, the most basic pathological response, helps protect the tissue from further injury and sets up the conditions that promote repair.

Taking a more detailed look at the inflammatory response, suppose that you have just cut your finger. It bleeds, but not for long because the blood clots (Fig. 4–4). Chemicals such as histamines are released by cells in the injured area, causing the blood vessels to dilate (increase in diameter) and become more permeable. As a result, large amounts of fluid may leave the blood and enter the injured area, causing **edema** (swelling). The excess fluid exerts pressure on nerves and other tissues, resulting in pain. Yet the fluid helps dilute harmful substances that may be present and brings large quantities of oxygen and nutrients needed in the repair process. Because of the unusually large amount of blood in the area the skin may feel warm and appear red. Clots form in the interstitial fluid, slowing the spread of bacteria and toxic materials. This mechanism serves to wall off the injured area.

A chemical produced by injured tissue is thought to trigger the release of large numbers of white blood cells from storage areas in the bone marrow. White blood cells easily pass out of the permeable blood vessels and phagocytize bacteria, dead cells, and other foreign material. When bacterial infection is present, **pus**, a creamy fluid containing dead white blood cells and bacteria, may be produced.

If the wound damages blood vessels, blood leaks out and a clot forms. Soon after it forms, the blood clot contracts and begins to dehydrate, forming a **scab**, a temporary covering that seals the defect in the skin. Basal cells in the epidermis multiply rapidly, and epithelial cells from the sides of the wound migrate beneath the scab, eventually covering the wound. When the scab finally falls off, new skin is fully formed beneath. Fibroblasts from the subcutaneous layer and dermis multiply and produce collagen, which accumulates slowly and eventually fills in the wound beneath the epithelium.

Gradually, **scar tissue** forms. The difference between scar tissue and normal dermis is that in scar

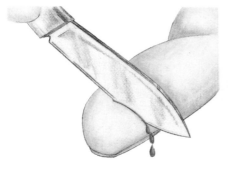

A typical cut or wound heals by a definite series of events.

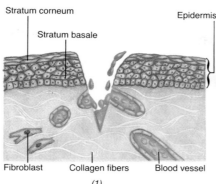

When injury occurs blood vessels may be severed, resulting in bleeding. Within seconds blood begins to clot.

*(1)*

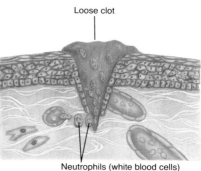

Several hours later blood has formed a loose clot. Large numbers of neutrophils (white blood cells) migrate into clot and nearby tissue, attracted by chemicals released by cells and bacteria in wounded area. Nearby blood vessels dilate. Epidermal cells have begun to divide and to migrate down over surface of injured tissue.

*(2)*

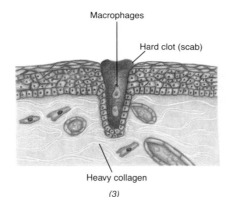

Within two days epidermal cells have covered injured tissue, or have covered area adjacent to them. Fibroblasts have migrated into area and begin producing collagen fibers necessary to reinforce repair. Macrophages (large janitor cells) have moved into area to clean up debris and bacteria. Developing collagen begins to force floor of wound upward. Clot hardens, forming scab.

*(3)*

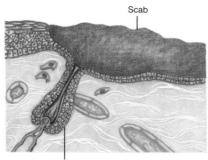

If wound is broad and shallow, healing may differ slightly in that epithelial cells derived from linings of hair follicles and sweat glands may spread over injured area much more quickly than adjacent surface cells could do by themselves.

*(3a)*

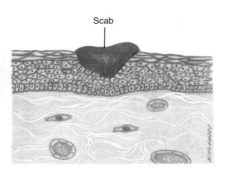

About a week after wound has occurred the scab has hardened and contracted, pulling walls of injury together. Epidermal cells have multiplied beneath it and thickening mass of collagen fibers has made wound shallower. Scab sloughs off but repair is not quite complete. Further production of dermis and thickening of epidermis must continue for some time before maximum strength is restored.

*(4)*

***Figure 4–4.** Repair of a wound.*

tissue the collagen is more dense, its fibers are arranged somewhat differently, and it contains fewer cells and blood vessels. Scar tissue may lack hair, sweat glands, and sensory receptors.

Formation of scar tissue is a process of collagen synthesis and collagen breakdown that continues for many months and even years after a wound appears to have healed. During this time the scar tissue is remodeled, that is, the collagen fibers are rearranged so as to impart maximum strength to the tissue.

## Burns

Burns are thermal injuries that may result from direct heat, certain chemicals, electricity, or radiation. Excessive heat denatures (coagulates) cell proteins, leading to injury or death of the cells. Of the 2 million people burned in the United States each year, about 12,000 die and 100,000 are hospitalized.

Least serious are first-degree burns, such as sunburn, in which the epidermis remains intact.

Blood vessels in the dermis dilate, causing inflammation, but the skin usually heals within a few days without scarring. First-degree burns require no special treatment but pain may be relieved by immersing the burned area in cold water.

Second-degree burns may be superficial or deep dermal burns. In superficial second-degree burns the epidermis and superficial dermis are damaged and excessive fluid between dermis and epidermis accumulates in blisters. Such burns usually heal in 2 to 3 weeks by outgrowth of epithelial tissue from hair follicles and other dermal appendages. In deep second-degree burns many dermal appendages are destroyed. This results in less capacity for regeneration and greater probability of scarring. After initial treatment with cold water, second-degree burns are treated by soaking in salt water.

In third-degree (or full-thickness) burns, portions of the epidermis, dermis, and subcutaneous tissue are destroyed. Nerve endings in the area may be destroyed, so that the victims feel little or no pain. Without its protective shield the body is in grave danger and the entire organism reacts profoundly to the crisis. Because the burned skin is unable to retain body fluids, large amounts of fluid may leave the body, resulting in shock. If this fluid (with its salts and protein) is not quickly replaced, the individual may die. Another serious threat is infection, as disease organisms can readily gain access to the exposed tissues. Third-degree burns require immediate skilled medical treatment, including intravenous replacement of lost fluids, treatment with antibiotics, and skin transplants (necessary in full-thickness burns because tissues are not able to repair themselves). If third-degree burns are extensive, the patient often dies despite heroic efforts to prolong his or her life.

Risk of death following extensive burns is roughly proportional to the percentage of body surface that has been damaged. When more than 20% of the body has been burned the injury may well be lethal but, of course, the depth of the injury affects the prognosis. Figure 4–5 illustrates the "rule of nines" used clinically to estimate the percentage of the body surface involved in burns.

## Skin Cancer

Skin cancer is most frequently linked to excessive, chronic exposure to the ultraviolet radiation of sunlight. This disease has also been associated with exposure to arsenic compounds, x-rays, and radioactive materials such as radium. Most forms of skin cancer progress relatively slowly; with skilled treatment there is a high rate of cure.

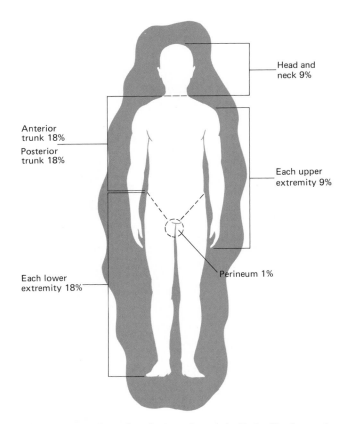

*Figure 4–5. The rule of nines is used clinically for estimating the extent of burns. When more than 20% of the body has been burned the injury is often fatal.*

The most common type of skin cancer is **basal cell carcinoma**, in which cells in the basal layer of the epidermis are altered and then malfunction (Fig. 4–6). They no longer honor the boundary between the epidermis and dermis. As they migrate into the dermis and subcutaneous tissues they erode normal tissue, causing erosive ulcers. Malignant basal cells appear to have lost their ability to form keratin and to mature normally. Because me-

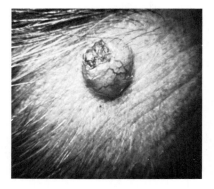

*Figure 4–6. Skin cancer. Photograph of a basal cell carcinoma on the forehead of a patient who had harbored the disease for 5 years. (Courtesy of Dr. Wilfred D. Little.) Also see Focus on Neoplasms—Unwelcome Tissues (Chapter 3) for a photomicrograph of basal cell carcinoma.*

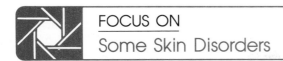

## FOCUS ON
## Some Skin Disorders

**Abscess:** a cavity formed in disintegrating tissue in which pus collects

**Callus:** a slightly thickened area of stratum corneum (the horny layer of the epidermis) that develops in response to constant friction or pressure

**Carbuncle:** a painful cluster of boils in the deep dermis and subcutaneous tissue; a type of infection with abscesses that discharge pus to the skin surface

**Corn:** similar to a callus but the thickened tissue is more separated and distinct from surrounding tissue; caused by friction and pressure

**Cyst:** a thick-walled sac that contains fluid or semisolid material

**Decubitus ulcer:** a bedsore; a pressure sore that develops in patients confined to bed for long periods of time, especially when they are unable to change position frequently

**Dermatitis:** inflammation of the skin

**Furuncle:** a boil; a localized infection (usually caused by staphylococcal bacteria) that develops into an abscess that drains to the skin surface;

**Hypodermic:** Under the skin

**Impetigo:** an acute bacterial infection of the skin characterized by lesions that rupture and develop distinct yellow crusts

**Intradermal:** Within the skin

**Miliaria:** heat rash; prickly heat; acute inflammation of the skin associated with blocked sweat gland ducts

**Nevus:** a lesion (disruption of normal tissue structure) containing melanocytes (pigment cells); a mole

**Nodule:** a solid mass larger than 1 cm that is formed from groups of cells or cell products within the dermis or subcutaneous tissue

**Papule:** a small, elevated solid lesion formed from cells, cell products, or accumulated fluid in the dermis or epidermis; usually smaller than 0.5 cm; a pimple

**Pediculosis:** a skin disease caused by infestation of blood-sucking lice

**Phthirus:** a species of louse that infects the pubic area and is most often spread by sexual contact (pubic lice are commonly referred to as "crabs")

**Pruritus:** itching of the skin when there is no visible lesion; may be due to irritation of a sensory nerve

**Psoriasis:** a genetically determined skin disease in which papules and plaques form, especially on the elbows and knees

**Pustule:** a small elevation (vesicle) of the skin containing pus

**Scabies:** a condition caused by infestation with itch mites, characterized by severe itching

**Shingles:** a viral disease characterized by painful blisters along certain nerve pathways; more formally called herpes zoster

**Wart:** an epidermal growth induced by infection by a specific virus

---

tastasis is uncommon in this type of cancer, there is a good chance for cure.

Two other types of skin cancer are **squamous cell carcinoma** and **malignant melanoma**. In squamous cell carcinoma the cells continue to form keratin and to differentiate. If the condition is untreated, metastasis occurs and leads to death. Malignant melanoma is a cancer of the pigment cells. Metastasis may occur and the chances for survival depend on early diagnosis and treatment.

## SUMMARY

I. The integumentary system consists of the skin and its hair, nails, and glands.

II. The integumentary system functions to
   A. Protect the body against mechanical and thermal injury.
   B. Prevent entrance of disease organisms.
   C. Prevent entrance of harmful chemicals.
   D. Prevent dehydration.
   E. Help maintain constant body temperature.
   F. Help excrete excess water and body wastes.
   G. Produce vitamin D.

III. As a basal cell moves outward through the layers of the epidermis it produces keratin, then dies, becoming scalelike, and finally is sloughed off the skin surface.

IV. The dermis consists of connective tissue containing large amounts of collagen. It gives substance to the skin, holds the blood vessels that bring nourishment to the epidermal cells, and contains sensory receptors and epidermal structures such as hair follicles and glands.

V. The subcutaneous layer consists of connective tissue, including adipose tissue. This tissue cushions underlying structures against mechanical injury, connects skin with tissues beneath, and stores energy in the form of fat.

VI. Hair follicles and sebaceous glands arise from epidermal cells that push down into the dermis during early development.

VII. Sweat glands release onto the skin surface a

dilute salt water, which evaporates, cooling the body.

VIII. Pigment cells in the basal layer produce pigment granules and pass them on to other epidermal cells, including those that form hair. Melanin absorbs ultraviolet rays from the sun, preventing damage to dermis and blood vessels.

IX. Inflammation is a reaction by the tissues that tends to protect them from further injury or irritation. Symptoms are redness, swelling, heat, and pain.

X. In first-degree burns there is inflammation but the epidermis remains intact; in second-degree burns epidermal cells and part of the dermis may be destroyed and inflammation and blistering occur; in third-degree burns the damage may extend into the subcutaneous tissue, resulting in significant fluid loss and infection.

XI. Skin cancer has been linked to excessive exposure to ultraviolet radiation from the sun, arsenic compounds, x-rays, and radioactive materials.

## POST TEST

1. The skin with its glands, hair, nails, and other structures makes up the _____ system.
2. The two main layers of the skin are the outer _____ and the inner _____.
3. The deepest stratum of the epidermis is the _____.
4. The tough waterproofing protein of the epidermis is _____.
5. The outermost layer of the epidermis is stratum _____.
6. The _____ _____ beneath the dermis consists of loose connective tissue.
7. The root of a hair together with its coverings is called a _____.
8. _____ glands are attached to each hair follicle by ducts; they secrete an oily substance called _____.
9. Sweat consists mainly of _____ with some _____ and a trace of urea.
10. Nails consist mainly of tough, compressed _____.
11. Granules containing melanin are produced by _____ _____.
12. The body's basic response to injury is _____.
13. The symptoms of inflammation are _____, _____, _____, and _____.
14. The least serious burns are _____ degree burns.
15. The rule of _____ is used clinically to estimate the percentage of the body surface involved in burns.
16. The most common type of skin cancer is _____ _____.

## REVIEW QUESTIONS

1. In what ways does the skin help preserve homeostasis?
2. Compare the structure of the epidermis with that of the dermis.
3. Which cells of the epidermis actively divide? Which are dead?
4. What are the functions of the dermis? The subcutaneous layer?
5. What is the function of the sebaceous glands? What happens when they malfunction?
6. Why is melanin important? How does it get into the skin cells?
7. What are the principal characteristics of inflammation?
8. Suppose you step on a nail. How does the body respond to the injury? Describe the healing process.

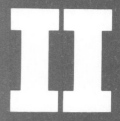

# SUPPORT AND MOVEMENT

# The Skeletal System

LEARNING OBJECTIVES

**After you study this chapter you should be able to**
1. List five functions of the skeletal system.
2. Label a diagram of a long bone and describe the microscopic structure of a bone.
3. Contrast endochondral with membranous bone development and describe the role of osteoblasts and osteoclasts in bone production.
4. List and describe the bones of the axial skeleton and identify each on a diagram or skeleton.
5. List and describe the bones of the appendicular skeleton and identify each on a diagram or skeleton.
6. Compare the main types of joints and describe the structure and functions of diarthroses.

When you first consider the skeletal system you may conjure up an image of the familiar dry, dead bones of the skeleton in your science laboratory. In life the skeletal system consists of bone, cartilage, and other connective tissues that respire, consume energy in their metabolism, and produce waste products.

## FUNCTIONS

The skeletal system serves several important functions.

1. It serves as a bony framework for the body, supporting the tissues and organs.
2. It protects delicate vital organs. For example, the skull encases the brain; the sternum (breastbone) and ribs protect the heart and lungs. For their weight, bones are nearly as strong as steel.
3. Bones serve as levers that transmit muscular forces. Muscles are attached to bones by bands of connective tissue called **tendons**. When muscles contract they pull on bones, thereby moving parts of the body. Bones are held together at joints by bands of connective tissue called **ligaments**. Most joints are movable. The interaction of bones and muscles also makes breathing possible.
4. The marrow within some bones produces blood cells.
5. Bones serve as banks for calcium and phosphorus. When the concentration of calcium in the blood increases above normal, calcium is deposited in the bones. When the concentration of calcium decreases, calcium is withdrawn from the bones and enters the blood.

## STRUCTURE OF A BONE

A bone is covered by a connective tissue membrane, the **periosteum** (per″-ee-**os**′-tee-um) (Fig. 5–1). At its joint surfaces the outer layer of a bone consists of articular cartilage. The main shaft of a long bone is known as its **diaphysis** (die-**af**′-i-sis). The expanded ends of the bone are called **epiphyses** (e-**pif**′-i-sees). In children, a disc of cartilage, the **metaphysis** (me-**taf**′-i-sis), is found between the epiphyses and the diaphysis. The metaphyses are growth centers that disappear at maturity, becoming vague **epiphyseal lines**. Within the long bone there is a central **marrow cavity** filled with a fatty connective tissue known as yellow bone marrow. The marrow cavity is lined with a thin membrane, the **endosteum** (en-**dos**′-tee-um).

Two types of bone tissue are compact bone and spongy bone. **Compact bone**, which is dense and hard, is found primarily near the surfaces of the bone, where great strength is needed. **Spongy bone** consists of a meshwork of thin strands of bone. The spaces within the spongy bone are filled with bone marrow. Spongy bone is found within the epiphyses and lining the marrow cavity.

Compact bone consists of interlocking, spindle-shaped units called **osteons** (**os**′-tee-ons), or **haversian systems** (Fig. 5–2). Within an osteon, **osteocytes** (**os**′-tee-o-sites″), the mature bone cells, are found in small cavities called **lacunae** (lah-**koo**′-nee). The lacunae are arranged in concentric circles around central **haversian canals**. Blood vessels that nourish the bone tissue pass through the haversian canals. Threadlike extensions of the cytoplasm of the osteocytes extend through narrow channels called **canaliculi** (kan″-ah-**lik**′-u-lie). These cellular extensions connect the osteocytes.

## BONE DEVELOPMENT

During fetal development bones form in two ways. The long bones develop from cartilage replicas, a process called **endochondral** (en″-dow-**kon**′-dral) **bone development**. The flat bones of the skull, the irregular vertebrae, and some other bones develop from a noncartilage connective tissue scaffold. This is known as **membranous bone development**.

**Osteoblasts** (**os**′-tee-o-blasts) are bone-building cells. They secrete the protein collagen, which forms the strong, elastic fibers of bone. A complex calcium phosphate called **apatite** (**ap**′-uh-tite) is present in the tissue fluid. This compound automatically crystallizes around the collagen fibers, forming the hard matrix of bone. As the matrix forms around them, the osteoblasts become isolated within the small spaces called lacunae. The trapped osteoblasts are referred to as osteocytes. The process of bone formation is called **ossification** (os″-i-fi-**kay**′-shun).

Bones are modeled during growth and remodeled continuously throughout life in response to physical stresses and other changing demands. As muscles develop in response to physical activity, the bones to which they are attached thicken and become stronger. As bones grow bone tissue must be removed from the interior, especially from the walls of the marrow cavity. This process keeps bones from getting too heavy. **Osteoclasts** are the

*Figure 5–1.* Anatomy of a bone. (a) The structure of a typical long bone. (b) Internal structure of a long bone.

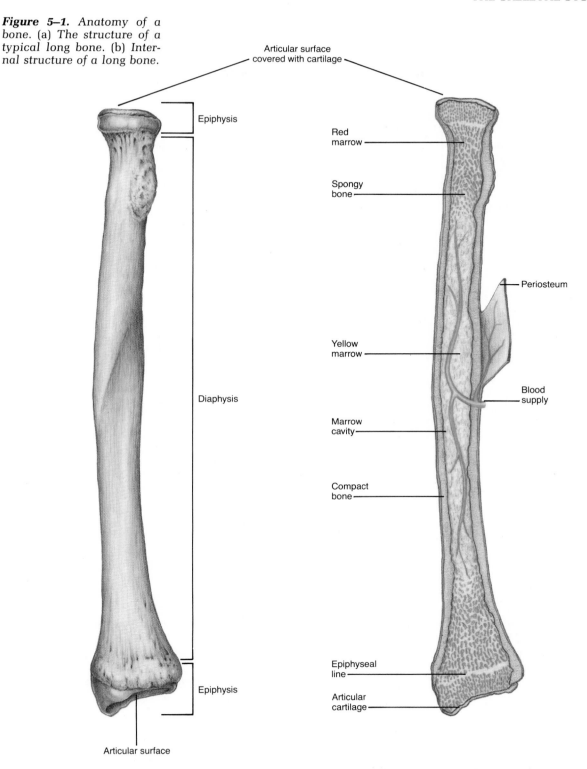

Articular surface covered with cartilage

Epiphysis

Diaphysis

Epiphysis

Articular surface

Red marrow

Spongy bone

Periosteum

Yellow marrow

Blood supply

Marrow cavity

Compact bone

Epiphyseal line

Articular cartilage

cells that break down bone, a process referred to as bone resorption. These bone-breaker cells are large cells that move about secreting enzymes that digest bone. Osteoclasts and osteoblasts work side by side to shape bones and to form the precise grain needed in the finished bone. Some important types of bone markings are described in Table 5–1.

## DIVISIONS OF THE SKELETON

The human skeleton (Figs. 5–3 and 5–4) may be divided into two groups of bones

1. The **axial** (ak'-se-al) **skeleton** consists of the skull, vertebral column, ribs, and sternum.
2. The **appendicular** (ap-en-**dik'**-u-lar) **skeleton**

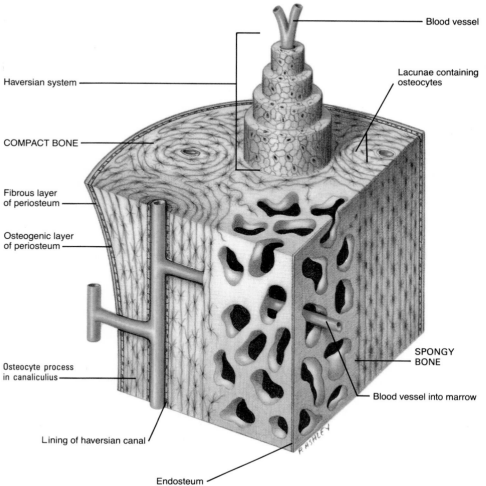

Haversian system

COMPACT BONE

Fibrous layer of periosteum

Osteogenic layer of periosteum

Osteocyte process in canaliculius

Lining of haversian canal

Endosteum

Blood vessel

Lacunae containing osteocytes

SPONGY BONE

Blood vessel into marrow

***Figure 5–2.*** *A three-dimensional diagram showing the microscopic appearance of both a cross section and a longitudinal section of the various components of compact bone.*

TABLE 5–1
## Bone Markings

**PROCESS: Any prominent bony projection**

### *Processes That Help Form Joints*

| | |
|---|---|
| Condyle (**kon**′-dil) | Rounded projection |
| Head | Rounded projection supported by narrow neck (constricted region); usually the upper or proximal extremity of a bone; often bears the ball of ball-and-socket joint |
| Facet | Smooth, flat surface; found on vertebrae for articulation with ribs |

### *Processes That Are Sites of Attachment for Tendons and Ligaments*

| | |
|---|---|
| Crest | Projecting line or ridge, often on long border of bone |
| Epicondyle | Bony bulge adjacent to condyle |
| Spine | Sharp projection; sometimes a long, strongly raised ridge |
| Trochanter (tro-**kan**′-ter) | Pulley-like process found only on femur |

| | |
|---|---|
| Tubercle (**too**′-ber-kul) | Small, rounded process |
| Tuberosity | Large, rounded, often roughened process |

### **DEPRESSIONS AND OPENINGS**

| | |
|---|---|
| Fissure (**fish**′-ur) | Narrow cleft or groove through which blood vessels and nerves pass |
| Foramen (foe-**ray**′-men) | Natural opening or passage into or through bony structure, often round; term means "hole" |
| Fossa | Trench or shallow depression; term means "basin-like depression" |
| Sulcus | Groove through which blood vessel or nerve may pass |
| Meatus (me-**a**′-tus) | Opening into some passageway in body, not necessarily bony; usually lengthy and tunnel-like |
| Sinus | Air-filled cavity (paranasal sinuses are connected to nasal cavity) |

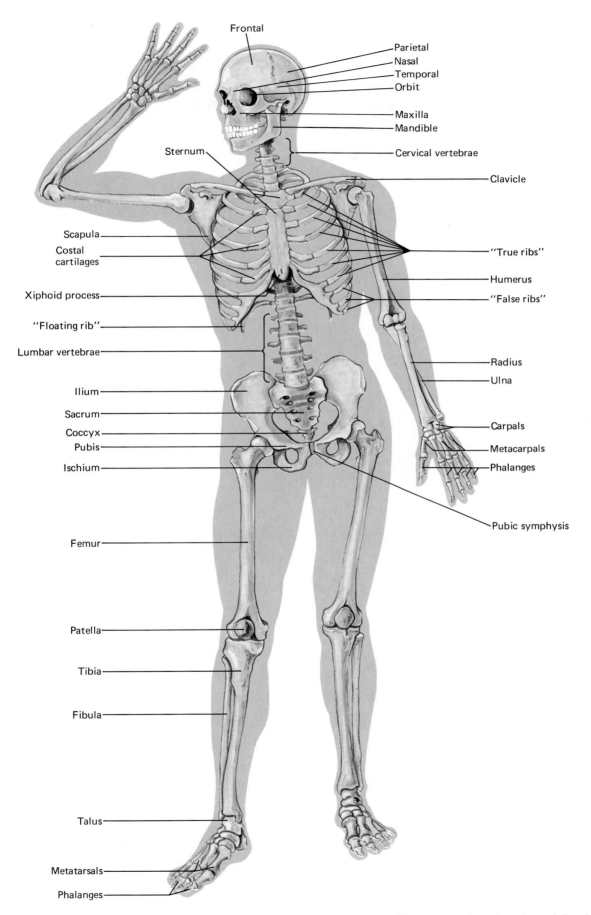

Frontal

Parietal
Nasal
Temporal
Orbit

Maxilla
Mandible

Cervical vertebrae

Sternum

Clavicle

Scapula

Costal
cartilages

"True ribs"

Humerus

"False ribs"

Xiphoid process

"Floating rib"

Lumbar vertebrae

Radius

Ulna

Ilium

Sacrum

Coccyx

Pubis

Ischium

Carpals

Metacarpals

Phalanges

Pubic symphysis

Femur

Patella

Tibia

Fibula

Talus

Metatarsals

Phalanges

*Figure 5–3.* Anterior view of the skeleton.

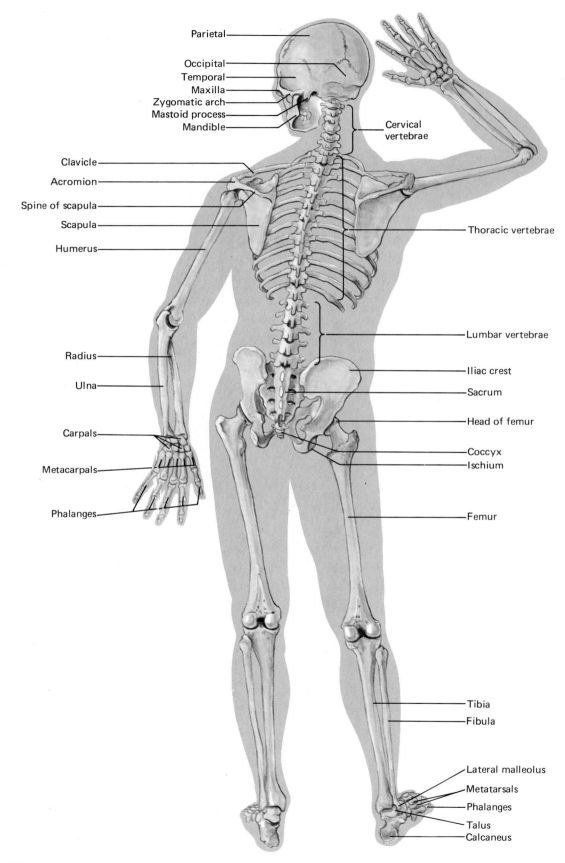

**Figure 5—4.** *Posterior view of the skeleton.*

consists of the upper and lower extremities (arms and legs), the shoulder girdle, and the pelvic girdle (with the exception of the sacrum).

## The Skull

The skull, the bony framework of the head, consists of the cranial and the facial bones. The eight cranial bones enclose the brain. Fourteen bones make up the facial portion of the skull. Also within the head are six small bones in the middle ears. The bones of the head are described in Table 5–2 and illustrated in Figures 5–5 through 5–8.

Most of the bones of the skull are joined by immovable joints called *sutures*. The **sagittal suture** is the joint between the two parietal bones. The **coronal suture** joins the parietal bones to the frontal bone. The **lambdoidal suture** is the joint between the parietal bones and the occipital bone.

*Text continued on page 83*

TABLE 5–2
**Bones That Make Up the Skeleton**

| Name of Bone (Number) | Function | Description |
|---|---|---|
| **Cranial Bones** | | |
| *Frontal (1)* | Forms forehead and front part of cranium floor; forms part of roof over eyes and nasal cavity | Large, curved bone<br>**Frontal sinuses:** air-filled cavities lined with mucous membrane<br>**Supraorbital ridge:** just below eyebrows |
| *Parietal (2)* | Form much of walls and roof of cranium | Curved, flattened bones that meet at midline of cranium just behind frontal bone |
| *Temporal (2)* | Helps form floor and lateral wall of cranial cavity; contains **external auditory meatus**, middle ear bones, and sensory portions of ear; bears temporomandibular joint (see mandible below) | Pointed **styloid process** serves as point of attachment for certain neck muscles; **mastoid process** contains air sinuses that may become infected when a middle ear infection spreads; **zygomatic process** helps form cheek |
| *Occipital (1)* | Forms most of floor and posterior part of skull; articulates with neck; many neck muscles attach to this bone | Contains **foramen magnum** through which spinal cord passes; **occipital condyles** articulate with first vertebra of spinal column |
| *Sphenoid (1)* | Forms floor of cranium; helps form eye orbits | Shaped like butterfly<br>**Sella turcica (sell'-ah-tur'-si-kah):** saddle-shaped depression on superior surface holds pituitary gland; also called Turkish saddle<br>**Sphenoid sinus:** air-filled spaces lined with mucous membrane |
| *Ethmoid (1)* | Forms roof of nasal cavity and part of medial walls of eye orbits | Has irregular shape<br>**Crista galli:** beak-shaped process to which an extension (falx cerebri) of outermost membrane surrounding brain attaches<br>**Cribriform plate:** area of ethmoid perforated by tiny holes through which fibers of olfactory nerves pass from nose to brain<br>**Superior and middle turbinates (conchae):** projections that form ledges along lateral walls of nasal cavity<br>**Ethmoid sinuses:** air spaces lined with mucous membrane |
| **Facial Bones** | | |
| *Mandible (1)* | Lower jawbone; joins with temporal bone on each side forming **temporomandibular joints** (only freely movable joints in the skull); used in many mouth movments, especially chewing; many muscles including some used in chewing and in facial expression attach to the mandible | U-shaped bone; its body (horizontal part) forms chin; its rami (vertical parts) have condyles (heads) that articulate with temporal bones<br>**Alveolar process:** bony ridge in which lower teeth are rooted |
| *Maxilla (2)* | Fuse to form upper jaw bone; form lateral walls of nose, floor of orbits, anterior part of hard palate (roof of mouth) | Very irregular shape; all facial bones except mandible touch maxilla<br>**Palatine processes:** form anterior part of hard palate<br>**Alveolar process:** bony arch in which upper teeth are rooted<br>**Maxillary sinuses:** largest sinuses; drain into nasal passages and throat<br>**Zygomatic process:** articulates with malar |

*Table continued on following page*

TABLE 5–2
**Bones That Make Up the Skeleton** Continued

| Name of Bone (Number) | Function | Description |
|---|---|---|
| **Facial Bones** Continued | | |
| *Palatine (2)* | Horizontal portion forms posterior part of hard palate; both portions help to form nasal cavity | Irregular shape; cleft palate occurs when these bones (or palatine processes) do not fuse |
| *Malar (zygomatic) (2)* | Cheekbones; form walls and floors of orbits | Curved, irregular shape |
| *Nasal (2)* | Form upper part of bridge of nose | Small, thin, triangular shape |
| *Lacrimal (2)* | Help form medial wall of orbit; contain a groove through which tears pass into nasal cavity | About size and shape of a fingernail |
| *Vomer (1)* | Forms inferior, back part of nasal septum | Trapezoid-shaped |
| *Inferior turbinate (2)* | Forms ledge along lateral walls of nose; increases surface area of nasal cavity | Scroll-shaped |
| **Ear Bones** | | |
| A chain of 3 tiny bones, or ossicles, in each middle ear cavity. | | |
| **Malleus** (2) | Transmits vibration from eardrum | Attached to eardrum; shaped somewhat like hammer |
| **Incus** (2) | Transmits vibration in middle ear | Shaped somewhat like anvil |
| **Stapes** (2) | Transmits vibration to oval window | Shaped like stirrup |
| *Hyoid (1)* | Important during swallowing | U-shaped, located in neck between mandible and larynx; does not articulate directly with any other bone |
| **Vertebral Column** | | |
| *Cervical vertebrae (7)* | | |
| **Atlas** (C1) | First cervical vertebra; forms joints with occipital condyles that allow head to nod "yes" | Has no centrum; no neural spine |
| **Axis** (C2) | Second cervical vertebra; its odontoid process serves as pivot for rotation of atlas and skull; permits you to shake your head "no" | **Odontoid process** (dens) projects upward from centrum |
| **Inferior cervical vertebrae** | **Spines** serve as points of attachment for neck and back muscles | Can be identified by its **transverse foramina** through which vertebral arteries and veins pass |
| *Thoracic vertebrae (12)* | Ribs attach to these vertebrae; part of thoracic cage | Have facets for articulation with ribs |
| *Lumbar vertebrae (5)* | Make up part of vertebral column in small of back; support most of body weight; responsible for much of flexibility of trunk; many of back muscles attach to them | Large, heavy vertebrae |
| *Sacrum (1)* | Part of pelvic girdle | 5 separate vertebrae in child; fuse to form a single bone in adult |
| *Coccyx (1)* | Several pelvic and hip muscles originate on coccyx | 3–5 separate vertebrae in child; fuse in adult |
| **Thoracic Cage** | | |
| *Ribs (24)* | Protect organs of thoracic cavity; form part of thoracic cage | Long, curved bones<br>**True ribs** Upper 7 pairs; attach directly to sternum by way of costal cartilages<br>**False ribs** Pairs 8, 9, and 10; attach to sternum by way of common bar of cartilage that joins costal cartilage of seventh ribs<br>**Floating ribs** Pairs 11 and 12; not connected to sternum |
| *Sternum (1)* | Breastbone; protects heart and anchors anterior ends of ribs; produces red blood cells in its marrow cavity | Consists of 3 parts: thick, superior **manubrium**; long **body**; inferior **xiphoid process** composed of cartilage (xiphoid process important landmark for CPR) |
| **Pectoral Girdle** | | |
| *Scapula (2)* | Shoulder blade | Somewhat flat, triangular bone<br>**Spine:** sharp ridge that runs diagonally across posterior surface of shoulder blade<br>**Acromion process:** helps hold head of humerus in place<br>**Coracoid process:** point of attachment for some upper arm muscles<br>**Glenoid fossa:** socket that receives head of humerus |
| *Clavicle (2)* | Collarbone; connects scapula with sternum; helps form shoulder joint | Small, curved bone |

TABLE 5–2
**Bones That Make Up the Skeleton** *Continued*

| Name of Bone (Number) | Function | Description |
|---|---|---|
| **Upper Extremities** | | |
| *Humerus (2)* | Upper arm bone | Longest, largest bone of upper extremity<br>**Head:** fits into glenoid process of scapula<br>**Greater and lesser tubercles:** projections where muscles attach<br>**Deltoid tuberosity:** rough elevation on shaft for attachment of muscles<br>**Trochlea:** spool-shaped projection at distal end for articulation with ulna at elbow joint<br>**Capitulum:** lateral process that articulates with radius<br>**Coronoid and olecranon fossae:** depressions that permit free movement of corresponding processes of ulna |
| *Radius (2)* | Bone on thumb side of lower arm | Curved with lengthwise ridge<br>**Head:** articulates with capitulum of humerus and with radial notch of ulna<br>**Styloid process:** on lateral surface at distal end<br>**Radial tuberosity:** area where tendon of biceps muscle attaches |
| *Ulna (2)* | Medial bone of forearm; main forearm bone in elbow joint | **Coronoid and olecranon processes:** join trochlea of humerus to form elbow<br>**Styloid process:** sharp projection at distal end |
| *Carpal bones (16)* | Wrist bones | Irregular bones at proximal end of hand |
| *Metacarpal bones (10)* | Form palm of hand | Heads of metacarpals are knuckles |
| *Phalanges (28)* | Bones of fingers; 3 in each finger, 2 in each thumb | |
| **Pelvic Girdle** | | |
| *Coxal (innominate) (2)* | Hipbone; supports weight of upper body | Formed by fusion of 3 bones: ilium, ischium, and pubis<br>**Acetabulum:** hip socket; receives head of femur |
| **Ilium** | Large flaring part of coxal bone; connects posteriorly with sacrum at sacroiliac joint | **Iliac crest:** upper edge of ilium (feels somewhat like a shelf)<br>**Anterior superior spine:** projection at anterior end of iliac crest |
| **Ischium** | Lower, posterior portion of coxal bone | **Ischial tuberosity:** large, rough area on which body rests when sitting erect<br>**Ischial spine:** superior to tuberosity; narrow pelvic outlet through which baby passes during delivery<br>**Greater sciatic notch:** permits sciatic nerve and blood vessels to pass from pelvis into thigh |
| **Pubis** | Most anterior part of coxal bone | **Obturator foramen:** largest foramen in body; formed by pubis and ischium |

**Pubic symphysis:** joint between pubic bones; made of fibrocartilage

**Pelvic brim (inlet):** opening within flaring parts of ilia that leads into true pelvis

**True (lesser) pelvis:** space inferior to pelvic brim; bounded by muscle and bone; pelvic organs located here; superior opening is **pelvic inlet**; inferior opening is **pelvic outlet** (true pelvis must be large enough in female to permit passage of infant's head during childbirth)

**False (greater) pelvis:** superior to true pelvis; actually part of abdominal cavity

| Name of Bone (Number) | Function | Description |
|---|---|---|
| **Lower Extremity** | | |
| *Femur (2)* | Thigh bone; largest bone in body | Slightly curved bone<br>**Head:** Ball-like upper end; fits into acetabulum<br>**Condyles:** rounded projections at distal end; articulate with tibia<br>**Greater trochanter:** prominent projection from upper part of shaft; large muscles (including gluteus maximus) attach here<br>**Lesser trochanter:** smaller projection located inferiorly and medially to greater trochanter |

*Table continued on following page*

TABLE 5–2
**Bones That Make Up the Skeleton** *Continued*

| Name of Bone (Number) | Function | Description |
|---|---|---|
| **Lower Extremity** *Continued* | | |
| *Patella (2)* | Kneecap | Largest sesamoid bone (one that occurs in a tendon or other soft tissue and does not articulate with any other bone) in body |
| *Tibia (2)* | Larger and more medial of the two shank bones | **Medial and lateral condyles:** articulate with condyles of femur, forming knee joint<br>**Anterior tibial border (crest):** ridge on anterior surface<br>**Medial malleolus:** medial, rounded process at distal end |
| *Fibula (2)* | Smaller bone of shank; foot muscles attach to it | Slender bone<br>**Lateral malleolus:** lateral, rounded process at distal end. The medial and lateral malleoli are popularly referred to as the anklebones; ligaments of the ankle are attached to them |
| *Tarsals (14)* | Ankle and proximal foot bones; 4 (3 cuneiforms and cuboid) articulate with long bones (metatarsals) of foot | 2 longitudinal and 1 transverse arch are formed by arrangement of tarsals and metatarsals; these bones are held in arched position by tendons and ligaments; arches permit bones and their ligaments to act as shock absorbers |
| **Talus** | Bears actual ankle joint, articulating with tibia and fibula and with some of the other tarsals | |
| **Calcaneus** | Heelbone; point of attachment for Achilles tendon | |
| *Metatarsals (10)* | Form middle part of foot | |
| *Phalanges (28)* | Toe bones; 3 in each toe; 2 in each great toe | |

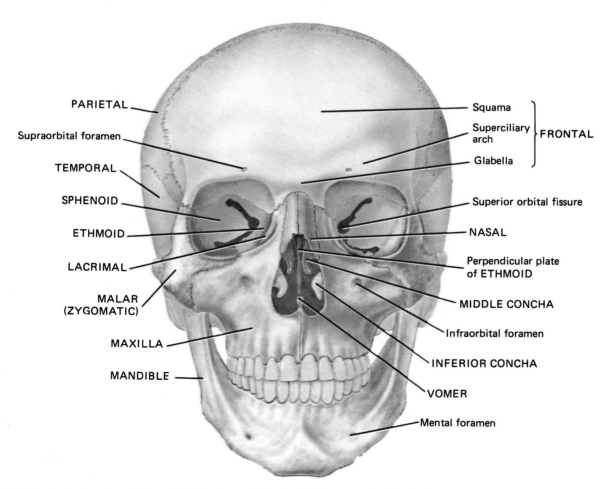

***Figure 5–5.*** *Anterior view of the skull. Regions of the frontal bone are indicated.*

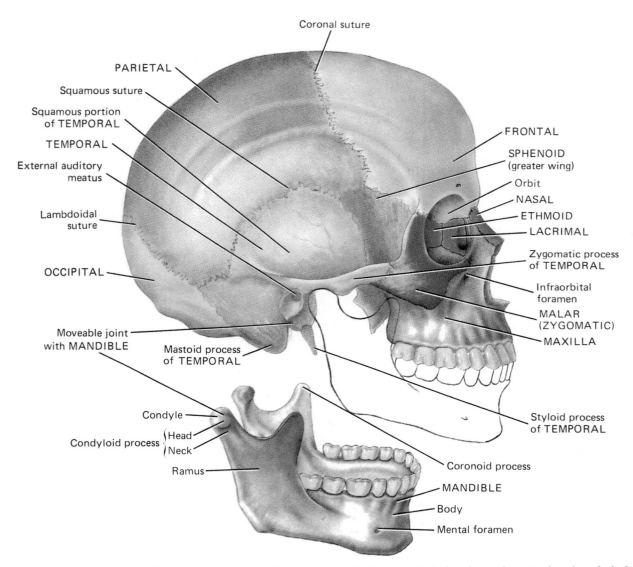

Coronal suture

PARIETAL

Squamous suture

Squamous portion
of TEMPORAL

TEMPORAL

External auditory
meatus

Lambdoidal
suture

OCCIPITAL

FRONTAL

SPHENOID
(greater wing)

Orbit

NASAL

ETHMOID

LACRIMAL

Zygomatic process
of TEMPORAL

Infraorbital
foramen

MALAR
(ZYGOMATIC)

MAXILLA

Moveable joint
with MANDIBLE

Mastoid process
of TEMPORAL

Condyle

Condyloid process { Head { Neck

Ramus

Coronoid process

MANDIBLE

Body

Mental foramen

Styloid process
of TEMPORAL

***Figure 5–6.*** *Lateral view of the skull; the mandible has been disarticulated and slightly turned.*

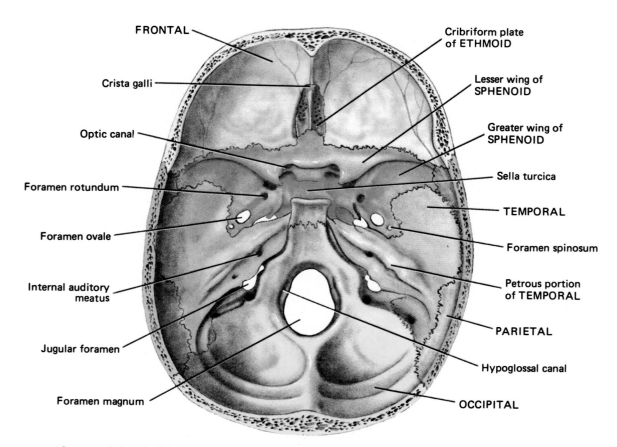

FRONTAL

Crista galli

Optic canal

Foramen rotundum

Foramen ovale

Internal auditory
meatus

Jugular foramen

Foramen magnum

Cribriform plate
of ETHMOID

Lesser wing of
SPHENOID

Greater wing of
SPHENOID

Sella turcica

TEMPORAL

Foramen spinosum

Petrous portion
of TEMPORAL

PARIETAL

Hypoglossal canal

OCCIPITAL

**Figure 5–7.** The top of the skull has been removed to expose the superior surface of the cranial floor. Portions of the superior views of the ethmoid and sphenoid bones can be seen in the floor of the cranial cavity.

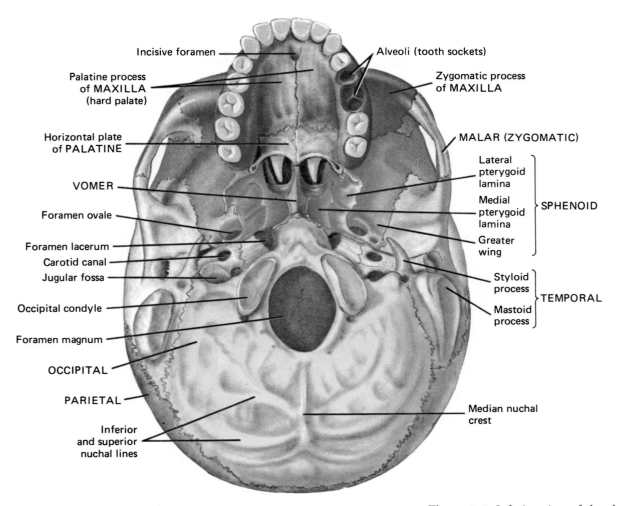

Incisive foramen

Palatine process
of MAXILLA
(hard palate)

Horizontal plate
of PALATINE

VOMER

Foramen ovale

Foramen lacerum

Carotid canal

Jugular fossa

Occipital condyle

Foramen magnum

OCCIPITAL

PARIETAL

Inferior
and superior
nuchal lines

Alveoli (tooth sockets)

Zygomatic process
of MAXILLA

MALAR (ZYGOMATIC)

Lateral
pterygoid
lamina

Medial
pterygoid
lamina        SPHENOID

Greater
wing

Styloid
process

Mastoid    TEMPORAL
process

Median nuchal
crest

*Figure 5–8. Inferior view of the skull.*

## The Vertebral Column

At birth ossification at the skull joints is not complete. Many of these bones are loosely joined by fibrous connective tissue or cartilage. Six such joints, called **fontanelles**, occur at the angles of the parietal bone. The largest is the anterior fontanelle at the junction of the sagittal, coronal, and frontal sutures. The fontanelles, popularly referred to as soft spots, permit the baby's head to be compressed slightly as it passes through the bony pelvis during birth. They also allow the infant's brain to grow during the latter weeks of prenatal development and permit growth of the skull bones.

**Sinuses** are air spaces lined with mucous membrane found in some of the cranial bones. Four pairs of sinuses, the paranasal sinuses (located in the frontal, maxillary, sphenoid, and ethmoid bones), are continuous with the nose and throat. In the familiar malady *sinusitis* (inflammation of the sinuses) the mucous membranes of the sinuses become swollen and inflamed.

The **vertebral column**, or spine, supports the body and bears its weight. It consists of 24 vertebrae and two fused bones, the **sacrum (say'-krum)** and **coccyx (kok'-six)** (Fig. 5–9). The regions of the vertebral column are the **cervical** (neck), composed of seven vertebrae; the **thoracic** (chest), which consists of 12 vertebrae; the **lumbar** (back), composed of five vertebrae; the **sacral** (pelvic), which consists of five fused vertebrae; and the **coccygeal**, also consisting of fused vertebrae.

The vertebral column is S-shaped because of four curves that develop before birth and during childhood. These curves impart strength and flexibility to the vertebral column.

Vertebrae articulate with each other by means of synovial joints and by means of **intervertebral discs** composed of cartilage (Fig. 5–10). The intervertebral discs are tiny pads that act as shock ab-

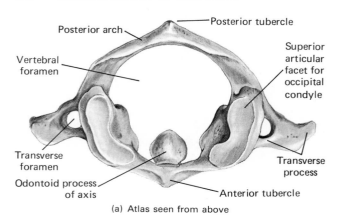

(a) Atlas seen from above

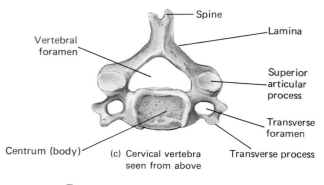

(b) Axis

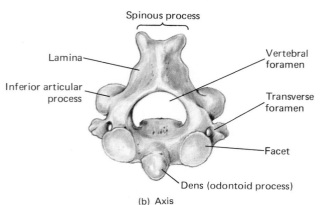

(c) Cervical vertebra seen from above

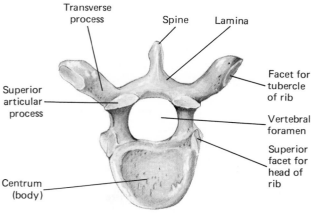

(d) Thoracic vertebra

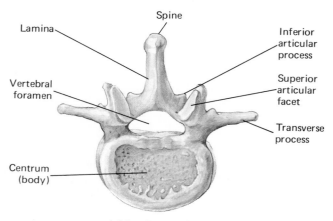

(e) Lumbar vertebra seen from above

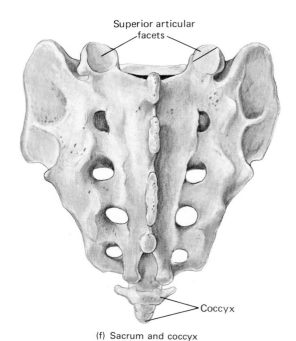

(f) Sacrum and coccyx

**Figure 5–9.** *The vertebrae. (a) The first cervical vertebra, the atlas, seen from above. (b) The second cervical vertebra, the axis. (c) A typical lower cervical vertebra seen from above. (d) A thoracic vertebra. (e) A lumbar vertebra. (f) The sacrum and coccyx. (g) The vertebral column. Note its normal curves.*

*Illustration continued on opposite page*

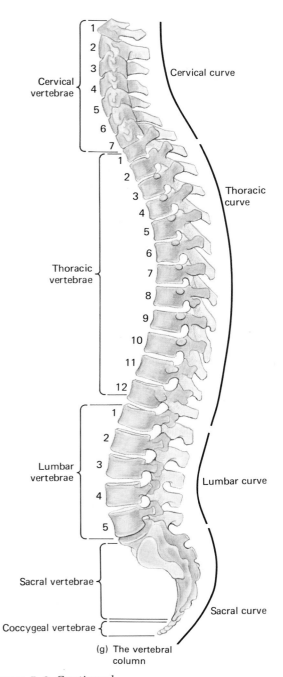

Cervical vertebrae
1
2
3
4
5
6
7

Cervical curve

Thoracic vertebrae
1
2
3
4
5
6
7
8
9
10
11
12

Thoracic curve

Lumbar vertebrae
1
2
3
4
5

Lumbar curve

Sacral vertebrae

Coccygeal vertebrae

Sacral curve

(g) The vertebral column

**Figure 5–9.** Continued

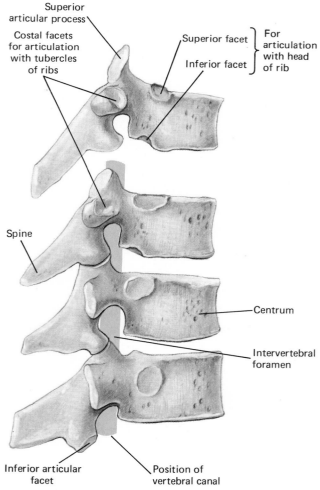

Superior articular process

Costal facets for articulation with tubercles of ribs

Superior facet

Inferior facet

For articulation with head of rib

Spine

Centrum

Intervertebral foramen

Inferior articular facet

Position of vertebral canal

**Figure 5–10.** *Lateral view of several vertebrae, showing how they articulate.*

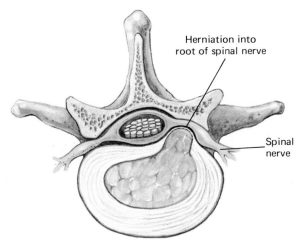

*Figure 5–11. How a herniated disc may press the root of a spinal nerve.*

sorbers. Occasionally an intervertebral disc herniates (ruptures) and puts pressure on the root of a spinal nerve (Fig. 5–11). This condition, popularly known as a slipped disc, can be extremely painful.

A "typical" vertebra has certain structural features (Fig. 5–9).

| | |
|---|---|
| **Centrum** (or body) | The bony central part of the vertebra that bears most of the body weight |
| **Lamina** | Arch |
| **Vertebral foramen** | Passageway through which the spinal cord passes |
| **Spinous process** | Posterior projection from the lamina; back muscles attach to this process |
| **Transverse processes** | Lateral projections from the centrum; provided with facetlike articular surfaces for joining with other vertebrae and ribs |
| **Superior and inferior articular processes** | Projections lateral to the vertebral foramen; where vertebra forms joints with adjacent vertebrae |

## The Thoracic Cage

The **thoracic cage**, or rib cage, is a bony cage formed by the **sternum** (breastbone) (Fig. 5–12), the thoracic vertebrae, and 12 pairs of ribs. It protects the internal organs of the chest, including the heart and lungs. The thoracic cage provides support for the bones of the pectoral girdle and upper extremities and also plays a role in respiration.

## The Pectoral Girdle

The **pectoral**, or shoulder, **girdle** attaches the upper extremities to the axial skeleton. Each pec-

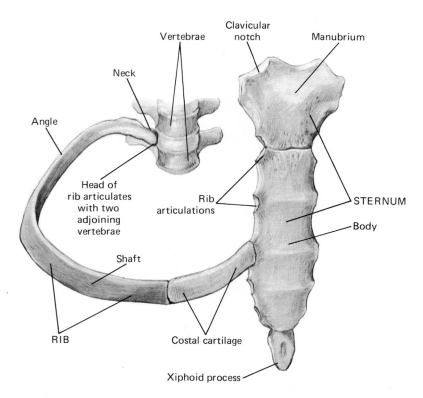

*Figure 5–12. The articulations of a rib with the vertebral column and with the sternum.*

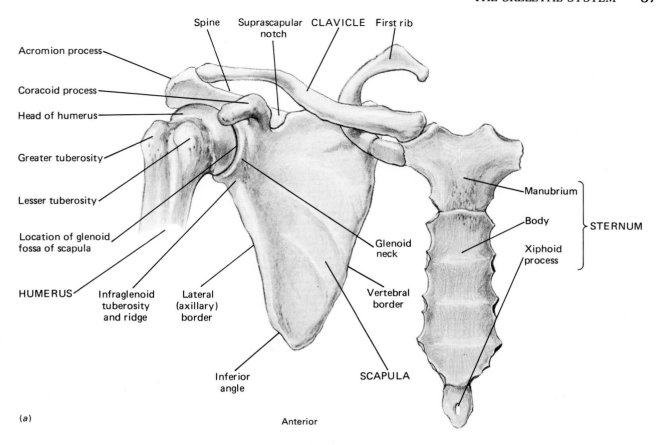

(a)                    Anterior

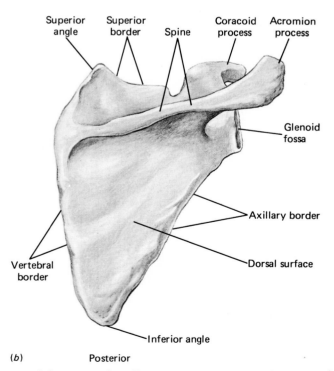

(b)        Posterior

**Figure 5–13.** *Bones of the pectoral girdle. (a) Anterior view of the scapula, sternum, and shoulder girdle. (b) The right scapula, posterior view.*

toral girdle consists of a **scapula** (skap'-u-la) (shoulderblade) and a **clavicle** (klav'-i-kul) (collarbone). The pectoral girdles articulate with the sternum but not with the vertebral column (Fig. 5–13).

## The Upper Extremity

Each upper extremity consists of 30 bones—the **humerus** (hu'-mer-us) in the upper arm (Fig. 5–14), **ulna** (ul'-nuh) and **radius** (ray'-de-us) in the forearm (Fig. 5–15), **carpal** (kar'-pal) **bones** in the

wrist, **metacarpals** in the palm of the hand, and **phalanges** in the fingers (Fig. 5–16).

## The Pelvic Girdle

The **pelvic girdle** is a broad basin of bone that encloses the pelvic cavity. The pelvic girdle supports the lower extremities and is the site of attachment of major muscles of the trunk and lower extremities. It supports the weight of the upper body and protects the organs that lie within the

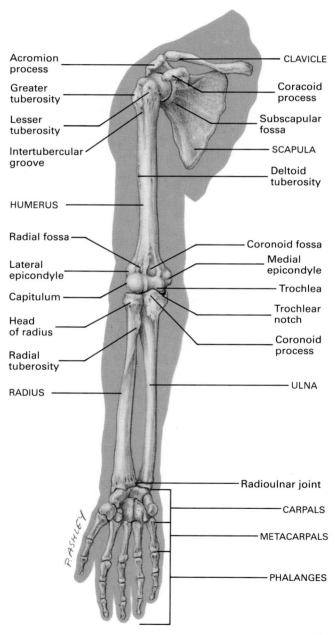

**Figure 5–14.** *The right humerus.*
*Illustration continued on opposite page*

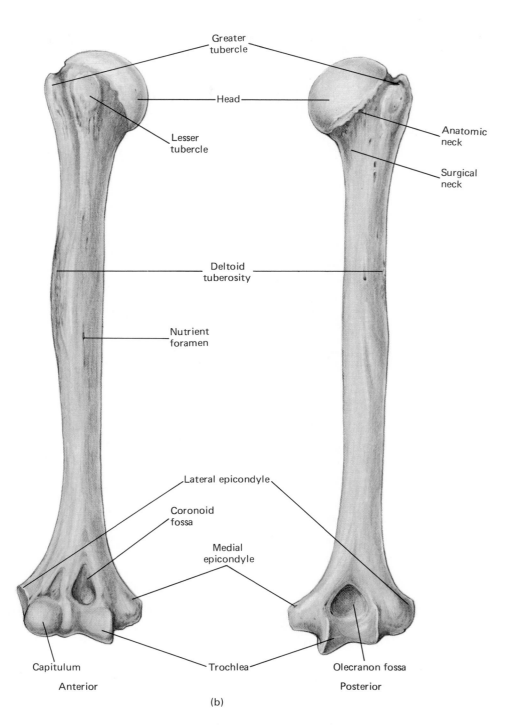

Greater
tubercle

Head

Lesser
tubercle

Anatomic
neck

Surgical
neck

Deltoid
tuberosity

Nutrient
foramen

Lateral epicondyle

Coronoid
fossa

Medial
epicondyle

Capitulum

Trochlea

Olecranon fossa

Anterior

Posterior

(b)

*Figure 5–14.* Continued

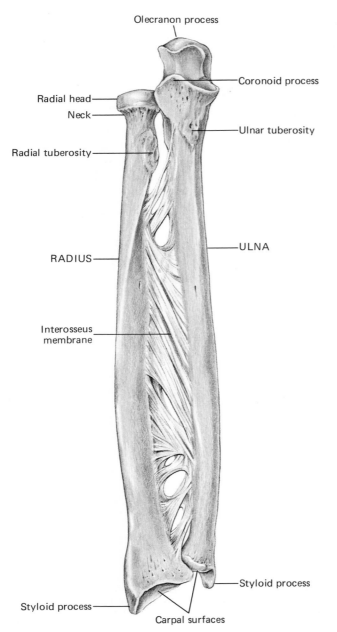

Olecranon process

Coronoid process

Radial head

Neck

Ulnar tuberosity

Radial tuberosity

RADIUS

ULNA

Interosseus membrane

Styloid process

Styloid process

Carpal surfaces

*Figure 5–15.* *Anterior view of the bones of the right forearm. The interosseous membrane extends as a sheet between the borders of the radius and the ulna. It is a broad, very thin ligament that unites the bones of the forearm.*

pelvic cavity—the reproductive organs, urinary bladder, and part of the large intestine. Two **coxal bones** (also called os coxae or innominate bones), together with the sacrum and coccyx, form the pelvic girdle.

Adapted for holding a developing baby and permitting its passage to the outside world at birth, the female pelvis is broader and more shallow than the male pelvis (Fig. 5–17). The pelvic inlet in the female is larger and more circular. The ischial spines of the female are shorter so that there is a greater relative distance between them. In the female there is also a greater angle between the pubic bones.

## The Lower Extremity

The lower extremity (Fig. 5–18) consists of 30 bones—the **femur** (**fee'**-mer) in the upper leg, or thigh; the **patella** (pah-**tel'**-uh), or kneecap; the **tibia** and **fibula** (**fib'**-u-lah) in the lower leg, or shin; the **tarsal bones** in the back part of the foot and heel; the **metatarsals** in main part of the foot; and the **phalanges** in the toes (Fig. 5–19).

## JOINTS (ARTICULATIONS)

An **articulation**, or **joint**, is the point of contact between two bones. Joints hold bones together and

*Text continued on page 95*

**Figure 5–16.** The skeleton of the hand.

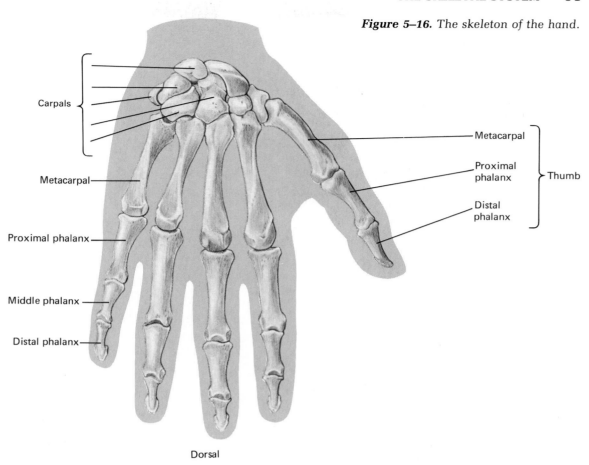

Carpals

Metacarpal

Proximal phalanx

Middle phalanx

Distal phalanx

Metacarpal

Proximal phalanx

Distal phalanx

Thumb

Dorsal

**Figure 5–17.** Generally, the male pubis is narrower than the female, and in the male the suprapubic angle also tends to be more acute. However, some pelves are hard to classify by sex. In this illustration extreme examples are shown. In the adult, the ilium, ischium, and pubis are fused with one another and should be considered regions of the coxal bone rather than separate bones.

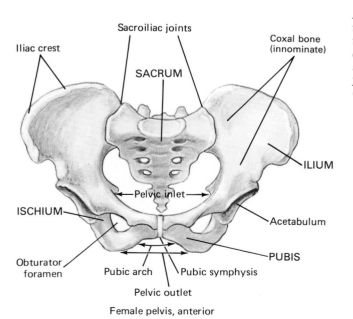

Iliac crest

Sacroiliac joints

SACRUM

Coxal bone (innominate)

ILIUM

ISCHIUM

Pelvic inlet

Acetabulum

PUBIS

Obturator foramen

Pubic arch

Pubic symphysis

Pelvic outlet

Female pelvis, anterior

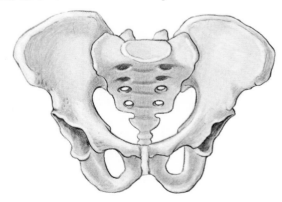

Male pelvis, anterior

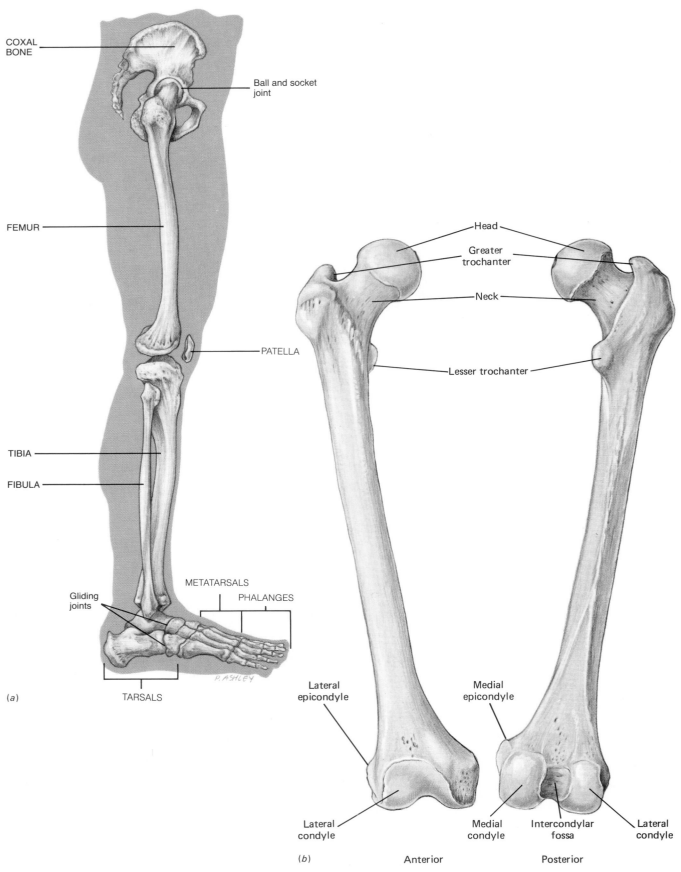

**Figure 5–18.** (a) Bones of the lower extremity. (b) The right femur. (c) Anterior view of the bones of the right shank.

*Illustration continued on opposite page*

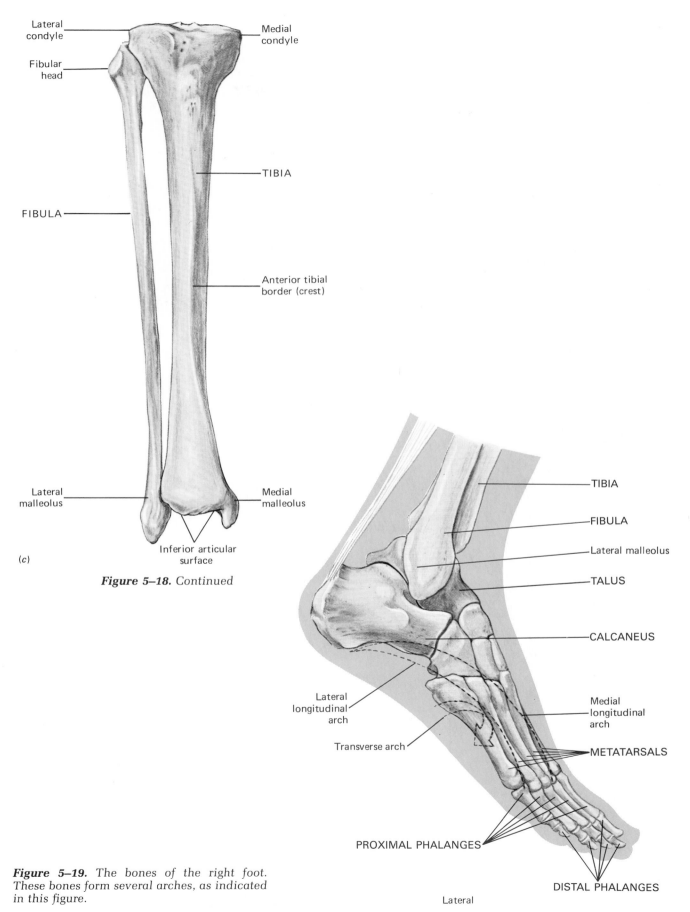

Lateral condyle

Medial condyle

Fibular head

FIBULA

TIBIA

Anterior tibial border (crest)

Lateral malleolus

Medial malleolus

Inferior articular surface

(c)

**Figure 5–18.** Continued

TIBIA

FIBULA

Lateral malleolus

TALUS

CALCANEUS

Medial longitudinal arch

Lateral longitudinal arch

Transverse arch

METATARSALS

PROXIMAL PHALANGES

DISTAL PHALANGES

Lateral

**Figure 5–19.** *The bones of the right foot. These bones form several arches, as indicated in this figure.*

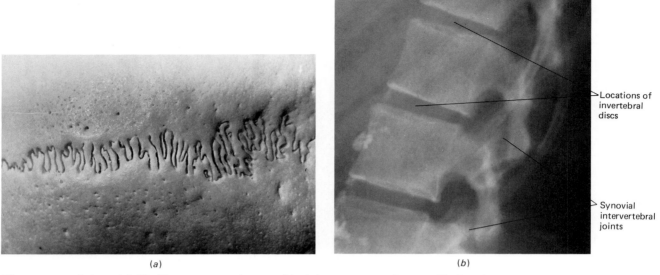

(a)    (b)

**Figure 5–20.** *Joints. (a) Skull sutures are immovable joints, or synarthroses. Notice the elaborate jigsaw puzzle–like interdigitations of this joint. (b) Intervertebral joints are amphiarthroses, or slightly movable joints.*

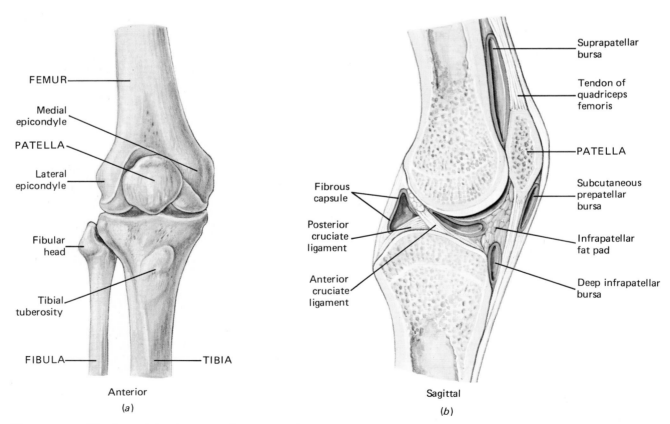

Anterior
(a)

Sagittal
(b)

**Figure 5–21.** *The knee joint is a complex synovial joint. (a) Anterior view of the knee joint. (b) Sagittal section of the knee joint.*

many of them permit flexibility and movement. Joints may be classified according to the degree of movement they permit: synarthroses do not permit movement; amphiarthroses permit slight movement; and diarthroses permit a high degree of movement.

## Synarthroses

**Synarthroses** (sin″-ar-**throw**′-sees) are immovable joints that connect bones with fibrous connective tissue. The sutures that join skull bones are synarthroses (Fig. 5–20).

## Amphiarthroses

**Amphiarthroses** (am″-fee-ar-**throw**′-sees) are slightly movable joints. They join bones to carti-

lage. The pubic symphysis of the pelvis and the intervertebral joints of the vertebral column are examples of amphiarthroses (Fig. 5–20b).

## Diarthroses

**Diarthroses** (die″-ar-**throw**′-sees), or synovial joints, are referred to as freely movable joints but their flexibility varies. Most of the body's joints are diarthroses.

The ends of the bones forming a diarthrodial joint are covered with hyaline cartilage that lacks any sort of covering membrane. This articular cartilage also lacks nerves and blood vessels. The joint is surrounded by a connective tissue capsule, the **joint capsule**, made of tough fibrous connective tissue (Fig. 5–21). This tissue is continuous with the periosteum of the bones but does not

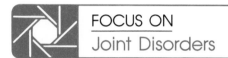

FOCUS ON
Joint Disorders

### Rheumatoid Arthritis

Rheumatoid arthritis is the most common cause of widespread inflammatory joint disease. Its cause is unknown. In rheumatoid arthritis the synovial membrane thickens and becomes inflamed. Synovial fluid accumulates, causing pressure and pain. An abnormal invasive tissue called pannus develops from the synovial membrane. The pannus may erode the articular cartilage. Over a period of time fibrous connective tissue, and then bone, may join the two bones, slowly reducing the range of movement of the joint.

The course of this progressive disease is whimsical. In about 25% of cases the disease seems suddenly to disappear within 2 years of onset. In the majority of cases the disease seems to come and go but there is a trend toward progressive deterioration. Rheumatoid arthritis is treated with a combination of education, physical therapy, and antiinflammatory drugs.

### Osteoarthritis (Degenerative Joint Disease)

The most common form of arthritis, osteoarthritis is characterized by loss of articular cartilage, abnormal proliferation of bone tissue at the joints, and mild inflammatory changes in the synovial membrane. Generally less damaging than rheumatoid arthritis, osteoarthritis develops when cartilage repair does not keep pace with degeneration. Although its primary cause is unknown, this disease sometimes occurs secondary to injury.

### Gouty Arthritis

Gouty arthritis is a recurrent inflammation of peripheral joints. It is thought to be an inherited disorder that results in a metabolic disturbance. Uric acid, a breakdown product of nucleic acid metabolism, is normally excreted in the urine. In the patient with gout, uric acid accumulates in the blood and crystals are deposited in the soft tissues, including in the joints. The crystals irritate the articular cartilage, causing inflammation and pain.

### Bursitis

Bursitis is an acute or chronic inflammation of a bursa. It is most common in the shoulder and may result from trauma, bacterial infection, gout, or inflammation caused by other disorders. People who spend a great deal of time kneeling sometimes develop bursitis of the knee; this is sometimes referred to as carpet layer's knee or housemaid's knee.

### Sprains

Twisting or wrenching of a joint can result in a sprain, a joint injury in which a ligament is ruptured but there is no dislocation of the bone. A sprain is more serious than a strain, which is the overstretching of a muscle or its tendon.

### Dislocation

A dislocation (luxation) is the displacement of a bone from its joint. Tendons and ligaments tear as the injury occurs.

TABLE 5–3
**Some Types of Synovial Joints**

| Type | Example | Shape of Joint Surface | Range of Movement |
| --- | --- | --- | --- |
| Gliding | Carpal joints of wrist; tarsal joints of ankle | Flat or slightly curved | One bone glides over another without circular movement |
| Saddle | Carpometacarpal joint of thumb | Saddle-shaped | Permits wide range of movement |
| Pivot | Atlantoaxial joint of first 2 cervical vertebrae; radioulnar joint of elbow | Small projection of one bone pivots in ring-shaped socket of another bone | Rotation |
| Hinge | Elbow; knee | Convex surface of one bone fits into concave surface of another bone | Motion in one plane only; permits only flexion and extension |
| Ball-and-socket | Shoulder; hip joint | Ball-shaped end of one bone fits into cup-shaped socket of another bone | Permits widest range of movement, including rotation |

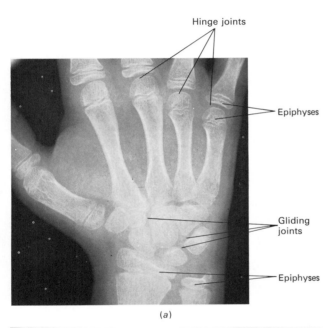

(a)

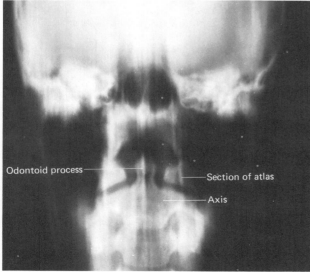

(b)

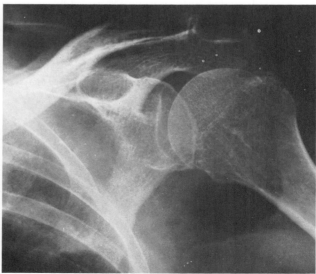

(c)

***Figure 5–22.*** *Synovial joints. (a) Gliding joints between the wrist bones, and hinge joints between the phalanges. (b) X-ray (tomogram) of the odontoid process of the axis. This illustration helps to clarify the pivot function of the odontoid process. (c) Ball-and-socket shoulder joint, one of the most freely movable joints and also the loosest joint in the body. The shoulder joint is held together partly by the steady contraction of the surrounding muscles.*

cover the articular cartilage. The joint capsule is lined with a smooth synovial membrane that secretes a lubricating **synovial fluid**. The joint capsule is generally reinforced with ligaments, bands of fibrous connective tissue that connect the bones and also limit movement at the joint.

Fluid-filled sacs called **bursae** are located between bone and tendons and between bone and some other tissues. Bursae cushion the movement of bone over other tissues. Inflammation of a bursa is a painful condition known as bursitis. (See Focus on Joint Disorders.)

There are six types of synovial joints: gliding, condyloid, saddle, pivot, hinge, and ball-and-socket. Some of these are described in Table 5–3 and shown in Figure 5–22. Some of the types of movement at the joints are described and illustrated in Table 5–4.

TABLE 5–4
**Types of Body Movements**

| Movement | Description | Illustration |
|---|---|---|
| *Flexion* | Bending of joint; usually a movement that reduces angle of joint and brings two bones closer together (when you crouch, your knees are flexed; when you touch your shoulder, your elbow is flexed) | A |
| *Extension* | Opposite of flexion; increases angle of joint, increasing distance between two bones; **hyperextension** occurs if angle of extension exceeds 180 degrees (as is possible when throwing back head); examples of extension include straightening the knee or the elbow | B |
| *Abduction* | Movement of bone or limb away from midline, or median plane of body; abduction in hands and feet is movement of digit away from central axis of limb (one abducts fingers by spreading them apart) | C |
| *Adduction* | Movement of bone or limb toward the midline of body or, for extremities, movement toward axis of limb; opposite of abduction | D |
| *Circumduction* | Combination of movements that makes body part describe a circle; characteristic of ball-and-socket joints such as shoulder | E |

*Table continued on following page*

TABLE 5–4
**Types of Body Movements** *Continued*

| Movement | Description | Illustration |
|---|---|---|
| *Rotation* | Pivoting of body part around its axis, as in shaking the head "no"; no rotation of any body part is complete (i.e., 360 degrees) | F |
| *Pronation* | Movement of forearm that in extended position brings palm of hand from upward-facing to downward-facing position; applies only to arm; this action moves distal end of radius across ulna | G |
| *Supination* | Opposite of pronation; when forearm is in extended position, this movement brings palm of hand upward | H |
| *Inversion* | Ankle movement that turns sole of foot medially; applies only to foot | Medial side  I |
| *Eversion* | Opposite of inversion; turns sole of foot laterally | Medial side  J |

## SUMMARY

I. The skeletal system supports and protects the body, transmits muscular forces, produces blood cells, and stores calcium and phosphorus.

II. A long bone consists of a diaphysis (shaft) with flared ends called epiphyses. It has a central marrow cavity and is covered by a periosteum.

III. Compact bone consists of osteons; spongy bone consists of thin strands of bone. The spaces within spongy bone are filled with bone marrow.

IV. Endochondral bones develop from a cartilage model; membranous bones develop from a noncartilage connective tissue replica.

V. Osteoblasts produce bone; osteoclasts break down bone.

VI. The axial skeleton consists of the skull, vertebral column, ribs, and sternum.
   A. The skull is formed by the cranial and facial bones. The cranial bones include the frontal, occipital, ethmoid, sphenoid, and the paired parietal and temporal bones. The facial bones include the maxilla, mandible, vomer, and the paired malars, palatines, nasals, lacrimals, and inferior turbinates.
   B. The vertebral column consists of seven cervical vertebrae, 12 thoracic vertebrae, five lumbar vertebrae, the sacrum, and the coccyx.
      1. The first cervical vertebra is the atlas; the second is the axis.
      2. A typical vertebra consists of a centrum, lamina, vertebral foramen, transverse processes, and superior and inferior articular processes.
   C. The thoracic cage is formed by the sternum, thoracic vertebrae, and 12 pairs of ribs.

VII. The appendicular skeleton consists of the upper and lower extremities, the pectoral girdle, and the pelvic girdle.
   A. The pectoral girdle attaches the upper extremities to the axial skeleton; it consists of the scapulae and clavicles.
   B. Each upper extremity consists of the humerus, ulna, radius, 8 carpal bones, 5 metacarpals, and 14 phalanges.
   C. The pelvic girdle consists of the coxal bones together with the sacrum and coccyx.
      1. Each coxal bone consists of three fused bones: ilium, ischium, and pubis.
      2. The female pelvis is broader and more shallow than the male pelvis; the pelvic inlet is larger and more circular.
   D. Each lower extremity consists of a femur, tibia, fibula, patella tarsal bones, 5 metatarsals, and 14 phalanges.

VIII. An articulation, or joint, holds bones together.
   A. Synarthroses are immovable joints, such as sutures in the skull.
   B. Amphiarthroses are slightly movable joints, such as the pubic symphysis.
   C. Diarthroses, also called synovial joints, are movable joints.
      1. In diarthroses, the articulating bone surfaces are covered with hyaline cartilage and enclosed in a joint capsule.
      2. Ligaments are bands of fibrous connective tissue that bind bones together at joints.
      3. There are several types of diarthroses. The ball-and-socket joint permits the greatest freedom of movement.

## POST TEST

1. The _____ within some bones produces blood cells.
2. Bone is covered by a connective tissue membrane, the _____.
3. The main shaft of a long bone is its _____.
4. Compact bone consists of spindle-shaped units called _____.
5. Osteocytes are found in small cavities called _____.
6. Osteoclasts are cells that _____ _____ _____.
7. The skull and ribs are part of the _____ skeleton.
8. The skull consists of the _____ and the _____ bones.
9. _____ are air spaces found in some of the cranial bones.
10. The vertebral foramen is a passageway for the _____ _____.
11. The scapula is part of the _____ _____.
12. The ribs are attached to the _____ vertebrae.
13. The bony central body of a vertebra is its _____.
14. Immovable joints are called _____.
15. _____ fluid is found in diarthroses.
16. The bending of a joint is known as _____; movement of a limb away from the midline of the body is _____.

17. A joint, like the elbow joint, that moves in one plane only is
a _____ joint.

*Select the most appropriate answer from Column B for each item in Column A. You may use an answer once, more than once, or not at all.*

| Column A | Column B |
|---|---|
| 18. _____ Lower jaw bone | a. atlas |
| 19. _____ Hip socket | b. mandible |
| 20. _____ Longest bone in body | c. calcaneus |
| 21. _____ Articulates with occipital condyles | d. acetabulum |
| | e. femur |
| 22. _____ Heelbone | f. glenoid fossa |
| 23. _____ Contains sella turcica | g. inferior turbinate |
| 24. _____ Forms ledge along lateral wall of nose | h. sphenoid |
| 25. _____ Receives head of humerus | |

## REVIEW QUESTIONS

1. What are the functions of the skeletal system? How does the skeletal system help maintain homeostasis?
2. How does spongy bone differ from compact bone?
3. How does the development of a skull bone differ from the development of a long bone such as the femur?
4. What is apatite?
5. How do osteoblasts and osteoclasts function together in bone remodeling?
6. Why are fontanelles important?
7. Describe the structure of the vertebral column. What are the advantages of a curved vertebral column rather than a straight one?
8. What are the functions of each of the following: (a) sella turcica (b) cribriform plate (c) occipital condyles (d) temporomandibular joint (e) olecranon process?
9. Locate each of the following: (a) metacarpals (b) malar (c) palatine (d) axis (e) incus (f) obturator foramen (g) talus.
10. How do false ribs differ from true ribs? How many pairs of ribs are there in a male? In a female?
11. Contrast the three main types of joints. What are ligaments? What are bursae?
12. What are the functions of (a) condyles (b) epicondyles (c) foramina (d) facets?

# The Muscular System

LEARNING OBJECTIVES

**After you study this chapter you should be able to**
1. Describe the structure of a skeletal muscle.
2. Trace the sequence of events that occur during muscle contraction.
3. Define muscle tone and tetanus and distinguish between isotonic and isometric contraction.
4. Explain how muscles work antagonistically to one another.
5. Locate and give the actions of the principal muscles as indicated in Table 6–1.

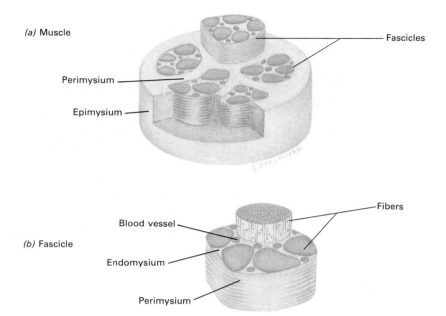

*(a)* Muscle

Fascicles

Perimysium

Epimysium

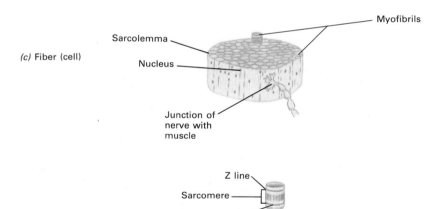

*(b)* Fascicle

Blood vessel

Endomysium

Perimysium

Fibers

*(c)* Fiber (cell)

Sarcolemma

Nucleus

Junction of nerve with muscle

Myofibrils

**Figure 6–1.** *Muscle structure. This diagram illustrates progressively smaller components of a muscle. (a) Cross section through a whole muscle. Note that the muscle consists of fascicles, bundles of muscle fibers, wrapped in connective tissue. (b) A single fascicle, a bundle of muscle fibers. (c) A single muscle fiber (a muscle cell). (d) A bundle of myofibrils. (e) Each myofibril consists of actin and myosin myofilaments.*

*(d)* Column of myofibrils

Z line

Sarcomere

Z line

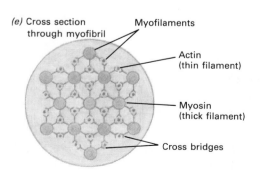

*(e)* Cross section through myofibril

Myofilaments

Actin (thin filament)

Myosin (thick filament)

Cross bridges

Running, speaking, chewing, circulating blood, moving food along the digestive tract—all body movements depend on the action of muscles. The three types of muscles—smooth, cardiac, and skeletal—were discussed in Chapter 4 (see Table 4–3). In this chapter we will focus on skeletal muscle, the voluntary muscles attached to bones. About 600 skeletal muscles working together permit us to move smoothly and precisely through our world.

## MUSCLE STRUCTURE

A skeletal muscle is an organ composed of hundreds of muscle cells, or **fibers**, and surrounded by a covering of connective tissue called the **epimysium** (ep″-i-**mis**′-ee-um) (Fig. 6–1). The muscle fibers are arranged in bundles known as **fascicles** (**fas**′-i-kuls). Each fascicle is wrapped by connective tissue, the **perimysium** (per″-i-**mis**′-ee-um). Finally, individual muscle fibers are surrounded by a connective tissue covering, the **endomysium** (en″-dow-**mis**′-ee-um).

The epimysium, perimysium, and endomysium are continuous. Extensions of epimysium form tough cords of connective tissue, the **tendons**, that anchor muscles to bones.

Each muscle fiber is a spindle-shaped cell with many nuclei (Fig. 6–2). The cell membrane,

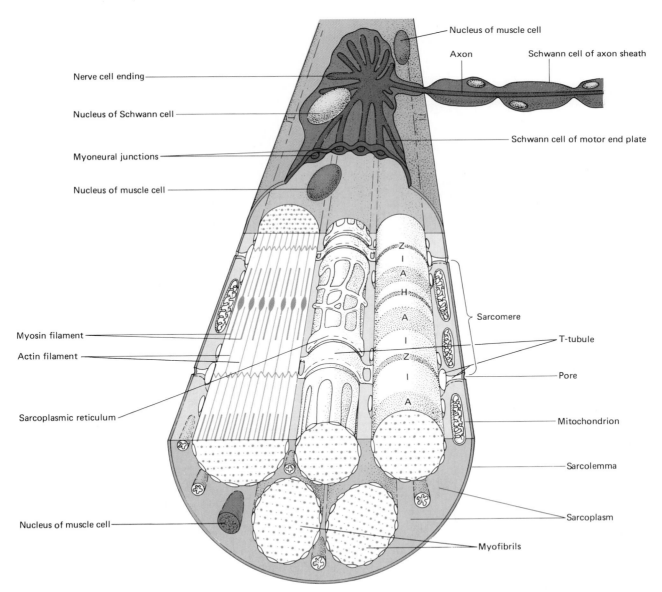

**Figure 6–2.** The structure of a skeletal muscle cell. A system of T tubules extends inward from the sarcolemma. Several nuclei are present and they are located just beneath the sarcolemma. The letters along the myofibril refer to the various bands within each sarcomere.

known in a muscle cell as the **sarcolemma** (sar-kow-**lem'**-ah), has multiple inward extensions that form a set of **T tubules** (transverse tubules). The cytoplasm of a muscle fiber is referred to as **sarcoplasm**, and the endoplasmic reticulum as **sarcoplasmic reticulum**.

Threadlike structures called **myofibrils** (my-o-**fye'**-brils) run lengthwise through the muscle fiber. The myofibrils are composed of two types of even tinier structures, the **myofilaments**. The thick myofilaments, called **myosin** (**my'**-o-sin) **filaments**, consist mainly of the protein myosin, whereas the thin **actin filaments** consist of the protein actin. Myosin and actin filaments are arranged lengthwise in the muscle fibers so that they overlap. Their overlapping produces a pattern of bands, or striations, characteristic of striated muscle. (These

are designated by specific letters as indicated in Figure 6–3.) A **sarcomere** is a unit of thick and thin filaments. Sarcomeres are joined at their ends by an interweaving of filaments called the *Z line*.

## MUSCLE CONTRACTION

During muscle contraction, the actin filaments are pulled inward between the myosin filaments. As this occurs the muscle shortens. We can summarize the process of muscle contraction as follows:

1. A motor neuron (a nerve cell that stimulates a muscle) releases a compound known as **acetylcholine** (as″-eh-til-**koe'**-lin) (Fig. 6–4).
2. The acetylcholine diffuses across the myo-

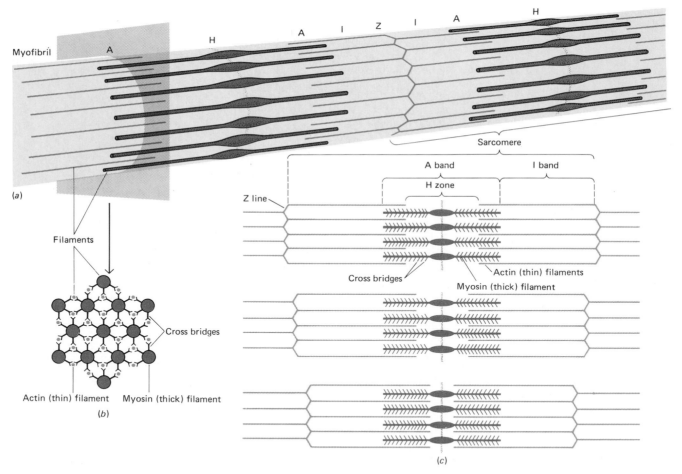

***Figure 6–3.*** *Structure of a myofibril. (a) View of a myofibril showing the overlapping actin and myosin filaments. The regular pattern of overlapping filaments gives skeletal and cardiac muscle their striated, or striped, appearance. Letters represent bands and zones along the myofibril. (b) Cross section of the myofibril shown in (a). Note the arrangement of the actin and myosin filaments. (c) Contraction of a myofibril. Actin and myosin filaments slide past each other during contraction. In the top diagram of (c), the myofibril is relaxed. In the middle diagram, the filaments have slid toward each other, increasing the amount of overlap. As the sarcomeres shorten in this way, the muscle cell shortens. In the bottom diagram, the sarcomere has shortened considerably. Contraction has occurred.*

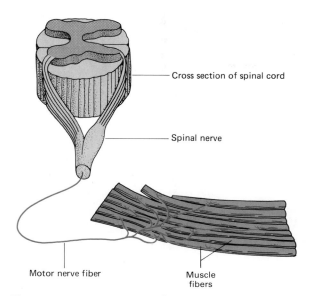

**Figure 6–4.** *Innervation of muscle fibers by a motor neuron.*

- Cross section of spinal cord
- Spinal nerve
- Motor nerve fiber
- Muscle fibers

neural (muscle-nerve) junction between the neuron and the muscle cell and combines with receptors on the surface of the muscle cell. This initiates an impulse (an electrical current) that spreads over the sarcolemma. The electrical current generated is known as an **action potential**. Excess acetylcholine is broken down by the enzyme **cholinesterase** (ko"-lin-**es'**-ter-ase).

3. The impulse spreads through the T tubules and stimulates the sarcoplasmic reticulum to release calcium ions into the sarcoplasm.
4. The calcium induces a process that uncovers binding sites on the actin filaments.
5. Cross bridges along the myosin filaments attach to the exposed binding sites on the actin filaments (Fig. 6–3). This process is powered by energy from ATP (adenosine triphosphate) molecules.
6. Cross bridges flex and attach to new binding sites. As this process continues, the actin filaments slide past the myosin filaments, shortening the muscle.

## Energy for Muscle Contraction

Muscle cells are often called on to perform strenuously and must be provided with large amounts of energy. Sufficient ATP can be stockpiled to store energy for only the first few seconds of strenuous activity. Muscles cells have another energy storage compound known as **creatine phosphate**. This compound *can* be stockpiled and as needed its stored energy is transferred to ATP.

However, the supply of creatine phosphate does not last long either during vigorous exercise. As ATP and creatine phosphate stores are depleted muscle cells must replenish their supply of these high-energy compounds. Stored glycogen is degraded, yielding glucose, which is then broken down in cellular respiration. When sufficient oxygen is available enough energy is captured from the glucose to produce needed quantities of ATP.

During strenuous exercise sufficient oxygen may not be available to meet the needs of the rapidly metabolizing muscle cells. Under these conditions muscle cells are capable of breaking down fuel molecules anaerobically (without oxygen) for short periods of time. However, anaerobic metabolism does not yield much ATP. The depletion of ATP results in weaker contractions and muscle fatigue. A waste product, called *lactic acid*, is produced during anaerobic breakdown of glucose. Lactic acid buildup contributes to *muscle fatigue*. During muscle exertion an *oxygen debt* develops, which is paid back during the period of rapid breathing that typically follows strenuous exercise.

## Muscle Tone

Even when we are not moving our muscles, they are in a state of partial contraction known as **muscle tone**. Because of messages from nerve cells, some muscle fibers are contracted at any given moment. Maintaining muscle tone is an unconscious process that helps to keep muscles prepared for action. When the motor nerve to a muscle is cut, the muscle becomes limp, or flaccid.

## Tetanus

Nerve impulses are generally delivered to a muscle at a rapid rate. With such rapidly repeated stimulation, the muscle contracts repeatedly without relaxing between each contraction. The individual contractions fuse into a single, smooth, sustained contraction. This type of muscle response is referred to as **tetanus**. (This type of tetanus is normal and has nothing to do with the disorder tetanus that causes muscles to go into uncontrollable spasms.)

## Isotonic and Isometric Contraction

When you lift a heavy object or bend your elbow, muscles shorten and thicken as they contract. Muscle tone remains the same. We usually think of muscle contraction in terms of this type of **isotonic** (i″-so-**ton**′-ik) **contraction**. However, if you push against a table or wall, no movement re-sults. Muscle length does not appreciably change but muscle tension may increase greatly. This type of muscle contraction is referred to as **isometric** (i″-so-**met**′-rik) **contraction**.

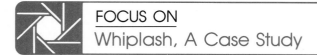

## FOCUS ON
## Whiplash, A Case Study

Five o'clock and the traffic on the interstate was bumper to bumper. Sherry was annoyed at being caught in the end of the day traffic. All of a sudden while Sherry was at a standstill she felt a terrible jarring and heard a loud crash. Someone had hit her car from behind with such an impact that her car was thrust against the car in front of her. Even though Sherry was wearing a seatbelt her body was thrust forward and the inertia of her head hyperextended her neck as it recoiled.

When she was seen at the emergency room, the doctors diagnosed a **whiplash** injury. The hyperextension and hyperflexion results in a severe muscle spasm, causing a sprain of the muscles and ligaments. Depending on the severity of the impact and the intensity of the trauma, the sprain can be mild, moderate, or severe.

At first Sherry experienced little discomfort but within an hour or so the affected muscles became more tender and painful. Sherry started to complain of an inability to hold her head upright when bending forward. The pain was generalized about her neck and referred to the scapula. She complained of a severe headache in the occipital area. Even though the x-ray films showed no fracture or dislocation Sherry experienced extreme tenderness over the cervical spine. The doctors ordered rest and heat over the tender areas to relieve the muscle spasm. A soft cervical collar was ordered to allow for additional rest of the muscles. Even though the accident was frightening and upsetting, Sherry will show steady improvement as the ligaments heal. For her moderate injury, noticeable improvement should occur within 3 to 6 weeks.

## Origin and Insertion

Skeletal muscles produce movements by pulling on tendons, which in turn pull on bones. Most muscles pass across a joint and are attached to the bones that form the joint. When the muscle contracts it draws one bone toward or away from the bone with which it articulates (forms a joint). The attachment of the muscle to the less movable bone is called its **origin**. The attachment of the muscle to the more movable bone is its **insertion**.

## Types of Muscle Action

Muscles can only pull; they cannot push. When you flex your elbow, your biceps muscle contracts pulling the radius (and thus, your forearm) upward so that you can touch your shoulder (Fig. 6–5). However, your biceps cannot push your radius back down. To move your forearm down again, the triceps muscle contracts, pulling on the ulna. Thus, the biceps and triceps can work **antagonistically** to one another. What one does, the other can undo.

The muscle that contracts to produce a particular action is known as the **agonist**, or **prime mover**.

The muscle that produces the opposite movement is the **antagonist**. When the agonist is contracting, the antagonist is relaxed. Generally, movements are accomplished by groups of muscles working together so that there may be several agonists and several antagonists in any action. Note that muscles that are agonists in one movement may be antagonists in another.

Synergists and fixators are muscles that help the agonist by reducing unnecessary movement. **Synergists** stabilize joints so that undesirable movement does not occur. **Fixators** stabilize the origin of an agonist so that its force is fully directed to the bone on which it inserts.

## SPECIFIC MUSCLES AND THEIR ACTIONS

Every muscle is important but including them all is beyond the scope of this book. Instead, some of the most prominent muscles are considered (Table 6–1) along with their actions, origins, and insertions (Fig. 6–6 and 6–7).

Several common shapes of muscles are shown in Figure 6–8.

*Text continued on page 115*

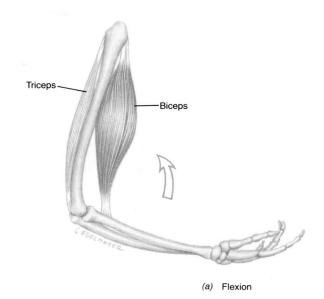

*(a)* Flexion

**Figure 6–5.** The antagonistic arrangement of biceps and triceps muscles. (a) In flexion, the biceps is the agonist and the triceps the antagonist. (b) In extension, the triceps is the agonist and the biceps the antagonist.

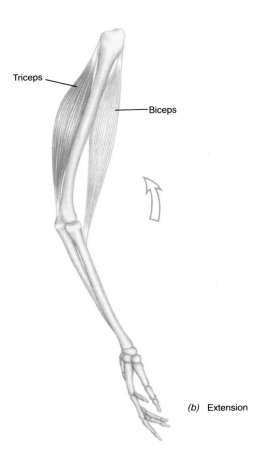

*(b)* Extension

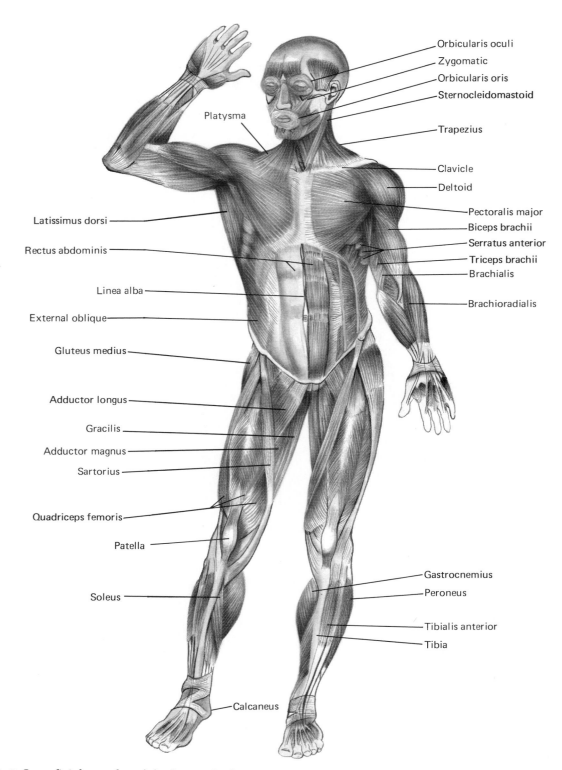

*Figure 6–6. Superficial muscles of the human body. Anterior view.*

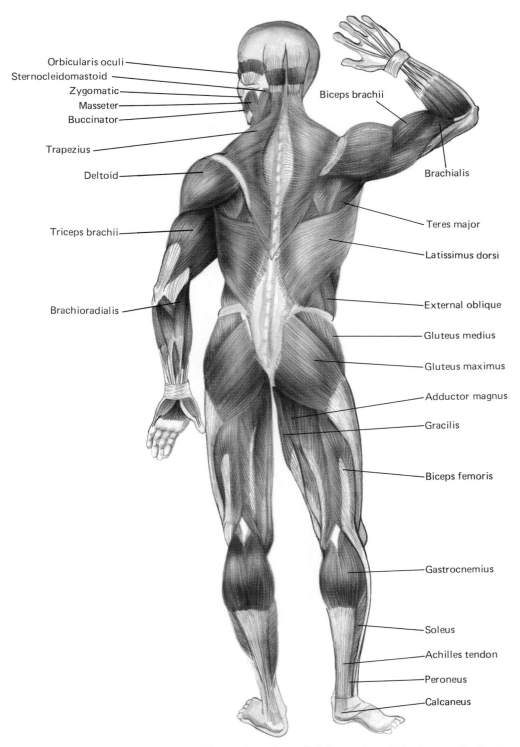

Orbicularis oculi

Sternocleidomastoid

Zygomatic

Masseter

Buccinator

Trapezius

Deltoid

Triceps brachii

Brachioradialis

Biceps brachii

Brachialis

Teres major

Latissimus dorsi

External oblique

Gluteus medius

Gluteus maximus

Adductor magnus

Gracilis

Biceps femoris

Gastrocnemius

Soleus

Achilles tendon

Peroneus

Calcaneus

*Figure 6–7. Superficial muscles of the human body. Posterior view.*

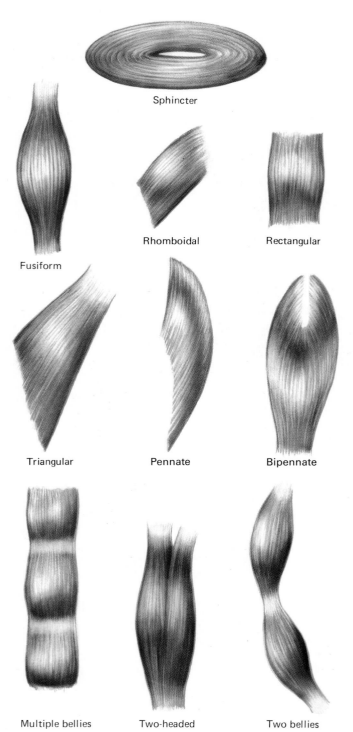

Sphincter

Fusiform

Rhomboidal

Rectangular

Triangular

Pennate

Bipennate

Multiple bellies

Two-headed

Two bellies

**Figure 6–8.** Some common muscle shapes.

TABLE 6–1
**Muscles**

| Muscle | Action | Origin | Insertion |
|---|---|---|---|
| **Facial Muscles** | | | |
| Orbicularis oculi (or-bik″-u-**lar**′-is **ok**′-u-li) | Closes eyes; these are sphincter muscles of eyelids | Frontal bone; maxilla | Eyelids |
| Frontalis (fron-**tal**′-is) | Raises brows; moves entire scalp backwards | Occipital | Skin of scalp and face |
| Orbicularis oris | Closes lips; protrudes lips | Tissue around lips | Lips |
| Zygomatic (zy-go-**mat**′-ik) | Elevates upper corners of mouth | Malar (zygomatic) | Corners of mouth |

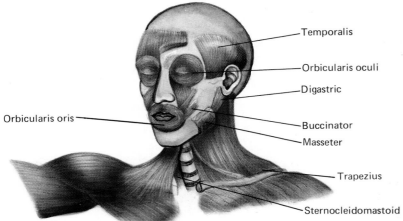

**Figure 6–9.** *Some muscles of the head and anterior neck.*

| Muscle | Action | Origin | Insertion |
|---|---|---|---|
| **Chewing Muscles** | | | |
| Digastric (di-**gas**′-trik) | Opens mouth; can elevate hyoid | Mastoid process of temporal | Hyoid; mandible |
| Buccinator (**buk**′-sih-nay″-tor) | Flattens cheek (as in whistling) | Lateral side of mandible | Maxilla |
| Masseter (mas-**see**′-ter) | Raises jaw; mastication | Maxilla (zygomatic arch) | Ramus of mandible |
| Temporalis (tem-po-**ra**′-lis) | Raises jaw; mastication | Temporal bone | Coronoid process of mandible |
| **Muscles of the Head and Trunk** | | | |
| Sternocleidomastoid (ster-no-kly-do-**mas**′-toid) (paired) | Contraction of both muscles flexes neck; contractions of one muscle rotates head to opposite side | Sternum and clavicle | Mastoid process of occipital |
| Trapezius (trah-**pee**′-zee-us) (paired) | Adducts scapula and rotates it; draws shoulder upward; extends, bends neck | Occipital bone and thoracic vertebrae | Scapula |
| External oblique | Contain the abdominal viscera; increase intraabdominal pressure (as in defecation); contraction of both compresses abdomen; contraction of one side bends vertebral column laterally | Lateral surface of lower 8 ribs | Linea alba (midline connective tissue), iliac crest |

*Table continued on following page*

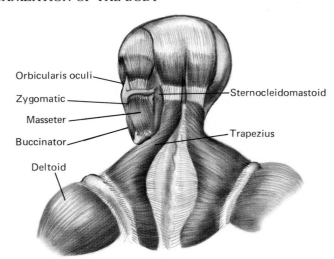

**Figure 6–10.** *Some superficial muscles of the head, neck, and back.*

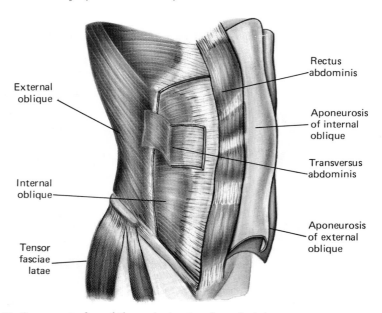

**Figure 6–11.** *Some muscles of the anterior trunk and abdomen.*

TABLE 6–1
**Muscles** *Continued*

| Muscle | Action | Origin | Insertion |
|---|---|---|---|
| **Muscles of the Head and Trunk** Continued | | | |
| Internal oblique | Contain the abdominal viscera; increase intraabdominal pressure (as in defecation); contraction of both compresses abdomen; contraction of one side bends vertebral column laterally | Pelvic structures | Last 4 ribs |

TABLE 6–1
**Muscles** *Continued*

| Muscle | Action | Origin | Insertion |
|---|---|---|---|
| **Muscles of the Head and Trunk** Continued | | | |
| Transversus abdominis | Compresses abdominal contents | Cartilages of lower 6 ribs; iliac crest | Linea alba, pubis, xiphoid process |
| Rectus abdominis | Flexes trunk; compresses abdominal contents | Pubis | Xiphoid process of sternum and costal cartilages of ribs 5 to 7 |
| Pectoralis minor | Pulls scapula forward and downward | Ribs 2 to 5 | Coracoid process of scapula |
| Serratus (ser-**ray'**-tus) anterior | Pulls scapula forward and downward | Upper 8 ribs | Scapula |
| **Muscles Used in Breathing** | | | |
| External intercostals | Elevate ribs | Inferior borders of ribs | Superior borders of ribs |
| Internal intercostals | Depress ribs | Inferior borders of ribs | Superior borders of ribs |
| Diaphragm | Increases volume of chest cavity | Xiphoid process, internal surfaces of lower 6 ribs, and first 3 lumbar vertebrae | Central tendon |
| **Muscles That Move the Arm** | | | |
| Pectoralis (pek-to-**ray'**-lis) major | Adducts, rotates arm medially | Clavicle, sternum | Humerus |
| Teres major | Adducts, rotates arm medially | Scapula | Humerus |
| Latissimus (lah-**tis'**-i-mus) dorsi | Adducts, rotates arm medially; lowers shoulder | Spines of thoracic vertebrae; ilium, ribs | Humerus |
| Deltoid | Abducts upper arm | Clavicle, scapula | Humerus |
| **Muscles That Move the Forearm** | | | |
| Biceps brachii (**bray'**-kee-i) | Flexes elbow; supinates forearm | Scapula | Radius |
| Brachialis | Flexes elbow | Humerus | Ulna |
| Brachioradialis | Flexes elbow | Humerus | Radius |
| Triceps brachii | Extends elbow | Scapula, humerus | Ulna |
| **Muscles That Move the Thigh** | | | |
| Iliacus | Flexes and rotates thigh | Ilium | Femur |
| Gluteus maximus (**gloo'**-te-us **mak'**-si-mus) | Extends and rotates thigh laterally; tilts pelvis | Sacrum, coccyx, ilium | Femur |
| Gluteus medius | Abducts, rotates thigh medially | Ilium | Femur |
| Gluteus minimus | Abducts, rotates thigh laterally | Ilium | Femur |
| Abductor longus and magnus | Adducts, flexes, rotates thigh | Symphysis pubis; pubis, ischium | Femur |
| Gracilis | Adducts thigh; flexes knee | Pubis | Tibia |
| **Muscles That Move the Leg** | | | |
| Sartorius | Flexes knee and thigh; abducts, rotates thigh laterally | Ilium | Tibia |
| Quadriceps femoris (**kwod'**-re-seps **fem'**-or-is) | Extends leg at knee | Ilium, femur | Tibia |
| Biceps femoris | Flexes knee; extends thigh | Ischium, femur | Tibia, fibula |

*Table continued on following page*

TABLE 6–1
**Muscles** *Continued*

| Muscle | Action | Origin | Insertion |
|---|---|---|---|
| **Muscles That Move the Foot and Ankle** | | | |
| Tibialis anterior (tib-ee-**a**'-lis) | Dorsiflexes foot | Tibia | Metatarsals |
| Peroneus (per-o-**nee**'-us) | Plantar-flexes and everts foot | Fibula, tibia | Metatarsals |
| Gastrocnemius (gas-trok-**nee**'-me-us) | Plantar-flexes foot; flexes knee | Femur | Calcaneus |
| Soleus (**so**'-lee-us) | Plantar-flexes foot | Tibia, fibula | Calcaneus |

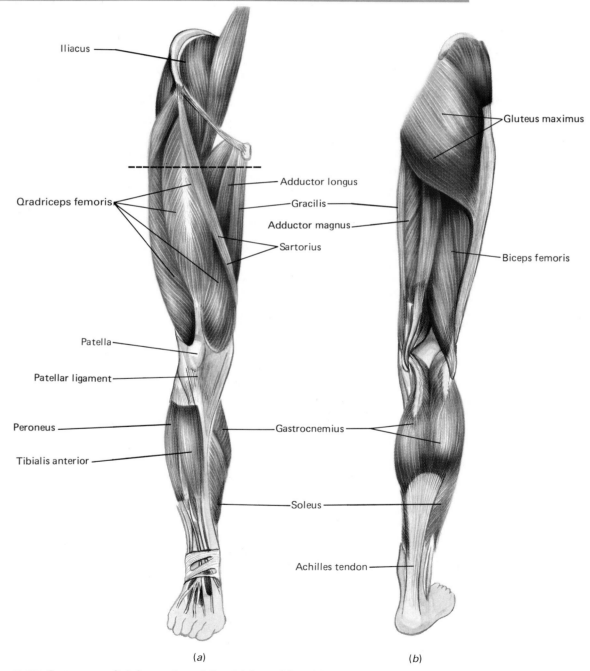

Iliacus

Gluteus maximus

Qradriceps femoris

Adductor longus

Gracilis

Adductor magnus

Biceps femoris

Sartorius

Patella

Patellar ligament

Peroneus

Gastrocnemius

Tibialis anterior

Soleus

Achilles tendon

(a)

(b)

***Figure 6–12.*** Some superficial muscles of the thigh and leg. (a) Anterior view. (b) Posterior view.

## SUMMARY

I. A skeletal muscle consists of hundreds of fibers arranged in fascicles.
   A. Each fiber is wrapped in an endomysium, the fascicle is surrounded by perimysium, and the entire muscle is covered by epimysium.
   B. Each muscle fiber contains thick myosin and thin actin filaments arranged in units called sarcomeres.
II. A muscle is signaled to contract by acetylcholine released by a motor nerve.
   A. The acetylcholine generates an action potential in the muscle fiber.
   B. The action potential spreads through the T tubules and stimulates the sarcoplasmic reticulum to release calcium ions.
   C. The calcium causes binding sites on the actin filaments to be uncovered.
   D. Cross bridges along the myosin filaments attach to the uncovered binding sites on the actin filaments. ATP is necessary for this to occur.
   E. Cross bridges flex and attach to new binding sites so that the actin filaments slide past the myosin filaments.
III. Creatine phosphate is an energy storage compound found in muscle cells; as needed its energy can be transferred to ATP.
IV. Muscle tone is the state of partial contraction that keeps muscles prepared for action.
V. Tetanus is a type of muscle response resulting from the fusion of rapid repeated contractions into a single, smooth, sustained contraction.
VI. In isotonic contraction muscles shorten and thicken as they contract; in isometric contraction muscle length does not change much, but muscle tension may increase greatly.
VII. Muscles work antagonistically to each other. The muscle that contracts to produce a particular action is the agonist; the muscle that produces the opposite movement is the antagonist.
VIII. Use Table 6–1 to review the specific muscles of the body.

## POST TEST

1. Muscle cells are called _____.
2. The connective tissue covering that surrounds each fascicle is the _____.
3. Thick myofilaments consist mainly of the protein _____; thin myofilaments consist of _____.
4. A muscle is stimulated to contract by acetylcholine released by a _____ _____.
5. The action potential stimulates the sarcoplasmic reticulum to release _____ _____.
6. The immediate source of energy for muscle contraction is _____.
7. Creatine phosphate is a compound that stores _____.
8. The state of partial contraction that exists in a muscle even when we are not moving it is called _____ _____.
9. A muscle that opposes an agonist is called an _____.
10. Muscles that stabilize joints are _____.

*Select the most appropriate answer from Column B for each item in Column A. You may use an answer once, more than once, or not at all.*

| **Column A** | **Column B** |
| --- | --- |
| 11. _____ Used in chewing | a. triceps brachii |
| 12. _____ Extends thigh | b. gluteus maximus |
| 13. _____ Flexes trunk | c. quadriceps femoris |
| 14. _____ Extends elbow | d. masseter |
| 15. _____ Extends shank at knee | e. rectus abdominis |
| 16. _____ Plantar-flexes foot | f. deltoid |
| 17. _____ Abducts upper arm | g. gastrocnemius |

18. Label the diagram below.

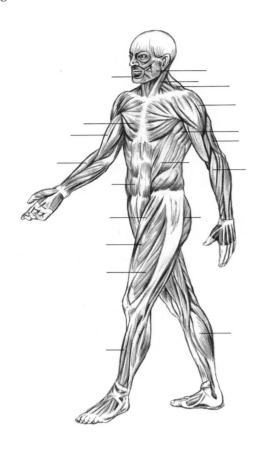

## REVIEW QUESTIONS

1. What are the functions of (a) cholinesterase (b) creatine phosphate (c) glycogen?
2. What is the function of the cross bridges along the myosin filaments?
3. What happens when the motor nerve to a muscle is cut?
4. Give an example of the antagonistic action of muscles.
5. List four abdominal muscles. What are their functions?
6. Which muscles function in breathing?
7. Identify two muscles that move the arm; identify three muscles that move the forearm.

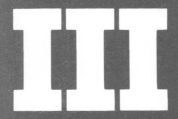

# REGULATION OF BODY ACTIVITIES

# The Nervous System: Basic Function and Central Nervous System

LEARNING OBJECTIVES

**After you study this chapter you should be able to**
1. List the divisions of the nervous system.
2. Draw a neuron, label its parts, and give the functions of each.
3. Distinguish between nerve and tract, ganglion and nucleus.
4. Briefly describe the four basic processes on which all neural responses depend— reception, transmission, integration, and response.
5. Diagram a withdrawal reflex pathway, identifying the essential components and indicating the direction of impulse transmission.
6. Describe the propagation of an action potential.
7. Describe synaptic transmission.
8. Describe how a postsynaptic neuron integrates incoming stimuli and "decides" whether or not to fire.
9. Label on a diagram the structures of the brain described in this chapter.
10. Describe the structure and functions of the

main parts of the brain: medulla, pons, midbrain, diencephalon (thalamus and hypothalamus), cerebellum, cerebrum.
11. Name the principal areas and functions associated with the lobes of the cerebrum.
12. Describe the actions of the limbic system and reticular activating system.
13. Review current theories regarding memory and cite experimental evidence linking environmental stimuli with demonstrable changes in the brain and its function.
14. List two functions of the spinal cord and describe its structure.
15. Describe the structures that protect the brain and spinal cord.

---

The nervous system directs the complex processes of the body's internal environment and serves as the body's link with the outside world. This system enables us to detect stimuli (changes within the body or in the outside world) and to respond to them. Together with the endocrine system, the nervous system works continuously to preserve homeostasis.

## ORGANIZATION OF THE NERVOUS SYSTEM

The two principal divisions of the nervous system are the **central nervous system (CNS)** and the **peripheral nervous system (PNS)** (Fig. 7–1). The CNS consists of the brain and spinal cord. Serving as a control center for the entire organism, these organs integrate incoming information and determine appropriate responses. The PNS is made up of the sense organs—eyes, ears, taste buds, olfactory receptors, and touch receptors—and the nerves, which are the communication lines. Twelve pairs of cranial nerves link the brain, and 31 pairs of spinal nerves link the spinal cord with sense organs, muscles, and other parts of the body. The peripheral nerves continually inform the CNS of changing conditions and then transmit its "decisions" to appropriate muscles and glands that effect the adjustments needed to preserve homeostasis.

For convenience the PNS may be subdivided into somatic and autonomic portions. Receptors and nerves concerned with changes in the external environment are **somatic**; those that regulate the internal environment are **autonomic**. Both systems

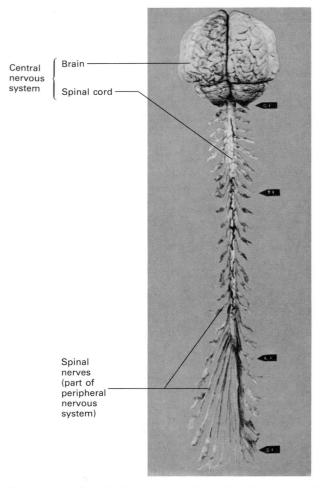

*Figure 7–1.* The brain and spinal cord with attached spinal nerve roots, photographed from the posterior aspect. The nerves that extend caudally from the lower region of the cord have been fanned out on the left. (Dissection by Dr. M.C.E. Hutchinson, Department of Anatomy, Guy's Hospital Medical School, London, England. From Williams, P., and Warwick, R. (eds.): Gray's Anatomy, 36th ed. Philadelphia, W.B. Saunders Company, 1980.)

have **afferent nerves**, also called **sensory nerves**, that transmit messages from receptors to the CNS, and **efferent nerves**, also called **motor nerves**, that transmit information back from the nervous system to the structures that must respond. In the autonomic system there are two kinds of efferent pathways—sympathetic and parasympathetic nerves. These will be discussed in Chapter 8.

## THE NEURON

Cell types unique to nervous tissue are glial cells and neurons. **Glial cells** protect and support the neurons. Highly specialized to receive and transmit messages in the form of neural impulses, the **neuron** is distinguished from all other cells by its long axon and dendrites; these are referred to as fibers (Fig. 7–2). A typical neuron has a prominent **cell body** that contains the nucleus and many of the other organelles.

**Dendrites** (**den′**-drites), highly branched fibers that project from the cell body, are specialized to receive neural impulses. Their surfaces are dotted with thousands of tiny **dendritic spines**, the sites

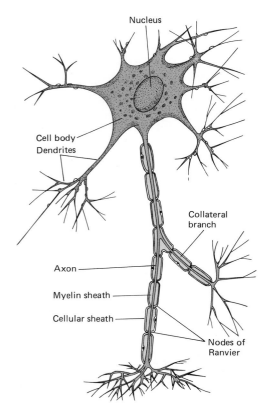

*Figure 7–2. Structure of a neuron. The axon of this neuron is myelinated, and therefore the myelin sheath is shown, as well as the cellular sheath. Cellular sheaths are found only around axons of peripheral neurons.*

of junctions with other neurons. The single **axon** transmits neural messages from the cell body toward another neuron (or toward a muscle or gland). Although microscopic in diameter, an axon may extend several feet in length. For example, neurons that exit from the lower portion of the spinal cord and innervate the foot may be almost a meter (more than 3 feet) long in a tall person.

At its distal end the axon branches extensively. These branches are studded with tiny enlargements called **synaptic knobs** that release **neurotransmitters**, chemical substances that transmit impulses from one neuron to another. Along its course an axon may give off branches known as **collaterals**.

Axons of many neurons of the PNS are covered by two sheaths—an inner **myelin sheath** and an outer **cellular sheath** (or neurilemma). Both sheaths are produced by glial cells known as **Schwann cells**. The cellular sheath is important in the regeneration of injured neurons.

Myelin, a white, lipid-rich substance, is an excellent electrical insulator and speeds the conduction of nerve impulses. Between successive Schwann cells, gaps called **nodes of Ranvier** occur in the myelin sheath. At these points myelin does not insulate the axon. Myelin is responsible for the white color of the white matter of the brain and spinal cord and of myelinated peripheral nerves.

> In **multiple sclerosis**, a neurological disease that affects some 300,000 persons in the United States alone, patches of myelin deteriorate at irregular intervals along neurons in the CNS. The myelin is replaced by glial cells, which form a hard matrix around the neurons. After the affected axons have lost their myelin sheaths, they are not able to conduct impulses effectively. Victims of this disease suffer from symptoms of impaired neural function, including loss of coordination, difficulty in seeing, tremor, and partial or complete paralysis of parts of the body.

## NERVES AND GANGLIA

A **nerve** is a large bundle of axons wrapped in connective tissue (Fig. 7-3). A nerve may be compared to a telephone cable. The axons of a nerve may be likened to the individual wires of a telephone cable, and the myelin, cellular, and connective tissue sheaths to the insulation.

The cell bodies attached to the axons of a nerve are often grouped together in a mass known as a **ganglion**. Many ganglia are located just outside the spinal cord. Within the CNS, the terminology is somewhat different. Collections of cell bodies are

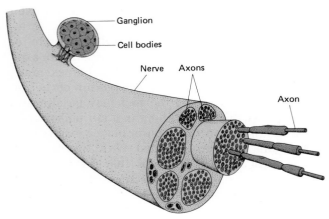

**Figure 7–3.** *Structure of a nerve and a ganglion. A nerve consists of bundles of axons held together by connective tissue. The cell bodies belonging to these axons are grouped together in a ganglion.*

referred to as **nuclei** rather than ganglia, and bundles of axons are known as **tracts** or **pathways** instead of nerves.

## HOW THE NERVOUS SYSTEM WORKS

The neurons of the nervous system are organized into sequences called **neural circuits**. Neurons are arranged so that the axon of one neuron in the circuit forms junctions with the dendrites of the next neuron in the circuit. A junction between two neurons is called a **synapse**. At a synapse neurons are separated by a tiny gap (less than one-millionth of an inch) known as the **synaptic cleft**.

A neuron that ends at a specific synapse is referred to as a **presynaptic neuron**; a neuron that begins at the synapse is known as the **postsynaptic neuron**. Note that these terms are relative to a specific synapse. A postsynaptic neuron with respect to one synapse may be presynaptic to the next synapse in the sequence.

## Reflex Action

The simplest example of a neural response in human beings is a **reflex action**, a predictable, automatic response to a specific stimulus. Most of the internal mechanisms of the body are regulated by reflex actions. For example, a change in body temperature acts as a stimulus, causing the temperature-regulating center of the hypothalamus to mobilize homeostatic mechanisms that bring body temperature back to normal.

Many responses to external stimuli, such as withdrawing from painful stimuli, are also reflex actions. Like all neural responses a reflex pathway depends on four processes: *reception of the stimulus, transmission of information, integration* (interpretation and determination of an appropriate response), and the *actual response*. Withdrawal reflexes require the participation of three sets of neurons (Fig. 7–4). Suppose you accidentally rest your hand on a hot stove. Almost instantly, and before you become consciously aware of the pain, you pull your hand away. Pain receptors (dendrites of sensory neurons) have sent messages through sensory neurons to the spinal cord. There each neuron synapses with an **association neuron**, a neuron within the CNS that links sensory and motor neurons. Integration takes place and impulses are sent via appropriate motor neurons to muscles in the arm and hand instructing them to contract, jerking the hand away from the harmful stimulus.

Obviously such withdrawal reflexes are protective. At the same time that the association neuron sends a message to the motor neuron it may also dispatch a message up neurons in the spinal cord to the conscious areas of the brain. Almost at the same time that you withdraw your hand you become aware of your plight and can make the conscious decision to hold your burned hand under cold water. None of this is part of the reflex action, however.

Some reflex actions (for example, the pupillary

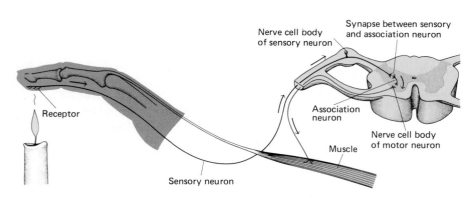

**Figure 7–4.** *The withdrawal reflex shown here involves a chain of three neurons. A sensory neuron transmits the message from the receptor to the CNS, where it synapses with an association neuron. Then an appropriate motor neuron (shown in color) transmits an impulse to the muscles that move the hand away from the flame (the response).*

reflex of the eye) do involve parts of the brain, but these are the so-called lower parts, functionally similar to the spinal cord, and have nothing to do with conscious thought. Sometimes, though, reflex actions are subject to conscious inhibition or facilitation (promotion). An example is the reflex that voids the urinary bladder when it fills with urine. In babies urination is effected by reflex whenever the bladder becomes full, but in early childhood we learn to facilitate the reflex by consciously stimulating it before the bladder pressure reaches the critical level. We also learn to inhibit the reflex consciously should the bladder become full at an inconvenient time or place.

## Transmission of Neural Impulses

Once a receptor has been stimulated, the message must be transmitted to the CNS and then back to appropriate effectors. Information must be conducted through a sequence of neurons. How is a neural message transmitted along an individual neuron? And how is it conducted from one neuron to the next in the sequence?

### Transmission Along a Neuron

Once a neuron has been stimulated sufficiently it transmits a neural impulse along the entire length of its axon. This transmission depends on changes in ion distribution.

**Resting Potential.** In a resting neuron, one that is not transmitting an impulse, the inner surface of the cell membrane is negatively charged compared with the tissue fluid surrounding it (Fig. 7–5). The resting neuron is said to be electrically **polarized**, oppositely charged along the inside of the membrane compared with the outside. When electrical charges are separated in this way, they have the *potential* of doing work should they be permitted to come together. The amount of work that can be performed may be expressed in volts, or in the case of electrically active cells, in millivolts. (A millivolt equals one-thousandth of a volt.)

The **resting potential** of a neuron is a direct result of a slight excess of positive ions outside the membrane. This results in part from efficient sodium pumps within the cell membrane that actively transport sodium out of the cell. (Recall that sodium ions are positively charged.) The same pumps may also actively transport potassium into the cell (some cells may have separate potassium pumps) but more positive ions are pumped out than in. The active transport of ions by these pumps is a kind of cellular work and requires the cell to expend energy.

**Action Potential.** Neurons are highly excitable cells. An electrical, chemical, or mechanical stimulus may alter the resting potential by increasing the permeability of the membrane to sodium. If the stimulus is sufficiently strong it may result in an **action potential**, that is, the transmission of a neural impulse.

Sodium gates are thought to be present within the neuron membrane. These are like tiny pores that are closed when the neuron is at rest but open, admitting sodium ions, when the neuron is stimulated. The greater the stimulation, the more sodium gates open. The more sodium ions that diffuse into the cell, the less negative the inner surface of the membrane becomes, and the lower the resting potential. The membrane begins to depolarize.

When the extent of depolarization reaches a critical point called the **threshold**, or **firing**, **level**, an almost explosive action occurs as the action potential is produced. The action potential is an electrical current of sufficient strength to induce collapse of the resting potential in the adjacent area of the membrane. The area of depolarization then spreads like a chain reaction down the length of the axon. Thus a neural impulse is transmitted as a **wave of depolarization** that travels down the neuron. The impulse moves along the axon at a constant velocity for each type of neuron.

Conduction of a neural impulse is somewhat analogous to burning a trail of gunpowder. Once the gunpowder is ignited at one end, the flame moves steadily along from one end of the trail to the other by igniting the powder particles ahead of it. Of course there is no way of restoring the gunpowder to its original condition after it has burned, but the nerve cell does restore itself!

As the wave of depolarization moves down the axon the normal polarized state is quickly reestablished behind it. By the time the action potential moves a few millimeters down the axon, the membrane over which it has just passed begins to repolarize (Fig. 7–5).

After an impulse has passed a particular point on the axon, that portion of the axon enters a **refractory period**. During the millisecond or so that it is depolarized, the neuron cannot transmit another impulse. However, even with the limits imposed by their refractory periods, most neurons can transmit more than 1000 impulses per second.

The smooth, progressive impulse transmission just described is characteristic of unmyelinated neurons. In myelinated neurons the myelin acts as an effective insulator around the axon except at

Stimulus

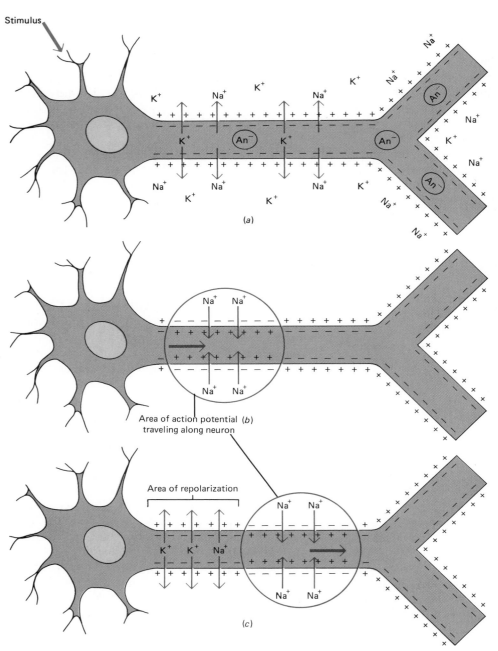

*(a)*

Area of action potential *(b)*
traveling along neuron

Area of repolarization

*(c)*

*Figure 7–5.* Transmission of an impulse along an axon. (a) The dendrites of a neuron are stimulated sufficiently to depolarize the cell membrane to firing level. The axon shown is still in the resting state and has a resting potential. (b) and (c) An impulse is transmitted as a wave of depolarization that travels down the axon. At the region of depolarization, sodium ions diffuse into the cell. As the impulse passes along from one region to another, resting conditions are quickly reestablished. ($Na^+$, Sodium ions; $K^+$, potassium ions; $An^-$, large ions within the neuron.)

the nodes of Ranvier, where the axon membrane makes direct contact with the surrounding tissue fluid. In these neurons depolarization jumps along the axon from one node of Ranvier to the next. The ion activity at the active node serves to depolarize the next node along the axon.

**The All-or-None Law.** Any stimulus too weak to depolarize the neuron to threshold level will not fire the neuron. It merely sets up a local response that fades and dies within a few millimeters from the point of stimulus. A stimulus strong enough to depolarize the neuron to its critical threshold level will result in the transmission of an impulse along

the axon. The threshold level varies with each type of neuron. Because the neuron either does or does not transmit an action potential, it is said to obey an **all-or-none law.** There is no variation in the strength of a single impulse.

### Transmission Between Neurons

When an impulse reaches the synaptic knobs at the end of a presynaptic axon, it stimulates the release of a **neurotransmitter** into the synaptic cleft (Fig. 7–6). This chemical messenger diffuses across the tiny gap and may combine with specific

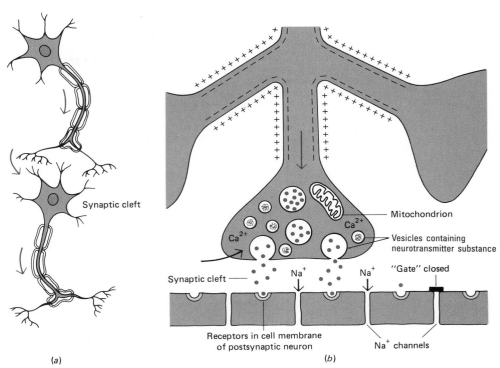

**Figure 7–6.** *Transmission of an impulse between neurons, or from a neuron to an effector. (a) The neural impulse must be transmitted across the synaptic cleft between the two neurons. (b) Neurotransmitter from vesicles within the synaptic knobs of the axon. The neurotransmitter diffuses across the synaptic cleft and may trigger an impulse in the postsynaptic neuron. It is thought that when the neurotransmitter combines with receptors in the membrane of the postsynaptic neuron, sodium gates open, permitting sodium to rush into the axon. (c) Electron micrograph of a synaptic knob and cleft (approximately ×125,000). In circled area, two synaptic vesicles are merging with the membrane of the synaptic knob and discharging neurotransmitter into the cleft. The membrane of a skeletal muscle cell synapsing with this knob is shown below. (SV, Synaptic vesicles; SC, synaptic cleft; neuron above cleft, muscle cell below.) (Courtesy of Dr. John Heuser.)*

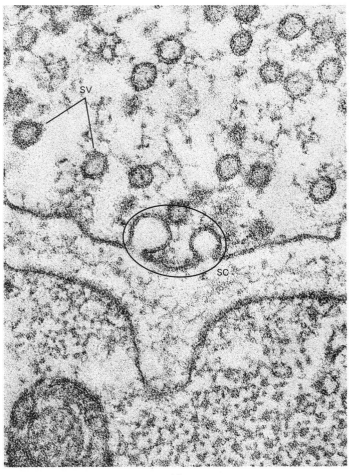

(c)

TABLE 7–1
**Some Neurotransmitters**

| Substance | Where Secreted | Comments |
|---|---|---|
| Acetylcholine | Myoneural (muscle-nerve) junctions; autonomic system[1]; parts of brain | Inactivated by cholinesterase |
| Norepinephrine | Autonomic system; reticular activating system and other areas of brain and spinal cord | Inactivated slowly by monoamine oxidase (MAO); mainly inactivated by reabsorption by vesicles in the synaptic knob; norepinephrine level in brain affects mood |
| Dopamine | Limbic system; cerebral cortex; basal ganglia; hypothalamus | Thought to affect motor function; may be involved in schizophrenia[2]; amount reduced in Parkinson's disease |
| Serotonin | Limbic system; hypothalamus; cerebellum; spinal cord | May play role in sleep; LSD antagonizes serotonin; thought to be inhibitory |
| GABA (gamma-aminobutyric acid) | Spinal cord, cerebral cortex, cerebellum | Acts as inhibitor; may play role in pain perception |
| Endorphins and enkephalins | Many parts of CNS | Groups of compounds that affect pain perception and other aspects of behavior |

[1]These and other structures listed in this table will be discussed in Chapter 8.
[2]Recent findings suggest that the brains of schizophrenics have more dopamine receptors than those of nonschizophrenics.

receptors on the dendrites or cell bodies of postsynaptic neurons. The postsynaptic membrane may then become more permeable to sodium, causing depolarization of the membrane. An action potential may result. Excess neurotransmitter is either reabsorbed into the synaptic vesicles or inactivated by enzymes. About 30 different substances are now known or suspected of being neurotransmitters (Table 7–1).

## Integration

When neurotransmitter combines with a receptor on the surface of a postsynaptic neuron the effect can either be excitatory, bringing the neuron closer to firing, or inhibitory, bringing it further away from firing. **Neural integration** is the process of sorting and interpreting incoming signals and determining an appropriate response. Each neuron synapses with hundreds of other neurons. It is the job of the dendrites and cell body of every neuron to integrate the hundreds of messages that continually bombard them. Because more than 90% of the neurons in the body are located in the CNS, most neural integration takes place there, within the brain and spinal cord. These neurons are responsible for making most of the "decisions."

## THE CENTRAL NERVOUS SYSTEM: THE BRAIN

Not even the most intricate computer begins to rival the complexity of the human brain. A soft, wrinkled mass of tissue weighing about 1.4 kg (3 pounds), the human brain is the most complex

mechanism known. Each of its 25 billion neurons is functionally connected to as many as 1000 others and there may be as many as $10^{14}$ synapses. No wonder that scientists have barely begun to unravel the tangled neural circuits that govern human physiology and behavior.

Although the brain accounts for only about 2% of the body weight, it receives about 20% of the blood pumped by the heart each minute and consumes about 20% of the oxygen used by the body. The brain is so dependent on its blood supply that, when deprived of it, consciousness may be lost quickly, and irreversible damage may occur within a few minutes. In fact, the most common cause of brain damage is a **cerebrovascular accident** (a stroke) in which a portion of the brain is deprived of its blood supply (often because a blood vessel has been blocked by a blood clot). (See Focus on Stroke, A Case Study.)

The main divisions of the brain are the medulla, pons, midbrain, diencephalon (which includes the thalamus and hypothalamus), cerebellum, and cerebrum (Figs. 7–7 and 7–8 and Table 7–2). The medulla, pons, and midbrain make up the **brain stem,** the elongated portion of the brain that looks like a stalk for the cerebrum.

## The Medulla

More formally known as the **medulla oblongata,** (meh-**dul'**-ah ob"-long-**gah'**-tuh), the medulla is the most inferior portion of the brain stem and is continuous caudally with the spinal cord. Its cavity, the **fourth ventricle** (Figs. 7–8 and 7–9), is continuous with the central canal of the spinal cord. Because of its position, all nerve tracts passing be-

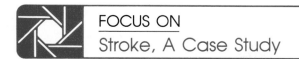

## FOCUS ON
## Stroke, A Case Study

Late one night John told his wife that he felt strange, a little dizzy, with some numbness on the left side of his mouth and some weakness in his left arm. The next morning when arising John fell backward on the bed unable to stand on his own. His left arm was limp and immobile.

John was taken to the emergency room where a physician did a neurological examination to determine the extent of neurological deficits. A CT scan was done immediately to identify any intracranial damage. The scan showed changes on the right side of the motor area in the precentral gyrus. John had suffered a cardiovascular accident (CVA), commonly referred to as a **stroke**.

The physician discussed the test results thoroughly with John telling him that the damage was most likely caused by a thrombus, a blood clot that formed within a blood vessel. He also explained that John would be starting with physical therapy within a few days to maintain the muscle tone of

his left arm and leg. Even with the support of the staff and his wife John was discouraged and depressed. The incident was overwhelming for him psychologically, as he had images of himself unable to move and confined to a wheelchair for the rest of his life. Within a few days the physical therapy had been started and John gradually learned to walk with assistance and move his arm. His improvement was slow but steady and his psychological outlook continued to improve. Occupational therapy was started to improve the muscle tone of the shoulder, arm, and hand. Improvement in his hand was slower and at times he was discouraged with the impaired movement of the fingers and hand.

Six months after the stroke John was able to walk freely and experienced return of much of his arm movement. Although motion of his fingers was still limited, he continued with strengthening exercises and noticed slow, but steady, improvement. He returned to work in his office within 6 months.

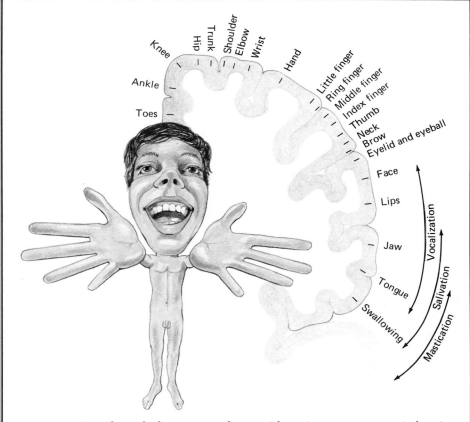

*A cross section through the precentral gyrus (the primary motor area) showing which area of cortex controls each body part. The figure (called a motor homunculus) shown here is proportioned according to the amount of cerebral cortex devoted to control of each part of the body. Note that more cortical tissue is devoted to regulating those body parts capable of skilled, complex movement.*

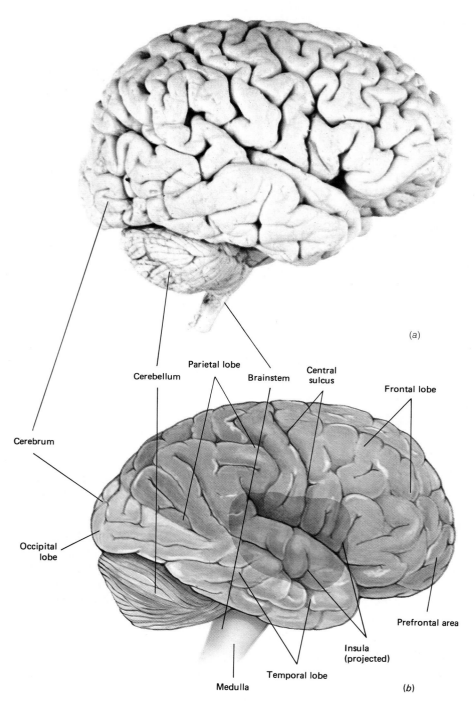

(a)

Cerebrum

Occipital
lobe

Cerebellum

Parietal lobe

Brainstem

Central
sulcus

Frontal lobe

Prefrontal area

Insula
(projected)

Temporal lobe

Medulla

(b)

**Figure 7–7.** *Structure of the human brain. (a) Photograph of the human brain, lateral view. Note that the cerebrum covers the diencephalon and part of the brain stem. (b) Lateral view of the human brain showing the lobes of the cerebrum. Part of the brain has been made transparent so that the underlying insular lobe can be located. ((a) from Williams, P., and Warwick, R. (eds.): Gray's Anatomy, 36th ed. Philadelphia, W.B. Saunders Company, 1980.)*

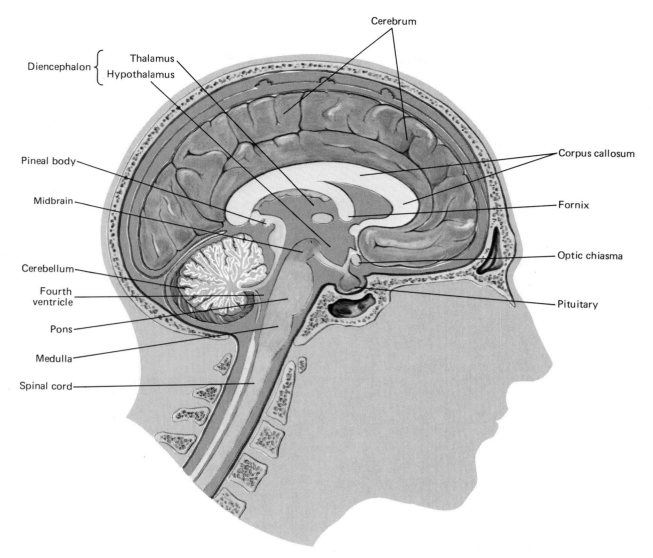

**Figure 7–8.** *A midsagittal section through the brain. Note that in this type of section half of the brain is cut away so that structures normally covered by the cerebrum are exposed.*

tween the spinal cord and the upper divisions of the brain must pass through the medulla.

The anterior surface of the medulla consists mainly of two prominent bulges of white matter known as the **pyramids.** The pyramids contain fibers of the **pyramidal tracts,** the major voluntary motor pathways between the cerebrum and spinal cord. Within the medulla about 80% of the pyramidal fibers cross (or decussate). Because these nerve fibers cross, the right side of the brain controls the movement of the left side of the body and the left side of the brain controls the movement of the right side of the body.

Within the medulla are several vital reflex centers. They include the **cardiac centers** that control heart rate, the **vasomotor centers** that control blood pressure, and the **respiratory centers** that regulate breathing. Centers for other reflex actions, such as vomiting, sneezing, coughing, and swallowing, are also found within the medulla. Centers for the reflexes mediated by cranial nerves IX through XII are located within the medulla.

## The Pons

The **pons,** a bulge on the anterior (ventral) surface of the brain stem, lies just above the medulla with which it is continuous. Its posterior surface is hidden by the cerebellum. The word pons means "bridge," and indeed the pons serves as a link connecting various parts of the brain. In fact, the pons consists mainly of nerve fibers passing between the medulla and other parts of the brain.

TABLE 7–2
**Divisions of the Brain**

| | Description | Functions |
|---|---|---|
| *Medulla* | Most inferior portion of the brain stem; continuous with spinal cord; its white matter consists of nerve tracts passing between the spinal cord and various parts of the brain; its gray matter consists of nuclei; the anterior portion consists mainly of the pyramids; contains nuclei of cranial nerves IX through XII[1]; its cavity is the fourth ventricle | Contains vital centers (within its reticular formation) that regulate heartbeat, respiration, and blood pressure; contains reflex centers that control swallowing, coughing, sneezing, and vomiting; relays messages to other parts of the brain |
| *Pons* | Consists mainly of nerve tracts passing between the medulla and other parts of the brain; forms a bulge on the anterior surface of the brain stem; contains a respiratory center and nuclei of cranial nerves V through VIII | Serves as a link connecting various parts of the brain; helps regulate respiration |
| *Midbrain* | Just superior to the pons; cavity is the cerebral aqueduct; posteriorly, tectum consists of corpora quadrigemina; within midbrain are nuclei of cranial nerves III and IV | Corpora quadrigemina mediate visual and auditory reflexes; cranial nerves III and IV control certain eye movements |
| *Diencephalon* | Consists of two parts: *Thalamus*—located on each side of the third ventricle; consists of two masses of gray matter partly covered by white matter and contains many important nuclei | Main relay center conducting information between spinal cord and cerebrum; incoming messages are sorted and partially interpreted within the thalamic nuclei before being relayed to the appropriate centers in the cerebrum |
| | *Hypothalamus*—forms ventral floor of third ventricle; contains many nuclei; optic chiasma mark the crossing of the optic nerves; infundibulum connects the pituitary gland to the hypothalamus | Contains centers for control of body temperature, appetite, and water balance; regulates pituitary gland and links nervous and endocrine systems; helps control autonomic system; involved in some emotional and sexual responses |
| *Cerebellum* | Second largest part of brain; superior to the fourth ventricle; consists of two lateral cerebellar hemispheres | Responsible for smooth, coordinated movement; maintains posture and muscle tone and helps maintain equilibrium |
| *Cerebrum* | Largest, most prominent part of the brain; longitudinal fissure divides the cerebrum into right and left hemispheres, each containing a lateral ventricle; each hemisphere is divided into six lobes; frontal, parietal, occipital, temporal, limbic, and insula | Center of intellect, memory, language, and consciousness; receives and interprets sensory information from all sense organs; controls motor functions |
| *Cerebral cortex* | Convoluted, outer layer of gray matter covering the cerebrum; functionally divided into: | |
| | (1) Motor areas | Control voluntary movement and certain types of involuntary movement |
| | (2) Sensory areas | Receive incoming sensory information from eyes, ears, touch, and pressure receptors, and other sense organs; sensory association areas interpret incoming sensory information |
| | (3) Association areas | Responsible for thought, learning, language, judgment, and personality; store memories; connect sensory and motor areas |
| *White matter* | Consists of fibers that connect the two hemispheres and fibers that are part of ascending and descending tracts; basal ganglia are located within the white matter | Links various areas of the brain |

[1]Cranial nerves are discussed in more detail in Table 8–1.

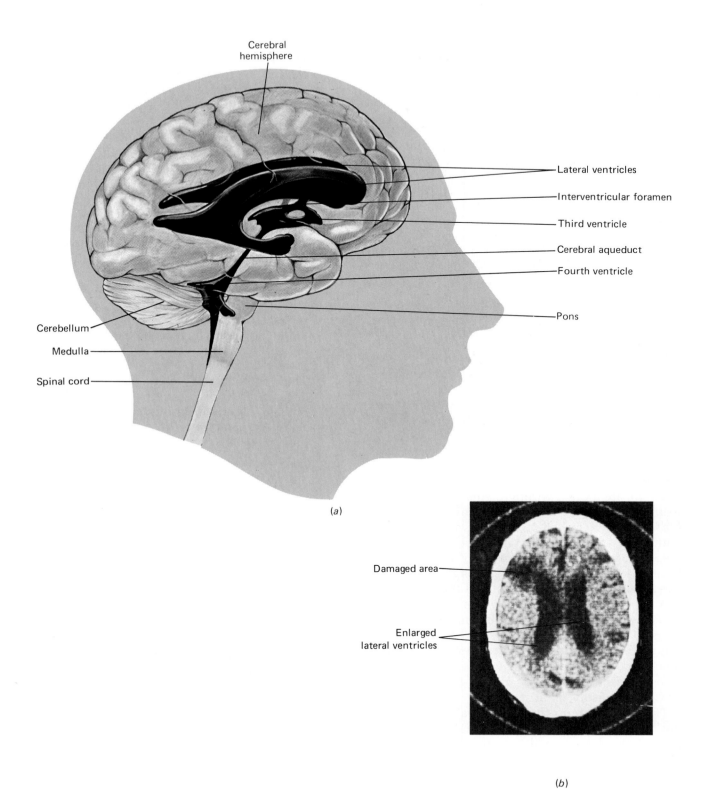

**Figure 7–9.** The ventricles of the brain. (a) Lateral view. (b) CT scan showing lateral ventricles. Note damaged area.

One of the respiratory centers is located within the pons. Centers for the reflexes mediated by cranial nerves V through VII are also located within the pons.

## The Midbrain

The **midbrain** (mesencephalon) extends from the pons to the diencephalon. Its cavity, the **cerebral aqueduct,** connects the third and fourth ventricles. The roof of the midbrain, called the **tectum,** lies posterior to the cerebral aqueduct. It consists of four rounded bodies, the **corpora quadrigemina.** The paired upper bodies serve as visual reflex centers for head and eyeball movements in response to certain types of visual and other stimuli. The lower bodies are relay centers for auditory information.

## The Diencephalon

The diencephalon (die″-en-**seph′**-ah-lon) is the part of the brain between the cerebrum and the midbrain. Its cavity is the **third ventricle** (Fig. 7–9). Among its important structures are the thalamus, hypothalamus, and pineal body (an endocrine gland).

The **thalamus** (**thal′**-ah-mus) consists of two oval masses, one located on each side of the third ventricle. Many nuclei, both sensory and motor in function, are located within the thalamus. Afferent neurons coming from all the sense organs (except the olfactory epithelium of the nose) synapse within these nuclei. Neural messages arriving from these afferent neurons are sent on into the cerebrum. Many neurons in descending motor pathways also synapse within nuclei of the thalamus.

A person becomes vaguely aware of sensory impulses when they reach the thalamus. If sensory areas of the cerebrum are destroyed, the person can still be conscious of pain, temperature, crude touch, and pressure. The thalamus also helps one associate feelings of pleasantness or unpleasantness with sensory impulses.

The **hypothalamus** (hy″-po-**thal′**-ah-mus), which lies inferior to the thalamus, forms the floor and part of the lateral walls of the third ventricle. Many nuclei are located within the hypothalamus. The **optic chiasma,** a prominent X-shaped structure in the floor of the hypothalamus, is formed by the crossing of part of each optic nerve. A stalk of tissue (the infundibulum) connects the pituitary gland to the hypothalamus.

A small but mighty part of the brain, the hypo-

thalamus helps to regulate an impressive number of mechanisms essential to maintaining homeostasis.

1. The hypothalamus connects the cerebral cortex and the lower autonomic centers. For example, stimulation of certain areas in the hypothalamus results in a decrease in heart rate. In this role the hypothalamus serves as an important link between "mind" (cognitive mechanisms) and "body" (physiological mechanisms).
2. The hypothalamus is the link between the nervous and endocrine systems. Wedded both anatomically and physiologically to the pituitary gland, the hypothalamus produces several releasing hormones that regulate the secretion of specific hormones from the anterior pituitary. In addition, the hypothalamus manufactures antidiuretic hormone (ADH), which helps maintain fluid balance. The hypothalamus also produces the hormone oxytocin, important in uterine contraction during childbirth and in release of milk from the breast.
3. The hypothalamus helps maintain fluid balance. In addition to producing ADH, the hypothalamus contains a thirst center.
4. Body temperature is regulated by the hypothalamus.
5. The appetite and satiety centers within the hypothalamus regulate food intake.
6. The hypothalamus influences sexual behavior and the affective (emotional) aspects of sensory input. Centers there help us decide whether something is pleasant or painful.

## The Cerebellum

The second largest part of the brain, the **cerebellum** (ser″-e-**bel′**-um), consists of two lateral masses called **hemispheres** and a connecting portion (the *vermis*). Fine coordination of muscle movements is the job of the cerebellum. Three functions may be listed:

1. The cerebellum helps make muscular movement smooth instead of jerky and trembling. When the cerebellum is damaged, movements essential to running, walking, writing, talking, and many other activities become incoordinated.
2. The cerebellum helps maintain muscle tone and, thus, posture.
3. Impulses from the vestibular apparatus (organ of balance) in the inner ear are continu-

ously delivered to the cerebellum, which uses that information to help maintain equilibrium.

When the cerebellum is damaged, movements become ataxic (incoordinated) because of errors in the direction, range, and rate of movement. A staggering, "drunken" gait is characteristic; speech may be slurred; and the patient, in attempting to touch an object, overshoots first to one side and then to the other (intention tremor). In one clinical diagnostic test for cerebellar damage the patient is asked to place a finger on his or her own nose. A patient with cerebellar damage will miss the mark and may miss several times before finding the target.

## The Cerebrum

More than 12 billion neurons are found within the **cerebrum** (seh-**ree'**-brum), the largest and most prominent part of the human brain. As governor of all higher mental processes, the cerebrum interprets sensation, controls motor activities, and serves as the center of intellect, reason, memory, language, and consciousness.

### Basic Structure

The thin, outer layer of the cerebrum consists of gray matter and is called the **cerebral cortex.** Beneath it lies white matter. The **basal ganglia,** paired nuclei that play an important role in movement, are located within the white matter of the cerebrum. The two cavities within the cerebrum are the **lateral ventricles.**

In the embryo the cerebrum grows rapidly, enlarging out of proportion to the rest of the brain. It grows backward over the brain stem and also folds upon itself, forming **convolutions** (kon-voe-**loo'**-shuns), or **gyri** (**jye'**-ree) (singular, gyrus). Grooves, called **sulci** (**sul'**-si) when shallow and **fissures** when deep, separate the gyri from one another.

The cerebrum is partially divided into right and left halves, the **right** and **left cerebral hemispheres,** by a deep groove called the **longitudinal fissure** (Fig. 7–10). The cerebrum is separated from the cerebellum by the **transverse fissure.**

Fissures and sulci divide each hemisphere into

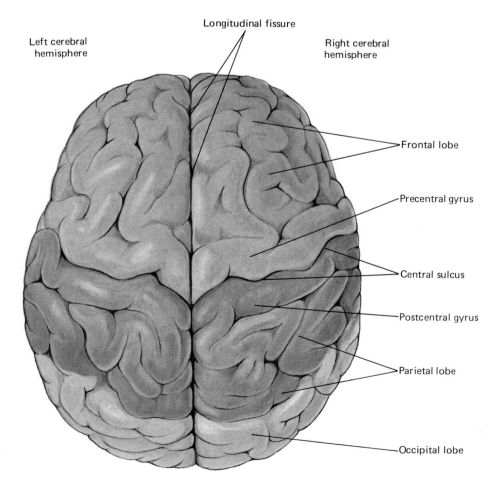

**Figure 7–10.** Superior view of the cerebrum.

six lobes: **frontal, parietal, occipital, temporal** (named after the bones that protect them), **central (insula),** and **limbic.** Each frontal lobe is separated from a parietal lobe by a **central sulcus.** Hidden from surface view, the central lobe is located deep within the cerebrum. The limbic lobe is the ring of cortex and associated structures that surrounds the ventricles of the cerebrum.

### White Matter of the Cerebrum

The white matter of the cerebrum is composed of myelinated fibers. These connect the cortical areas with one another and with other parts of the nervous system. A large band of white matter, the **corpus callosum,** connects the right and left hemispheres (Fig. 7–8). The **fornix** connects the cortex with the thalamus.

### Functions of the Cerebrum

Human beings differ from other organisms in the intricate development of the cerebral cortex. The neural basis of those human qualities that we cherish so highly—abilities to reason, communicate by language, make intellectual and moral judgments, create poetry and art, invent computers and artificial hearts—resides within this soft gray mass of tissue.

For convenience we may divide the functions performed by the cerebrum into three categories:

1. **Sensory functions.** The cerebrum receives information from the sense organs and then interprets these messages so that we "know" what we are seeing, hearing, tasting, smelling, or feeling. These functions are carried out by certain areas of the cerebrum known as **sensory areas.**
2. **Motor functions.** The **motor areas** of the cerebral cortex are responsible for all voluntary movement and for some involuntary movement.
3. **Association functions. Association areas** are responsible for the intellectual activities of the cerebral cortex. These include learning and reasoning, memory storage and recall, language abilities, and even consciousness. Association areas also link sensory with motor areas.

Investigators have attempted to draw maps of the brain, indicating which area is most responsible for each function. Brodmann's classification, one of the most widely used, is shown in Figure 7–11.

### Lobes of the Cerebrum

As already mentioned, each cerebral hemisphere is divided into six lobes. The anterior portion of each **frontal lobe** is an association area known as the **prefrontal area.**

Prefrontal lobotomies were performed on psychiatric patients prior to the advent of psychotropic medications to make them less aware of the hallucinations and delusions to which they reacted. The tracts were severed to the prefrontal area, which decreased psychotic behavior but left the patient with little affect and minimal emotional response to the environment. Frontal lobotomies are now performed mainly in patients suffering from severe chronic pain. Although such patients still feel the pain, they no longer seem to mind it. Instead, they experience a false feeling of euphoria (well-being).

Just anterior to the central fissure lies the **precentral gyrus** of the frontal lobe. Because voluntary movements of skeletal muscles are controlled from this area, it is known as the **motor cortex** or **primary motor area.** One part of the premotor area, known as **Broca's speech area,** is concerned with directing the formation of words.

The **parietal lobe** has a primary sensory area, the **postcentral gyrus,** that receives information from the sensory receptors in the skin and joints. This information is relayed to the parietal lobe by way of the thalamus. Important sensory association areas, also located within the parietal lobe, integrate information received by the primary sensory area and also receive and integrate information about visual, auditory, and taste sensations from other areas of the cortex and thalamus. Through this integration process persons become aware of themselves in relation to their environments. They are able to interpret characteristics of objects that they feel with their hands and to comprehend spoken and written language.

The **occipital lobe** receives information from the thalamus about what we see and integrates the information to formulate an appropriate response. The area that receives the visual information is known as the **primary visual area;** the portion that integrates the information is the **visual association area.**

The **temporal lobe** is concerned with reception and integration of auditory messages. Part of the temporal lobe is concerned with emotion, personality, and behavior as a result of its connections with limbic and frontal lobes.

The **limbic lobe** is thought to be a link between emotional and cognitive (thought) mechanisms.

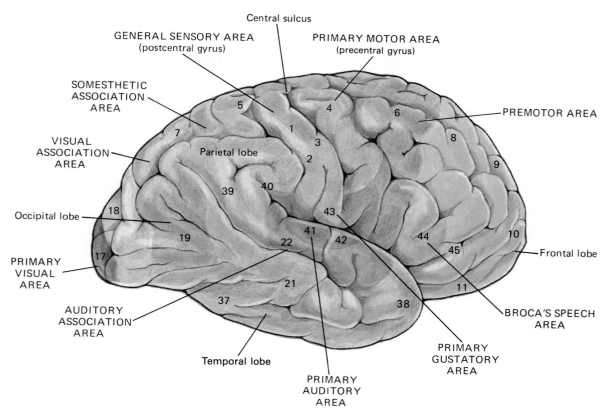

**Figure 7–11.** Map of the lateral surface of the cerebral cortex showing some of the functional areas. Areas 4, 6, and 8 are motor areas; areas 1, 2, 3, 17, 41, 42, and 43 are primary sensory areas; and areas 9, 10, 11, 18, 19, 22, 38, 39, and 40 are association areas.

This lobe is an important part of the limbic system.

Neural pathways of the **insula** (central lobe) are not understood but this lobe is thought to be involved in both autonomic and somatic activities.

## The Limbic System

The **limbic system** is an action system in the brain that plays a role in emotional responses, autonomic responses, subconscious motor and sensory drives, sexual behavior, biological rhythms, and motivation, including feelings of pleasure and punishment. Certain structures of the cerebrum and diencephalon make up the limbic system.

When an electrode is implanted in the so-called reward center of the limbic system, a rat will press a lever that stimulates this area 10,000 to 15,000 times per hour. Stimulation of this area is apparently so rewarding that an animal will forego food and drink and may continue to press the lever until it drops from exhaustion.

## The Reticular Activating System

The **reticular activating system (RAS)** is a complex pathway of neurons in the brain stem. It receives messages from neurons in the spinal cord and from many other parts of the nervous system and communicates with the cerebral cortex by complex circuits. The RAS is ultimately responsible for maintaining consciousness and the extent of its activity determines the state of alertness. When the RAS bombards the cerebral cortex with stimuli, you feel alert and are able to focus your attention on specific thoughts. When its activity slows, you begin to feel sleepy. If the RAS is severely damaged, the victim may pass into a deep, permanent coma.

## Electrical Activity of the Brain

Continuous electrical activity within the brain can be measured by placing electrodes on the sur-

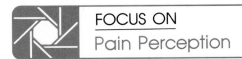

## FOCUS ON
## Pain Perception

Pain is a protective mechanism that signals us to react to remove the source of the damage. When stimulated, pain receptors send messages to the spinal cord. Within the cord the sensory neurons synapse with an association neuron that relays the message to at least one more association neuron. The message is transmitted to the opposite side of the spinal cord and then sent upward via the spinothalamic tract to the thalamus (see figure), where awareness of pain begins. From the thalamus messages are sent to the primary sensory and sensory association areas in the parietal lobe. At that time the individual becomes fully aware of the pain and can analyze the situation. How intense is the pain? How threatening is the situation? What can be done about it? From the thalamus, messages are also sent to the limbic system, where the affective (emotional) aspects of the discomfort can be evaluated.

Pain can be inhibited or facilitated at many levels. Fear and anxiety tend to intensify the perception of pain. The intensity of perceived pain depends partly on how one has learned to deal with

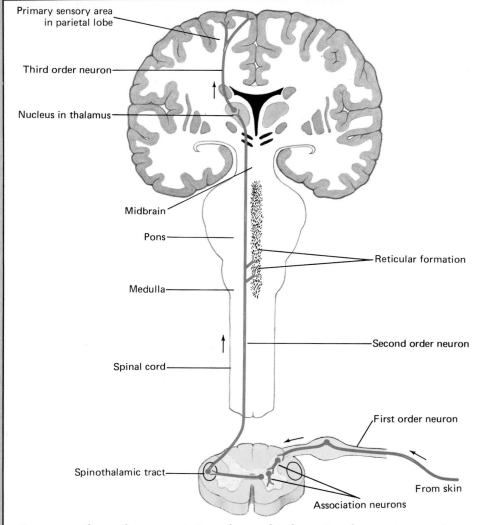

*Sensory pathway for transmission of neural information from pain receptors. The first-order neurons are sensory neurons that synapse with neurons of the spinothalamic pathway within the spinal cord. The second-order neurons cross to the opposite side of the spinal cord and then pass upward through the brain stem to a nucleus within the thalamus. There they synapse with the third-order neurons, which transmit impulses to the sensory areas in the parietal lobe.*

pain. Thus, a child with a bruised knee may heighten the feeling of pain emotionally. How adults respond to a child's pain is also important. Making a fuss over a hurt child teaches the child to magnify the discomfort to increase the reward. Diverting the child's attention from the discomfort, on the other hand, tends to minimize pain perception. Intensity of perceived pain also depends on the particular situation. A professional fighter may virtually ignore a long series of well-delivered blows.

Most visceral organs are poorly supplied with pain receptors, which explains why pain from visceral structures is often difficult to locate. In fact, pain is often **referred** to a superficial area that may be some distance from the organ involved. The area to which the pain is referred generally receives its innervation from the same level of the spinal cord as does the visceral organ involved. A headache is sometimes referred pain from the blood vessels or meninges beneath the surface of the skull. A person with angina who feels cardiac pain in his or her left arm is experiencing referred pain. The pain originates in the heart as a result of ischemia (insufficient oxygen) but it is felt in the arm. One explanation is that neurons from both the heart and the arm converge on the same neurons in the central nervous system. The brain interprets the incoming message as coming from the body surface because somatic pain is far more common than visceral pain; the brain acts on the basis of its past experience. When visceral pain is felt both at the site of the distress and as referred pain it may seem to spread, or *radiate*, from the organ to the superficial area.

Sometimes when a limb is amputated the patient feels **phantom pain,** that is, pain from the missing limb. This is because, when stimulated, the severed nerve reports impulses to the CNS, which "remembers" the nerve only in conjunction with its original site of innervation, the missing limb.

The physiology of pain is not completely understood. A peptide known as **substance P** is thought to function as a neurotransmitter (or perhaps as a modulator of neural activity) in neurons that transmit pain impulses to the spinal cord and brain. Opiates, such as morphine, are analgesic drugs (drugs that relieve pain). They work by blocking the release of substance P. The body has its own pain control system. Morphinelike peptides, the **endorphins** and **enkephalins,** are produced by the CNS and pituitary gland. Like the opiate drugs, these peptides are thought to work by suppressing the release of substance P from pain-transmitting neurons. The transmitter substance gamma-aminobutyric acid (GABA) is also thought to inhibit release of substance P in some parts of the brain.

Stimulation of large numbers of touch receptors also seems to depress transmission of pain signals. You may have had the experience of rubbing the body surface near a painful area to relieve pain.

Some neurologists now feel that endorphins may explain the mechanisms of action of *acupuncture*. For thousands of years acupuncture has been used to relieve pain but how it works has remained a mystery. There is now some evidence that acupuncture needles stimulate nerves deep within the muscles, which in turn stimulate the pituitary gland and parts of the brain to release endorphins. The endorphins may inhibit neurons in the brain that normally fire in response to pain.

Various clinical methods have recently been developed for relieving pain. Stimulation of the skin over the painful area with electrodes has been successful in some patients. This procedure is called *transcutaneous electrical nerve stimulation*. In a few patients, electrodes have been implanted in appropriate areas of the brain so that the patient can stimulate her or his own brain at will. This procedure is thought to relieve pain by stimulating the release of endorphins.

face of the scalp and recording differences in electrical potentials. Patterns of activity called **brain waves** can be traced, producing a record called an **electroencephalogram (EEG).**

Brain waves are produced primarily from the cerebral cortex. The wavelike patterns arise from synchronized cyclical activity of groups of neurons. One's EEG is as unique as one's fingerprints but the EEG changes with the state of consciousness or emotion.

Although brain waves are often irregular, four main kinds of wave patterns have been distinguished. **Alpha wave** patterns are associated with resting and relaxed activity. **Beta waves** are characteristic of states of heightened mental activity, such as problem solving or information process-

ing. **Delta waves** are slow, large waves associated with normal sleeping. **Theta waves** are recorded mostly in children but are also produced in some adults when they are under emotional stress.

The EEG is used as a diagnostic tool to determine certain disease states such as epilepsy. Electrical activity of the brain is also used as a criterion of life or death. When electrical activity in the brain ceases for a specific time, a patient may be pronounced dead.

Subjects have had some success in controlling their brain wave patterns by the use of biofeedback machines, which permit them to see and listen to their brain waves. With such continuous feedback they are able to condition themselves to produce the relaxed alpha state.

## Learning and Memory

Despite extensive research, mechanisms by which the brain thinks, learns, and remembers are still poorly understood. The human brain differs most markedly from the brains of other animals by the remarkable development of its association areas within the cerebral cortex. Damage to association areas can prevent a person from thinking logically, even though he or she may still be able to hear or even read.

In order to learn, the brain must be able to (1) focus attention on specific stimuli, whether they be the words on this printed page or the color of a traffic light; (2) compare incoming sensory stimuli with stimuli it has encountered before; (3) store information. **Memory** is the ability to recall stored information.

Just how the brain stores information and retrieves the memory on command has been the subject of much speculation and is not settled to this day. According to current theory there are several levels of memory. Short-term memory involves recalling information for a few seconds or minutes. Usually when you look up a phone number you remember it only long enough to dial. Should you need the same number the next day, you would have to look it up again. One theory of short-term memory suggests that it is based on reverberating neural circuits. A memory circuit may continue to reverberate for several minutes until it fatigues or until new signals are received that interfere with the old.

Researchers have methodically removed portions of the brains of experimental animals without finding specific regions where information is stored. As more cerebral cortex tissue is destroyed, more information is lost but no specific area can be labeled the "memory bank."

Several minutes are required for information to become consolidated within long-term memory. Should a person suffer a brain concussion or undergo electroconvulsive therapy, memory of what transpired immediately prior to the incident may be completely lost. When parts of the limbic system are injured or removed, a person can recall information stored in the past but is no longer able to store new information.

Retrieval of information stored in the long-term memory bank is of considerable interest—especially to students! Some researchers think that once information is deposited in long-term storage it remains in the brain permanently. The only problem is finding the information when we need it! When we seem to forget a particular bit of information it may be because we have not searched for it effectively.

## Does Environmental Experience Affect the Brain?

Experiments have shown that environmental experience may cause physical as well as chemical changes in brain structure. When rats are provided with a stimulating environment and given the opportunity to learn, neurons in their brains increase in size. They develop a greater number of glial cells and show increased concentration of synaptic contacts. Some investigators have reported that the cerebral cortex actually becomes thicker and heavier. Characteristic biochemical changes also take place. Other experiments indicate that animals reared in a complex environment may be able to process and remember information more quickly than animals deprived of stimulation and social interaction.

During early life there are apparently certain critical or sensitive periods of nervous system development that are influenced by environmental stimuli. For example, when the eyes of young mice first open, large numbers of dendritic spines form on neurons in the visual cortexes. When the animals are kept in the dark and deprived of visual stimuli, fewer dendritic spines form. If the mice are exposed to light later in life, some new dendritic spines form but never in the number that develop in a mouse reared in a normal environment.

Such studies linking the development of the brain with environmental experience suggest that early stimulation is extremely important for the neural, motor, and intellectual development of children. Hence the rapidly expanding educational toy market and widespread acceptance of early education programs.

## THE CENTRAL NERVOUS SYSTEM: THE SPINAL CORD

The spinal cord has two main functions: (1) it controls many reflex activities of the body and (2) it transmits information back and forth from peripheral nerves to the brain via its ascending and descending tracts. A slightly flattened hollow cylinder, the spinal cord emerges from the base of the brain at the level of the foramen magnum of the occipital bone and extends caudally to the level of the second lumbar vertebra (Fig. 7–12). The average length of the spinal cord is about 45 cm (17 inches), although this varies somewhat with the length of the trunk; its diameter is about that of a finger. Generally, the spinal cord tapers from its cranial to its caudal end. However, it has two bulges, the **cervical** and **lumbar enlargements.**

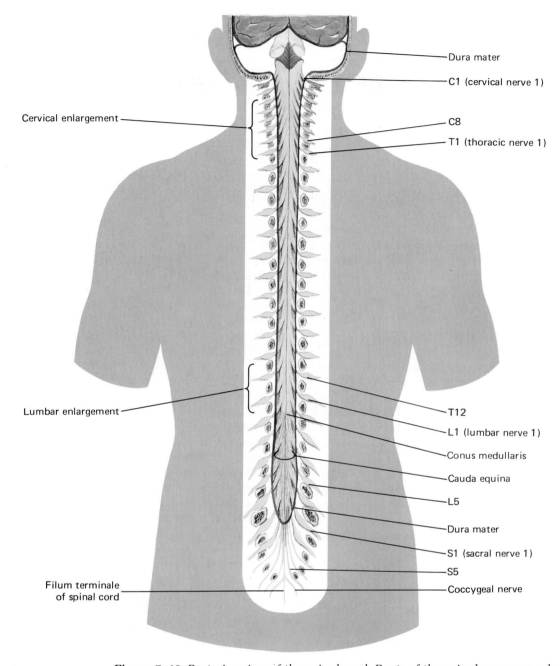

Dura mater

C1 (cervical nerve 1)

Cervical enlargement

C8

T1 (thoracic nerve 1)

Lumbar enlargement

T12

L1 (lumbar nerve 1)

Conus medullaris

Cauda equina

L5

Dura mater

S1 (sacral nerve 1)

S5

Filum terminale
of spinal cord

Coccygeal nerve

**Figure 7–12.** *Posterior view of the spinal cord. Roots of the spinal nerves are shown. Spinal nerves are named for the general region of the vertebral column from which they originate, and they are numbered in sequence.*

The large spinal nerves that supply the upper and lower extremities emerge in these regions.

At its caudal end the spinal cord narrows to a sharp tip called the **conus medullaris.** From the end of the conus an extension of the inner connective tissue covering (pia mater) known as the **filum terminale** continues to the end of the vertebral column, where it attaches to the coccyx.

Thirty-one pairs of spinal nerves exit from successive levels of the cord. Nerves from the lower region of the cord pass caudally to below the level of the conus medullaris before they leave the vertebral canal. Because they resemble a horse's tail they are aptly known as the **cauda equina** (Fig. 7–6).

Several longitudinal grooves, called **fissures,** divide the spinal cord into regions. The deepest groove, the **anterior** (ventral) **median fissure** lies in the midanterior line. Opposite on the posterior (dorsal) surface is the more shallow **posterior (dorsal) fissure.**

A cross section through the spinal cord reveals a small **central canal** surrounded by an area of gray matter shaped somewhat like the letter H (Fig. 7–13). Outside the gray matter the cord is composed of white matter.

## Gray Matter

The **gray matter** of the spinal cord is subdivided into sections called **columns,** or **horns.** The right and left halves of the H-shaped area are connected by a bar of gray matter. The anterior (ventral) portions of the letter H are the **anterior columns;** the posterior (dorsal) segments are the **posterior columns.**

## White Matter: The Spinal Tracts

**White matter** consists of myelinated axons arranged in bundles, called **tracts** or **pathways.** Long **ascending tracts** carry sensory impulses upward to the brain, while **descending tracts** conduct impulses (the "decisions") from the brain back down the cord toward the efferent neurons.

For example, the **spinothalamic tracts** consist of axons of neurons that receive pain and temperature information from sensory neurons reporting from the skin. Spinothalamic tract axons convey this information to the brain. The **pyramidal tracts** are descending tracts that convey voluntary motor impulses from the cerebrum to spinal nerves at various levels in the cord.

## PROTECTION OF THE CENTRAL NERVOUS SYSTEM

The soft, fragile brain and spinal cord are the most carefully protected organs in the body. Both are encased in bone, covered by the **meninges,** three layers of connective tissue, and bathed in cushioning fluid, the **cerebrospinal fluid.**

## The Meninges

The outermost of the meninges is the **dura mater,** a tough, double-layered membrane (Fig. 7–14). In some regions the two layers of the dura mater are separated by large blood vessels called sinuses. These vessels drain blood leaving the brain and deliver it to the jugular veins in the neck (Fig. 7–14). The dura mater forms four partitions (septa) that subdivide the cranium into compartments. In the region of the spinal cord the **epidural space** lies between the bone and the dura mater. A potential space, the **subdural space,** separates the dura mater from the arachnoid in both cranial and spinal cord regions.

The **arachnoid** is a thin delicate membrane. Projections from the arachnoid extend like the threads of a web to the innermost meningeal layer, the pia mater. The **pia mater,** a thin, vascular membrane, adheres closely to the brain and spinal cord.

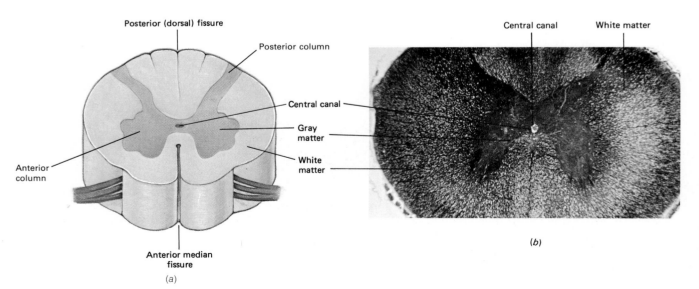

*Figure 7–13.* The spinal cord consists of gray matter and white matter. (a) Cross section through the spinal cord. (b) Photomicrograph of a cross section through the spinal cord (approximately ×25).

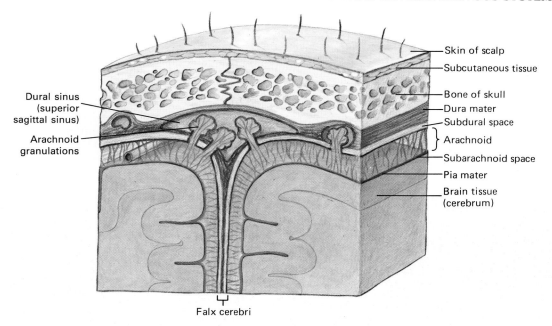

**Dural sinus (superior sagittal sinus)**

**Arachnoid granulations**

Skin of scalp
Subcutaneous tissue
Bone of skull
Dura mater
Subdural space
Arachnoid
Subarachnoid space
Pia mater
Brain tissue (cerebrum)

Falx cerebri

***Figure 7–14.*** *The protective coverings of the brain. Note the large blood sinus shown between two layers of the dura mater. Blood leaving the brain flows into such sinuses and then circulates to the large jugular veins in the neck.*

The dura and arachnoid layers extend below the level of the cord. The subarachnoid space extends to the level of the second sacral vertebra. This is of clinical importance because a hollow needle can be safely inserted into the subarachnoid space between the neural arches of the third and fourth lumbar vertebrae. Known as a **spinal tap** or **lumbar puncture,** this procedure can be used to withdraw small amounts of cerebrospinal fluid without damaging the cord itself. Analysis of this fluid can be helpful in diagnosing certain CNS disorders. For example, blood in the cerebrospinal fluid may provide a clue in the diagnosis of cerebral hemorrhage. When indicated, lumbar puncture is often followed by computed tomography (CT) scanning or magnetic resonance imaging (MRI), considered more dependable methods for diagnosing cerebral hemorrhage and brain tumors.

Injections of an anesthetic into the subarachnoid space blocks neural transmission from sensory neurons. This type of anesthesia is commonly called a spinal or, if administered low in the subarachnoid space, a saddle block. Injection of a local anesthetic into the epidural space above the dura mater is called a caudal block. Epidural anesthesia is commonly administered to women during childbirth.

**Meningitis,** an inflammation of the meninges, is usually due to infection by bacteria or viruses. Viral meningitis is usually a self-limited disease from which the patient recovers fully. However, some viruses that cause meningitis can spread, causing inflammation of the brain itself. This more serious illness is **encephalitis.**

## The Cerebrospinal Fluid

The shock-absorbing cerebrospinal fluid (CSF) fills the ventricles, the cavities within the brain, and the subarachnoid spaces around the brain and spinal cord (Fig. 7-15). Most of the CSF is produced by clusters of capillaries, the **choroid plexuses,** which project from the pia mater into the ventricles. The CSF circulates through the ventricles, then passes through small apertures into the subarachnoid space. Finally it is reabsorbed into the blood through structures called **arachnoid granulations** that project from the arachnoid layer into large blood sinuses within the dura mater.

The brain actually floats in the CSF and this buoyancy protects against mechanical injury. CSF also dissolves and transports substances filtered from the blood and serves as a medium for the exchange of nutrients and waste products between the blood and the brain.

Many substances do not easily pass from the blood into the tissue fluid of the brain. Complex **blood-CSF barriers** and **blood-brain barriers** are thought to exist that slow or prevent certain materials from entering brain tissues. Some substances (for example, arsenic and gold) are almost completely blocked out. Certain drugs such as penicillin can enter the brain only to a limited extent, whereas other drugs (for example, erythromycin) enter readily.

## FOCUS ON
## Effects of Drugs on the Nervous System

About 25% of all prescribed drugs are taken to alter psychological conditions and almost all the drugs commonly abused regulate mood. Many of these drugs act by altering the levels of neurotransmitter within the brain. In particular, levels of norepinephrine, serotonin, and dopamine are thought to influence affective behavior. For example, when excessive amounts of norepinephrine are released in the RAS, we feel stimulated and energetic, whereas low concentrations of this neurotransmitter reduce anxiety. Several commonly used and abused drugs and their effects are given below.

Habitual use of almost all mood drugs may result in psychological dependence, in which the user becomes emotionally dependent on the drug. When deprived of it the user craves the feeling of **euphoria** (well-being) that the drug induces. Some drugs induce **tolerance** when they are taken continuously for several weeks. This means that an increasingly larger amount is required to obtain the desired effect. Tolerance often occurs because the liver cells "learn" to break down the drug more rapidly. Use of some drugs (such as heroin) also results in **physical dependence (addiction),** in which tolerance develops and physiological changes take place. When the drug is withheld, the addict suffers physical illness and characteristic withdrawal symptoms.

### Effects of Some Commonly Used Drugs

| Name of Drug | Effect on Mood | Actions on Body | Dangers Associated with Abuse |
|---|---|---|---|
| Barbiturates (e.g., Nembutal, Seconal) | Sedative-hypnotic[1]; "downers" | Inhibit impulse conduction in RAS: depress CNS, skeletal muscle, and heart; depress respiration; lower blood pressure; cause decrease in REM sleep | Tolerance, physical dependence, death from overdose, especially in combination with alcohol |
| Methaqualone (e.g., Quaalude, Sopor) | Hypnotic | Depresses CNS; depresses certain polysynaptic spinal reflexes | Tolerance, physical dependence, convulsions, death |
| Meprobamate (e.g., Equanil, Miltown; "minor tranquilizers") | Antianxiety drug[2]; induces calmness | Causes decreases in REM sleep; relaxes skeletal muscle; depresses CNS | Tolerance, physical dependence; coma and death from overdose |
| Valium, Librium ("mild tranquilizers") | Reduce anxiety | May reduce rate of impulse firing in limbic system; relax skeletal muscle | Minor EEG abnormalities with chronic use; very large doses cause physical dependence |
| Phenothiazines (chlorpromazine; "major tranquilizers") | Antipsychotic; highly effective in controlling symptoms of psychotic patients | Affect levels of catecholamines in brain (block dopamine receptors, inhibit uptake of norepinephrine, dopamine, and serotonin); depress neurons in RAS and basal ganglia | Prolonged intake may result in Parkinson-like symptoms |
| Antidepressant drugs (e.g., Elavil) | Elevate mood; relieve depression | Block uptake of norepinephrine, so more is available to stimulate nervous system | Central and peripheral neurological disturbances; incoordination; interfere with normal cardiovascular function |
| Alcohol | Euphoria; relaxation; release of inhibitions | Depresses CNS; impairs vision, coordination, judgment; lengthens reaction time | Physical dependence; damage to pancreas; liver cirrhosis; possible brain damage |

Table continued on opposite page

| Name of Drug | Effect on Mood | Actions on Body | Dangers Associated with Abuse |
|---|---|---|---|
| Narcotic analgesics (e.g., morphine, heroin) | Euphoria; reduction of pain | Depress CNS; depress reflexes; constrict pupils; impair coordination; block release of substance P from pain-transmitting neurons | Tolerance; physical dependence; convulsions; death from overdose |
| Cocaine | Euphoria; excitation followed by depression | CNS stimulation followed by depression; autonomic stimulation; dilates pupils; local anesthesia; inhibits re-uptake of norepinephrine | Mental impairment; convulsions; hallucinations; unconsciousness; death from overdose |
| Amphetamines (e.g., Dexedrine) | Euphoria; stimulant; hyperactivity; "uppers," "pep pills" | Stimulate release of dopamine and norepinephrine; block re-uptake of norepinephrine and dopamine into neurons; inhibit monoamine oxidase (MAO); enhance flow of impulses in RAS: increase heart rate; raise blood pressure; dilate pupils | Tolerance; possible physical dependence; hallucinations; death from overdose |
| Caffeine | Increases mental alertness; decreases fatigue and drowsiness | Acts on cerebral cortex; relaxes smooth muscle; stimulates cardiac and skeletal muscle; increases urine volume (diuretic effect) | Very large doses stimulate centers in the medulla (may slow the heart); toxic doses may cause convulsions |
| Nicotine | Psychological effect of lessening tension | Stimulates sympathetic nervous system; combines with receptors in postsynaptic neurons of autonomic system; effect similar to that of acetylcholine, but large amounts result in blocking transmission; stimulates synthesis of lipid in arterial wall | Tolerance; physical dependence; stimulates development of atherosclerosis |
| LSD (lysergic acid diethylamide) | Overexcitation; sensory distortions; hallucinations | Alters levels of transmitters in brain (may inhibit serotonin and increase norepinephrine); potent CNS stimulator; dilates pupils sometimes unequally; increases heart rate; raises blood pressure | Irrational behavior |
| Marijuana | Euphoria | Impairs coordination; impairs depth perception and alters sense of timing; inflames eyes; causes peripheral vasodilation; exact mode of action unknown | In large doses, sensory distortions, hallucinations; evidence of lowered sperm counts and testosterone (male hormone) levels |

[1]Sedatives reduce anxiety; hypnotics induce sleep.
[2]Antianxiety drugs reduce anxiety but are less likely to cause drowsiness than the more potent sedative-hypnotics.

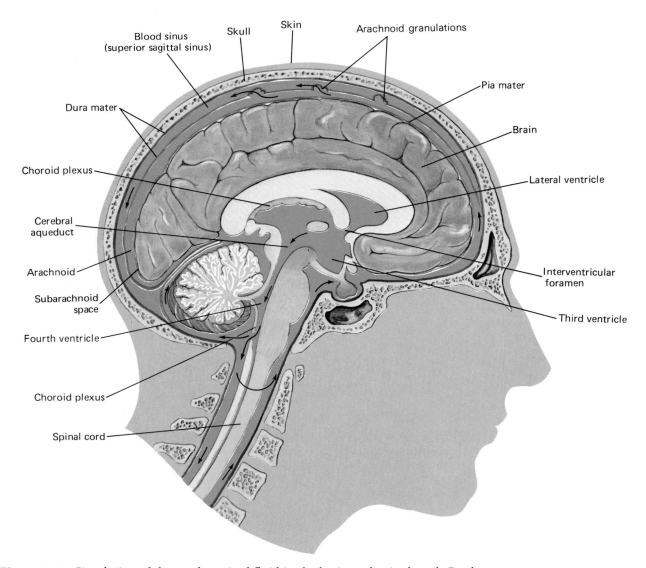

**Figure 7–15.** Circulation of the cerebrospinal fluid in the brain and spinal cord. Cerebrospinal fluid is produced by the choroid plexuses located in the ventricles. The fluid circulates through the ventricles and subarachnoid space. It is continuously produced and continuously reabsorbed into the blood of the dural sinuses through the arachnoid granulations.

A normal volume of CSF is essential to normal nervous system function. Blockage of CSF flow or abnormally rapid production can result in **hydrocephalus,** which means literally "water in the head." As CSF accumulates, the resulting pressure can cause enlargement of the skull in children and, eventually, brain damage; in severe cases, mental retardation may result. Hydrocephalus occasionally occurs in adults but is most common as a birth defect in infants and children. Surgical placement of a shunt permits excess fluid to drain into a vein in the neck region.

## SUMMARY

I. The two principal divisions of the nervous system are the central nervous system (CNS) and the peripheral nervous system (PNS).
 A. The CNS consists of the brain and spinal cord.
 B. The PNS may be divided into somatic and autonomic systems; the efferent portion of the autonomic system is divided into sympathetic and parasympathetic systems.

II. Glial cells are the supporting cells of nervous tissue; neurons transmit messages.
 A. The main structures of a neuron are the cell body, the axon, and the dendrites.
 B. Synaptic knobs at the ends of axons release neurotransmitter.
 C. Axons may be covered by both a cellular sheath and a myelin sheath; in the PNS these sheaths are produced by Schwann cells.

III. Every neural response involves a sequence of several steps.
 A. Reception—a stimulus must be received by receptors.
 B. Transmission—information must be transmitted to the CNS.
 C. Integration—information must be sorted and interpreted so that an appropriate response can be determined.
 D. Transmission—a message must be delivered from the CNS to the appropriate effectors.
 E. Actual response—the effector contracts (or secretes), producing the actual response to the stimulus.

IV. In a reflex pathway, a stimulus results in a predictable, automatic response. In a withdrawal reflex, an association neuron is interposed between a sensory neuron and a motor neuron.

V. Transmission of neural messages along a neuron is an electrochemical process.
 A. When a neuron is not conducting an impulse it has a resting potential owing in part to the action of sodium pumps.
 B. An action potential is initiated when sufficient numbers of sodium ions are allowed to diffuse into the neuron to depolarize the axon to a critical threshold level.
 C. According to the all-or-none law, an impulse cannot be transmitted unless the threshold level is reached, and any stimulus strong enough to fire the neuron either sends a message or it does not; there is no variation in the intensity of a single impulse.

VI. Transmission of an impulse from one neuron to another across a synapse generally depends on the release of neurotransmitter.
 A. Presynaptic neurons release neurotransmitter from their synaptic knobs.
 B. Molecules of neurotransmitter diffuse across the synaptic cleft and combine with receptors on postsynaptic neurons. Excess neurotransmitter may be inactivated by enzymatic action or reabsorbed into the synaptic vesicles.

VII. The surface of a postsynaptic neuron is continually exposed to excitatory and inhibitory neurotransmitters and responds by tabulating them, the process of neural integration. When sufficient excitatory neurotransmitter is present to depolarize the membrane, an impulse is transmitted.

VIII. The medulla is the lowest portion of the brain stem. It contains nerve tracts passing from the spinal cord to the brain and tracts descending from the brain to the spinal cord. The medulla contains vital centers that control respiration, heart rate, and blood pressure and centers that control reflex actions, such as swallowing, vomiting, sneezing, and coughing.

IX. The pons serves as a bridge connecting various parts of the brain and helps to regulate respiration.

X. The tectum (roof) of the midbrain consists of the corpora quadrigemina, which serve as visual and auditory reflex centers.

XI. The thalamus, part of the diencephalon, is a major relay station for impulses going to and from the cerebrum. It contains many nuclei. When sensory impulses reach the thalamus, one becomes vaguely aware of them.

XII. The hypothalamus, which is part of the diencephalon, forms the floor of the third ventricle.
 A. It serves as a link between the nervous and endocrine systems.
 B. It serves as a link between the cerebrum and the lower autonomic centers.
 C. It helps regulate temperature.
 D. It helps maintain fluid balance.
 E. It influences emotional and sexual behavior.
 F. It regulates satiety and appetite.

XIII. The cerebellum consists of two hemispheres connected by the vermis. It makes muscular movements smooth and coordinated, maintains posture, and maintains equilibrium.

XIV. The cerebrum is divided into right and left hemispheres by the longitudinal fissure. The cerebral cortex consists of gyri separated by sulci or fissures. The white matter of the cerebrum contains the basal ganglia.

    A. Each hemisphere is divided into six lobes.
        1. The frontal lobes contain the motor cortex and the premotor area, which includes Broca's speech area.
        2. The parietal lobes receive sensory information and integrate it.
        3. The occipital lobes receive and interpret visual information.
        4. The temporal lobes receive and interpret auditory information and are also involved in emotion, personality, behavior, and memory storage.
        5. The limbic lobes are concerned with olfaction and with emotional behavior; they are part of the limbic system.
        6. The insula is thought to function in autonomic and somatic activities.

    B. The functions of the cerebrum may be divided into three groups: sensory, motor, and association.

XV. Some of the types of drugs that affect the nervous system are amphetamines, barbiturates, meprobamate, phenothiazines, antidepressants, narcotic analgesics, and alcohol.

XVI. The spinal cord is continuous with the medulla and extends to the level of the second lumbar vertebra.

    A. Below the conus medullaris, the filum terminale and cauda equina extend caudally.
    B. In cross section the spinal cord reveals a central canal surrounded by gray matter and an outer portion of white matter.
    C. The spinal cord functions as a reflex control center and transmits information back and forth between the brain and the peripheral nerves.

XVII. The brain and spinal cord are protected by bone, cerebrospinal fluid, and three connective tissue coverings called meninges—dura mater, arachnoid, and pia mater.

## POST TEST

1. The CNS consists of the _____ and the _____.
2. Sense organs (receptors) and nerves belong to the _____ nervous system.
3. Sensory nerves are also called _____ nerves.
4. The supporting cells of nervous tissue are called _____ cells.
5. Cells that are specialized to transmit impulses are called _____.
6. The nucleus of a neuron is located within the _____.
7. The process of a neuron specialized to transmit impulses away from the cell body is the _____.
8. Synaptic knobs release _____.
9. A mass of cell bodies outside the CNS is termed a _____; within the CNS it is called a _____.
10. The first step in any type of neural action is _____ of a stimulus.
11. The junction between two neurons is called a _____.
12. The three types of neurons in a typical withdrawal reflex pathway are _____, _____, and _____.
13. Any stimulus that increases the permeability of the neuron to _____ may result in transmission of an impulse.
14. After an impulse has passed a particular point on the axon, that portion of the axon enters a brief _____ _____.
15. Sodium is actively transported out of the resting neuron by _____ _____.
16. The outermost of the meninges is the tough _____ _____.

17. The subarachnoid space contains _____ _____.
18. The cavities within the brain are called _____.
19. The medulla, pons, and midbrain make up the _____ _____.

*Select the most appropriate answer from column B for each item in column A. You may use an answer once, more than once, or not at all.*

| | **Column A** | | **Column B** |
|---|---|---|---|
| 20. ____ | Vital centers found here | a. | cerebrum |
| 21. ____ | Contains the corpora quadrigemina | b. | cerebellum |
| | | c. | midbrain |
| 22. ____ | Helps maintain posture and equilibrium | d. | medulla |
| 23. ____ | Controls voluntary movement | e. | pons |
| | | f. | hypothalamus |
| 24. ____ | Link between nervous and endocrine systems | g. | thalamus |

| | **Column A** | | **Column B** |
|---|---|---|---|
| 25. ____ | Contains Broca's speech area | a. | occipital lobes |
| 26. ____ | Contains auditory areas | b. | frontal lobes |
| 27. ____ | Contains visual areas | c. | temporal lobes |
| | | d. | parietal lobes |

28. Label the diagram below. Refer to Figure 7–8 for correct labels.

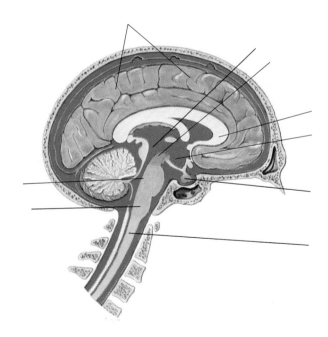

## REVIEW QUESTIONS

1. Imagine that you have just burned your finger with a match. Describe the events that occur. Draw a diagram of a withdrawal reflex pathway, label its parts, and relate the diagram to your description.
2. Give examples of reception, conduction, integration, and response.
3. Describe the transmission of an impulse along an axon.

4. How does the nervous system signal intense pain as opposed to minor pain?
5. How is neural function affected by the presence of a myelin sheath?
6. How are neural messages generally conducted from one neuron to another?
7. Suppose that a postsynaptic neuron receives both excitatory and inhibitory impulses simultaneously. How does it "decide" whether or not to fire?
8. What are the functions of the spinal cord?
9. How does the crossing of the pyramidal fibers affect neural function?
10. How do the right and left cerebral hemispheres communicate?
11. Identify the part of the brain most closely associated with each of the following functions:
    a. Regulation of body temperature
    b. Regulation of heart rate
    c. Reflex center for pupil constriction
    d. Link between nervous and endocrine systems
    e. Interpretation of language
    f. Maintenance of posture.
12. In which part of the cerebrum would you find (a) the basal ganglia (b) Broca's speech area (c) primary motor area (d) primary visual area?
13. How are EEGs used clinically?
14. What is the RAS? What does it do?
15. How does environmental experience influence brain development?
16. What structures protect the brain and spinal cord?

# The Nervous System: Peripheral Nervous System

LEARNING OBJECTIVES

**After you study this chapter you should be able to**
1. List the cranial nerves and give the functions of each.
2. Describe the structure of a typical spinal nerve and describe a plexus.
3. Summarize what is meant by segmental innervation.
4. Contrast the somatic and autonomic systems.
5. Describe the components of a reflex pathway in the autonomic system.
6. Describe the efferent pathway of the sympathetic system.
7. Compare and contrast the sympathetic with the parasympathetic system.
8. Compare the effect of sympathetic with parasympathetic stimulation on several specific organs, such as heart, digestive tract, and bronchial tubes.

The peripheral nervous system (PNS) is made up of the sense organs, the nerves that link the sense organs with the central nervous system (CNS), and the nerves that link the CNS with the effectors. That portion of the PNS that keeps the body in balance with the outside world is the somatic system, whereas the nerves and receptors that maintain internal balance make up the autonomic system.

## THE SOMATIC SYSTEM

The **somatic system** includes the sense organs that react to changes in the external world (Chapter 9), the sensory neurons that keep the CNS informed of the changes, and the motor neurons that adjust the positions of skeletal muscles to respond homeostatically to changes in the outside world. The sensory and motor neurons of the somatic system, as well as those of the autonomic system, are part of the cranial and spinal nerves.

### Cranial Nerves

Twelve pairs of nerves emerge from the brain (Fig. 8–1). These **cranial nerves** transmit information to the brain from sense receptors; bring orders from the CNS to the voluntary muscles that control movements of the eyes, face, tongue, and throat; and provide communication between the CNS and the visceral organs.

Cranial nerves are designated by Roman numerals as well as by name. The numbers indicate the sequence in which the nerves emerge from the brain. Table 8–1 lists the cranial nerves, their distributions, and functions. Some cranial nerves consist only of sensory fibers but most are mixed nerves, consisting of both sensory and motor neurons.

### Spinal Nerves

Thirty-one pairs of **spinal nerves** emerge from the spinal cord. They are all mixed nerves, transmitting sensory information to the cord through their afferent neurons and motor information from the central nervous system to the various parts of the body through their efferent neurons.

Spinal nerves are named for the general region of the vertebral column from which they originate and are numbered in sequence. There are eight pairs of cervical spinal nerves, numbered C1 to C8; 12 pairs of thoracic spinal nerves, numbered T1 to T12; five pairs of lumbar spinal nerves, numbered L1 to L5; five pairs of sacral spinal nerves, numbered S1 to S5; and one pair of coccygeal spinal nerves (Fig. 8–2). The first cervical nerve exits from the vertebral canal between the occipital bone and the atlas. The other spinal nerves exit from the vertebral column through intervertebral foramina. For example, the fourth cervical nerve passes through the intervertebral foramen between the third and fourth cervical vertebrae.

Each spinal nerve has two points of attachment with the cord. The **dorsal (posterior) root** consists of sensory (afferent) fibers that transmit information from the sensory receptors to the spinal cord (Fig. 8–3). Just before the dorsal root joins with the cord it is marked by a swelling, the **spinal ganglion**, which consists of the cell bodies of the sensory neurons. The **ventral root** consists of motor (efferent) fibers leaving the cord. Cell bodies of the motor neurons are located within the gray matter of the cord. Dorsal and ventral roots unite to form the **spinal nerve** (Fig. 8–3).

#### Branches

Just after a spinal nerve emerges from the vertebral column, it divides into four branches called **rami (ray'-me)**. The **dorsal ramus** of each nerve consists of fibers that supply the muscles and skin of the posterior portion of the body in that region. The dorsal ramus branches, giving rise to various nerves. The **ventral ramus** consists mainly of fibers that innervate the anterior and lateral body trunk in that area as well as the extremities.

#### Plexuses

Except for the branches of nerves T2 to T11, the ventral rami of the spinal nerves do not pass directly to the body structures they innervate. Instead, the ventral rami of several spinal nerves form networks called **plexuses**. Each plexus is a tangled network of fibers from all of the spinal nerves involved. Within a plexus the fibers of a spinal nerve may separate and then regroup with fibers that originated in other nerves. Thus, nerves emerging from a plexus consist of neurons that originated in several different spinal nerves. Peripheral nerves that emerge from a plexus may be named for the region of the body that they innervate. Each of these peripheral nerves may give rise to smaller nerve branches. The main plexuses are the cervical plexus, the brachial plexus, the lumbar plexus, and the sacral plexus (Fig. 8–2 and Table 8–2).

*Text continued on page 155*

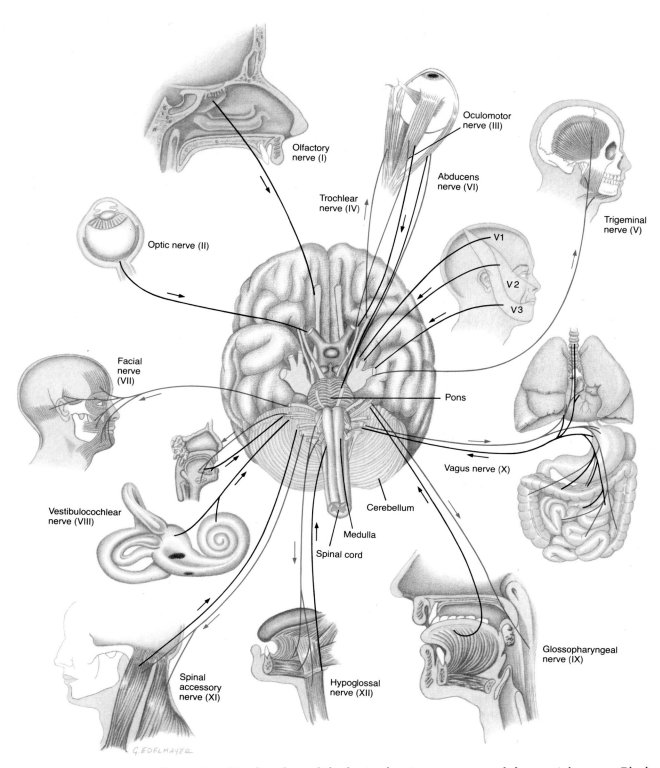

Olfactory
nerve (I)

Oculomotor
nerve (III)

Abducens
nerve (VI)

Trochlear
nerve (IV)

Trigeminal
nerve (V)

Optic nerve (II)

V1

V2

V3

Facial
nerve
(VII)

Pons

Vagus nerve (X)

Vestibulocochlear
nerve (VIII)

Cerebellum

Medulla

Spinal cord

Glossopharyngeal
nerve (IX)

Spinal
accessory
nerve (XI)

Hypoglossal
nerve (XII)

G. EDELMAYER

**Figure 8–1.** *Basal surface of the brain showing emergence of the cranial nerves. Black indicates sensory; color indicates motor fibers.*

TABLE 8–1
**The Cranial Nerves**

| Name | Function | Distribution |
|---|---|---|
| I. Olfactory | Sensory: smell | Transmit messages from olfactory mucosa to olfactory bulbs of cerebrum |
| II. Optic | Sensory: vision | Transmit messages from retina of eye to thalamus and midbrain, where they synapse with neurons that convey messages to visual areas of occipital lobes |
| III. Oculomotor | Mixed, but mainly motor: movement of eyeball and eyelid; regulation of pupil size; accommodation of lens for near vision | Midbrain to eye muscles (superior rectus, medial rectus, inferior rectus, inferior oblique) |
| | Sensory: messages regarding condition of innervated muscles | Convey messages from eye muscles to brain |
| IV. Trochlear | Mixed, but mainly motor: movement of eyeball | Midbrain to superior oblique eye muscle |
| | Sensory: messages regarding condition of innervated muscles | Superior oblique muscle to midbrain |
| V. Trigeminal | Mixed. Sensory: sensations of head and face | Face and scalp to pons |
| | Motor: chewing | Pons to muscles of mastication |
| Ophthalmic branch | Sensory | Conveys messages from upper eyelid, surface of eye, tear glands, part of nose, scalp, and forehead |
| Maxillary branch | Sensory | Conveys messages from upper teeth, upper gum, upper lip, palate, and skin of face |
| Mandibular branch | Sensory | Conveys messages from lower teeth, lower gum, lower lip, skin of jaw, and part of scalp |
| | Motor | Pons to muscles of mastication |
| VI. Abducens | Mixed, but mainly motor: eye movement | Pons to lateral rectus muscle of the eye |
| | Sensory: messages regarding condition of lateral rectus | Lateral rectus muscle to pons |
| VII. Facial | Mixed. Sensory: taste | Taste buds on tongue to medulla |
| | Motor: facial expression, secretion of saliva and tears | Pons-medulla junction to muscles of the face and scalp, and to salivary and tear glands |
| VIII. Vestibulocochlear | Sensory: hearing and equilibrium | Cochlea and semicircular canals of inner ear to pons-medulla junction |
| Vestibular branch | Equilibrium | Organs of equilibrium of inner ear to vestibular nuclei |
| Cochlear (auditory) branch | Hearing | Organ of hearing in cochlea of inner ear to medulla, then to inferior colliculi of midbrain |
| IX. Glossopharyngeal | Mixed. Sensory: taste | Taste buds in tongue to medulla; receptors in carotid arteries to medulla |
| | Motor: swallowing, saliva secretion | Medulla to muscles of pharynx; medulla to parotid salivary gland |
| X. Vagus | Mixed. Sensory: sensation from larynx, trachea, heart, and other thoracic and abdominal organs | Various organs to medulla |
| XI. Spinal accessory | Mixed, but mainly motor: movement of shoulders and head | Medulla and spinal cord to muscles of shoulder and neck; and to muscles of pharynx and larynx |
| | Sensory: messages regarding condition of innervated neck and shoulder muscles | Muscle spindles of shoulder and neck muscles to spinal cord |
| XII. Hypoglossal | Mixed, but mainly motor: tongue movement | Medulla to tongue muscles |
| | Sensory: messages regarding condition of tongue | Muscle spindles in tongue to medulla |

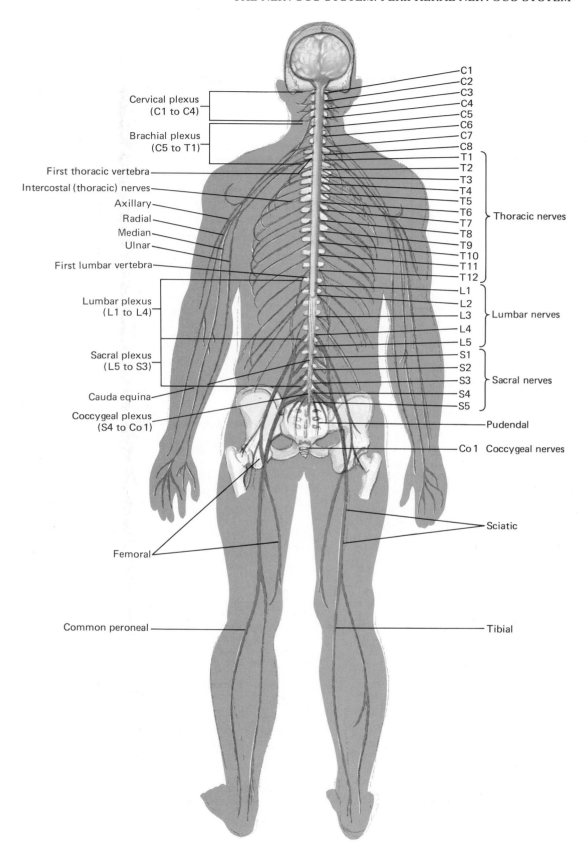

**Figure 8–2.** The spinal nerves and some of their major branches and plexuses.

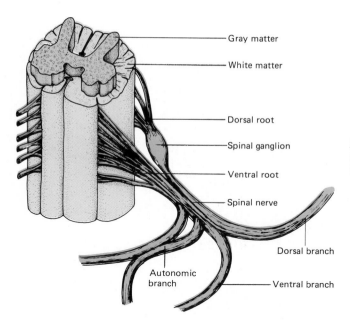

**Figure 8–3.** Dorsal (posterior) and ventral (anterior) roots merge to form a spinal nerve. The spinal nerve divides into several branches.

TABLE 8–2
**Spinal Nerves and Their Branches[1]**

| Spinal Nerve[2] | Plexus Formed | Principal Spinal Nerve Branches From Plexus | Parts of Body Supplied |
|---|---|---|---|
| C1 | | Lesser occipital | Skin over back of head |
| C2 | | Greater auricular | Skin over lower part of ear and anterior to ear |
| | Cervical plexus | | |
| C3 | | Transverse cervical | Skin over ventral part of neck |
| C4 | | Supraclavicular | Skin of shoulder and upper chest |
| | | Ansa cervicalis | Muscles of neck and shoulders |
| | | Phrenic | Diaphragm |
| | | Axillary | Shoulder; arm |
| C5 | | Musculocutaneous | Arm |
| C6 | | Median | Forearm |
| C7 | Brachial Plexus | Ulnar (crazy bone) | Forearm |
| C8 | | Radial | Arm; forearm; hand |
| T1 | | | |
| T2–T12 | None | Intercostal (thoracic) nerves | Intercostal (between ribs) and abdominal muscles |
| L1 | | Iliohypogastric | Skin and muscles of abdominal wall; skin over buttock |
| L2 | | | |
| L3 | Lumbar plexus | Ilioinguinal | Muscles of abdominal wall; skin over base of penis and scrotum |
| L4 | | Genitofemoral | Skin of thigh; base of penis and scrotum |
| | | Femoral | Skin and muscles of thigh |
| | | Obturator | Skin and muscles of thigh |
| L5 | | | |
| S1 | Sacral plexus | Sciatic | Skin and muscles of leg and foot |
| S2 | | | |
| S3 | | Pudendal | Perineal region |
| S4 | | | |
| S5 | Coccygeal plexus | Coccygeal | Sensory fibers from skin in coccygeal region |
| Co1 | | | |

[1]See Figure 8–2.
[2]C, cervical; T, thoracic; L, lumbar; S, sacral; Co, coccygeal.

## Segmental Innervation of the Body Surface

The entire body surface below the neck is innervated by the spinal nerves. The area of skin supplied by any one spinal nerve through both of its rami is called a segment, or **dermatome** (der′-mah-tome). Each dermatome is named for the principal spinal nerve that serves it. (Regions of the head are supplied by branches of the trigeminal nerve, cranial nerve V.) Fortunately, there is sufficient overlap of innervation so that if a single spinal nerve is injured the dermatome will still be supplied by nerves that serve segments on either side of it. Figure 8–4 illustrates the dermatomes on the anterior body surface. Muscles are also segmentally innervated; muscle segments are termed **myotomes**.

Knowledge of the segmental innervation of the body is useful clinically, because this information enables one to determine which nerve has been damaged. For example, if the skin of the upper thigh is stimulated and the patient does not perceive sensation, the physician will have reason to think that the L2 nerve is not functioning. When movement is affected, the physician can similarly trace the malfunction to a specific spinal nerve. On the other hand, if the level of the lesion is known, one can predict which areas of the body and which functions will be affected.

## THE AUTONOMIC SYSTEM

Whereas the somatic portion of the nervous system operates to preserve the integrity of the organism with reference to the external environment, the **autonomic system** acts to maintain a steady state within the internal environment (Table 8–3). For instance, it functions to maintain a constant body temperature and to regulate the rate of the heartbeat.

The autonomic system works automatically and without voluntary input. Its effectors are smooth cardiac muscles and glands. Like the somatic system, it is functionally organized into reflex pathways. Receptors within the viscera relay information via afferent nerves to the CNS, the information is integrated at various levels, and the "decision" is transmitted along efferent nerves to the appropriate muscles or glands. The efferent portion of the autonomic system is subdivided into sympathetic and parasympathetic systems.

Although both sympathetic and parasympathetic systems function continuously, the sympathetic system dominates during stressful times, whereas the parasympathetic system is most active

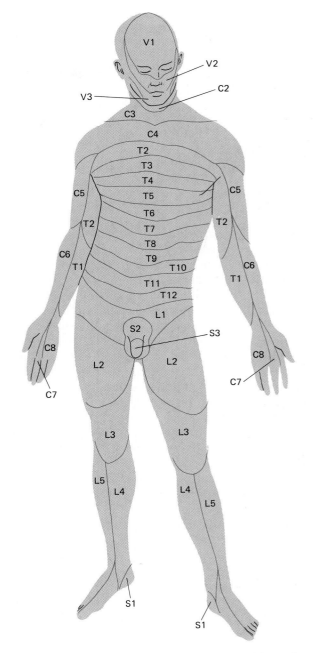

**Figure 8–4.** *Distribution of spinal nerves and branches of the trigeminal nerve to segments of the body surface. Each segment is named for the principal spinal nerve that serves it. (C, Cervical segments; T, thoracic segments; L, lumbar segments; S, sacral segments; V, trigeminal segments.) (Anatomists do not entirely agree on the designation of specific segments. This is due in part to the extensive overlap of neurons that supply them.)*

during periods of emotional calm and physical rest (Table 8–4). Thus the sympathetic system dominates when you are rushing to class or taking a test, whereas the parasympathetic system is in control after you have finished a relaxing dinner and are sitting down in front of the television set.

TABLE 8–3
**Comparison of Efferent Components of Somatic and Autonomic Nervous Systems**

|  | Somatic System | Autonomic System |
|---|---|---|
| **Structures Innervated** | Skeletal (voluntary) muscle | Smooth (involuntary) muscle, cardiac muscle, glands |
| **Effect on Effector** | Excitatory | Excitatory or inhibitory |
| **General Role** | Adjustments to external environment | Adjustments within internal environment (homeostasis) |
| **Number of Neurons from CNS to Effector** | One | Two |
| **Ganglia Outside CNS** | None | Chain ganglia, collateral ganglia, or terminal ganglia (near effector) |
| **Neurotransmitter** | Acetylcholine | Acetylcholine; norepinephrine by sympathetic postganglionic neurons |
| **Effect of Nerve Destruction on Effector** | Paralysis and atrophy | Effector remains functional but is not able to respond to changing needs of body. |

Many organs are innervated by both sympathetic and parasympathetic nerves and may be stimulated by one type of nerve and inhibited by the other. For example, sympathetic nerves increase both the rate and force of contraction of the heart, increasing its effectiveness as a pump. Parasympathetic (vagus) nerves cause the opposite effects, decreasing the heart's pumping effectiveness and allowing it some measure of rest (Fig. 8–5). The digestive system is mainly under parasympathetic control. Parasympathetic stimulation increases peristalsis (waves of muscle contraction) so that food is moved along more quickly. Sympathetic stimulation is not necessary for the normal function of the digestive system, but strong sympathetic stimulation does inhibit the movement of food through the digestive tract. Table 8–5 summarizes some autonomic effects on various organs (see also Fig. 8–6).

Instead of utilizing a single efferent neuron, as in the somatic system, the autonomic system utilizes two efferent neurons between the spinal cord and the effector. The first neuron, called the **preganglionic neuron**, has a cell body and dendrites within the CNS. Its axon, part of a peripheral nerve, ends by synapsing with a **postganglionic neuron**. The dendrites and cell body of the post-ganglionic neuron are located within a ganglion outside the CNS. Its axon terminates near or on the effector organ.

## The Sympathetic System

The **sympathetic system** is referred to as the **thoracolumbar outflow** of the spinal cord because its neurons emerge through the ventral roots of the thoracic and two upper lumbar spinal nerves. Efferent sympathetic neurons pass through the branch of each spinal nerve known as the **white rami communicantes** (called white because the preganglionic sympathetic neurons are myelinated). After passing through the white rami communicantes, these neurons pass into the ganglia of the **paravertebral sympathetic ganglion chain**. This chain is a series of ganglia located along the length of the vertebral column (Figs. 8–6 and 8–7). Most of the preganglionic neurons end within the ganglia and synapse there with postganglionic efferent neurons.

Axons of some of the postganglionic neurons leave the ganglion as various sympathetic nerves and as plexuses around major blood vessels. They innervate blood vessels and organs in the head,

TABLE 8–4
**Comparison of Sympathetic with Parasympathetic System**

|  | Sympathetic System | Parasympathetic System |
|---|---|---|
| **General Effect** | Mobilization of energy (especially during stress situations) | Conservation and restoration of energy |
| **Extent of Effect** | Widespread throughout body | Localized |
| **Neurotransmitter Released at Synapse with Effector** | Norepinephrine (usually) | Acetylcholine |
| **Duration of Effect** | Lasting | Brief |
| **Outflow from CNS** | Thoracolumbar levels | Craniosacral levels |
| **Location of Ganglia** | Chain and collateral ganglia | Terminal ganglia |
| **Number of Postganglionic Fibers with Which Each Preganglionic Fiber Synapses** | Many | Few |

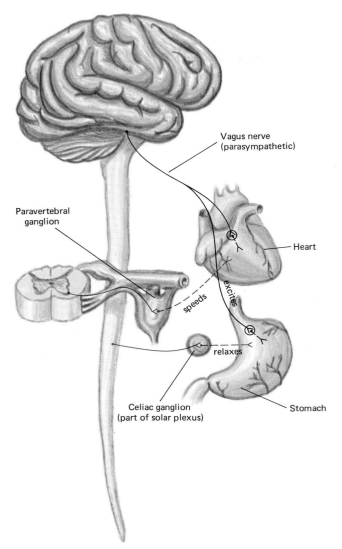

neck, and thoracic region. Axons of other postganglionic neurons reenter the spinal nerves by way of the **gray rami communicantes** (called gray because the postganglionic fibers are not myelinated). These fibers travel with the other fibers of the spinal nerve and eventually branch off to innervate smooth muscle and sweat glands (Fig. 8–7).

Some preganglionic neurons do not end in the ganglia of the paravertebral chain but instead pass on to ganglia located in the abdomen close to the aorta (the largest artery in the body) and its major branches. These ganglia are collectively known as **collateral ganglia** and are individually named after the blood vessels with which they are associated. (The celiac ganglia and the nerves associated with them are called the **solar plexus.**) Postganglionic neurons from the collateral ganglia innervate smooth muscles and glands of the abdominal and pelvic viscera and their blood vessels. These include organs of the digestive, urinary, and reproductive systems.

Preganglionic sympathetic neurons are referred to as cholinergic fibers because they secrete acetylcholine as a neurotransmitter. Most sympathetic postganglionic neurons release norepinephrine as the neurotransmitter at the effector synapse; these are known as adrenergic fibers.

## The Parasympathetic System

Because they emerge from the brain (as part of cranial nerves) and from the sacral region of the spinal cord, neurons of the **parasympathetic system** are referred to as the **craniosacral outflow**. About 75% of all parasympathetic fibers are in the vagus nerves.

**Figure 8–5.** Dual innervation of the heart and stomach by sympathetic and parasympathetic nerves. Sympathetic nerves are shown in red. Postganglionic fibers are shown as dotted lines.

TABLE 8–5
**Comparison of Sympathetic and Parasympathetic Actions on Selected Effectors[1]**

| Effector | Sympathetic Action | Parasympathetic Action |
| --- | --- | --- |
| Heart | Increases rate and strength of contraction | Decreases rate; no direct effect on strength of contraction |
| Bronchial tubes | Dilates | Constricts |
| Iris of eye | Dilates (pupil becomes larger) | Constricts (pupil becomes smaller) |
| Sex organs | Constricts blood vessels; ejaculation | Dilates blood vessels; erection |
| Blood vessels | Generally constricts | No innervation for many |
| Sweat glands | Stimulates | No innervation |
| Intestine | Inhibits motility | Stimulates motility and secretion |
| Liver metabolism | Stimulates glycogen breakdown | No effect |
| Adipose tissue | Stimulates free fatty acid release from fat cells | No effect |
| Adrenal medulla | Stimulates secretion of epinephrine and norepinephrine | No effect |
| Salivary glands | Stimulates thick, viscous secretion | Stimulates profuse, watery secretion |

[1]Refer to Figure 8–6 as you study this table. Note that many other examples could be added to this list.

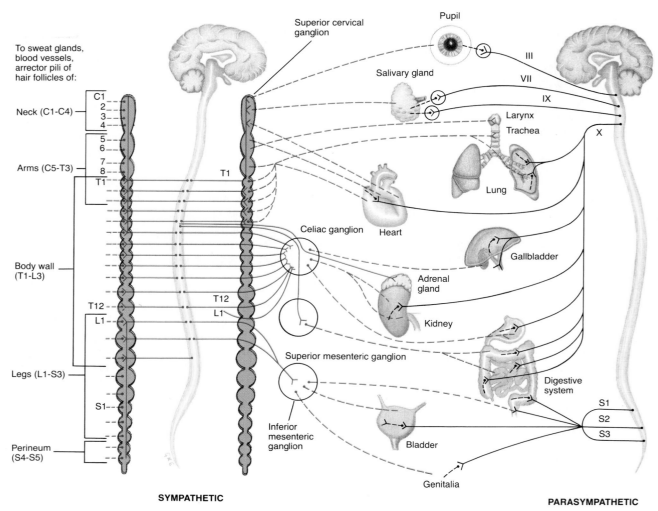

***Figure 8–6.*** *Sympathetic and parasympathetic nervous systems. For clarity, peripheral and visceral nerves of the sympathetic system are shown on separate sides of the cord. Complex as it appears, this diagram has been greatly simplified. (Colored lines represent sympathetic nerves, black lines represent parasympathetic nerves, and dotted lines represent postganglionic nerves.)*

Preganglionic fibers synapse with postganglionic neurons in **terminal ganglia** located near or within the walls of the organs that they innervate. Neurons from the cranial region innervate the eye, structures of the head, and thoracic and abdominal viscera. Branches of the vagus innervate the heart, lungs, liver, pancreas, esophagus, stomach, small intestine, and upper portion of the large intestine. The sacral parasympathetic fibers form the pelvic nerves; they innervate the lower portion of the large intestine, urinary system, and reproductive system. The parasympathetic nerves do not innervate the blood vessels or sweat glands.

In the parasympathetic system, both preganglionic and postganglionic fibers release the neurotransmitter acetylcholine. For this reason the parasympathetic system is known as a **cholinergic**

**system** and its postganglionic fibers are referred to as cholinergic fibers.

## Alpha and Beta Receptors

There are two main types of adrenergic receptors, **alpha receptors** and **beta receptors**, on the cell membranes of effector cells. Norepinephrine has a more pronounced effect on the alpha receptors, whereas epinephrine (released by the adrenal glands) activates both types of receptors equally. Stimulation of alpha receptors causes vasoconstriction (narrowing) of blood vessels, whereas beta receptor stimulation causes dilation of blood vessels. Stimulation of either alpha or beta receptors, however, causes relaxation of the intestine.

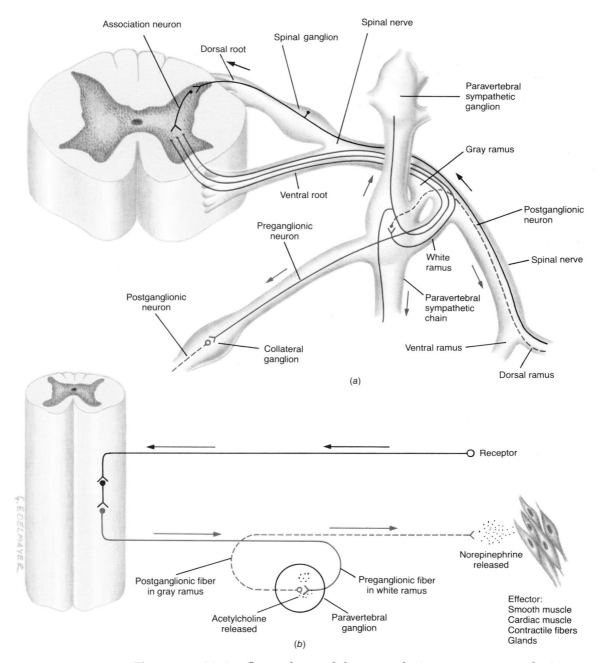

**Figure 8–7.** (a) A reflex pathway of the sympathetic nervous system. (b) Diagrammatic representation of the sympathetic reflex pathway. Dark line represents afferent component, solid colored line represents preganglionic efferent component, and dotted colored line represents postganglionic efferent component in both parts of the figure.

An understanding of the different types of receptors is important clinically because certain drugs are used to stimulate or to block certain types of receptors. For example, the bronchial constriction that occurs in asthma can be countered by stimulation of beta receptors of the bronchial smooth muscle using such drugs as theophyllin or caffeine. (See Focus on Pharmacology of the Autonomic System.)

## FOCUS ON
## Pharmacology of the Autonomic System

| Drug | Mode of Action | Clinical Uses |
|------|----------------|---------------|
| *Sympathomimetic Drugs* | | |
| Also called adrenergic drugs. These stimulate physiological responses similar to those produced by the sympathetic adrenergic nerves and mimic the action of norepinephrine. | | |
| Epinephrine | Acts directly on both alpha and beta receptors | Used in asthma and other allergic diseases; stimulates relaxation of constricted respiratory passageways and reduction of swelling |
| Isoproterenol | Acts directly on beta receptors | Drug of choice in cardiac resuscitation |
| Phenylephrine (Neo-synephrine) | Acts directly on alpha receptors; constricts small blood vessels in lining of nose, thus relieving nasal congestion | Used as a decongestant |
| Ephedrine | Causes release of norepinephrine from synaptic vesicles | Ephedrine and epinephrine were the original adrenergic drugs; many of the drugs currently in use for treating asthma and other allergic disorders, and used to stimulate the heart, are derivatives of ephedrine |

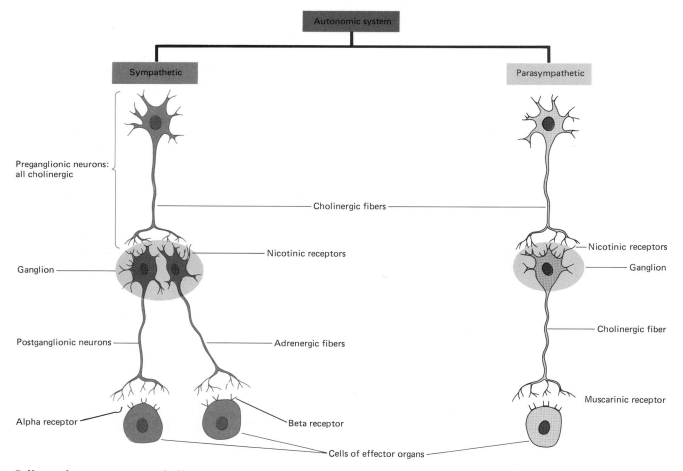

*Cell membrane receptors of effector cells of the autonomic system.*

| Drug | Mode of Action | Clinical Uses |
|------|----------------|---------------|
| *Sympathomimetic Drugs Continued* | | |
| Amphetamine | Causes accumulation of norepinephrine in synaptic clefts | No longer in widespread clinical use; sometimes used to treat narcolepsy and hyperkinetic symptoms in children |
| *Adrenergic Blocking Drugs* | | |
| Reserpine | Blocks synthesis and storage of norepinephrine | Used in management of some types of hypertension (high blood pressure); used in some psychotic patients unable to tolerate phenothiazines |
| Propranolol (e.g., Inderal) | Blocks beta receptors | Used to relieve pain in angina (a heart disease discussed in Chapter 12); by decreasing sympathetic stimulation it reduces heart rate and strength of contractions; useful in controlling some tremors and preventing migraine headaches |

*Cholinomimetic Drugs*

Also called parasympathomimetic drugs. These drugs stimulate physiological responses similar to those produced by acetylcholine or activation of the parasympathetic system. Acetylcholine activates two types of cholinergic receptors (see figure) in the cell membranes of effector cells. **Muscarinic receptors** were so named because they are activated by muscarine, a poison found in toadstools. Muscarinic receptors are present in all effector cells stimulated by postganglionic parasympathetic neurons and also in those stimulated by postganglionic sympathetic neurons that release acetylcholine. Nicotine, a poisonous drug obtained from tobacco, activates the **nicotinic receptors** but not the muscarinic. Nicotinic receptors are found on the postganglionic neurons of both sympathetic and parasympathetic systems, as well as in the cell membranes of skeletal muscle fibers. (Many of the effects of tobacco use on the body can be explained by the effects of nicotine on the autonomic system.)

| | | |
|------|----------------|---------------|
| Pilocarpine | Acts directly on the muscarinic receptors | Used in ophthalmology to constrict iris of the eye |

*Cholinergic Blocking Drugs*

Also called anticholinergic drugs.

| | | |
|------|----------------|---------------|
| Atropine | Blocks action of acetylcholine on muscarinic receptors of cholinergic effector cells | Used to prepare patients for surgical anesthesia; inhibits salivary, nasal, and bronchial secretions that might block respiratory passages; used in treatment of poisoning with anticholinesterase agents, e.g., nerve gases or organophosphate pesticides |
| Scopolamine | Blocks action of acetylcholine on muscarinic receptors of cholinergic effector cells | In low oral doses used as a remedy for motion sickness; in obstetrics, used to promote drowsiness with amnesia (twilight sleep) during labor |

## SUMMARY

I. The somatic system is the part of the PNS that keeps the body in adjustment with the external environment. It consists of sensory receptors and nerves.

II. Twelve pairs of cranial nerves link the brain with many sensory receptors and effectors. Table 8–1 summarizes the cranial nerves.

III. Thirty-one pairs of spinal nerves link the spinal cord with sensory receptors and effectors. Table 8–2 summarizes the spinal nerves.

A. Each spinal nerve has a dorsal root consisting of sensory fibers and a ventral root consisting of motor fibers. Within the intervertebral foramen, the roots unite to form a spinal nerve.

B. Each spinal nerve divides to form four

branches. The dorsal ramus supplies the skin and muscles of the dorsal part of the body; the ventral ramus supplies the ventral and lateral body trunk; the gray rami communicantes consist of sympathetic fibers.

 C. The ventral rami of several spinal nerves may join to form a plexus. The principal plexuses are the cervical, brachial, lumbar, and sacral.

 D. The area of skin supplied by a spinal nerve is a dermatome; the area of muscle innervated by a spinal nerve is a myotome.

IV. The autonomic system of the PNS works to maintain a steady state within the internal environment.

 A. Afferent fibers of the autonomic system run through cranial and spinal nerves along with somatic fibers.

 B. The efferent portion of the autonomic system is divided into sympathetic and parasympathetic systems; their neurons also are components of certain spinal and cranial nerves.

 C. The sympathetic system emerges from the spinal cord at the thoracic and lumbar regions.

  1. The sympathetic system regulates activities that mobilize energy and is especially important when the body is under stress.

  2. A typical sympathetic pathway might consist of the following: a preganglionic fiber emerges from the cord, passes through the white ramus communicans, and ends in a sympathetic chain ganglion. A postganglionic fiber then passes through a gray ramus communicans and reenters a spinal nerve. Eventually this fiber branches off, forming a visceral nerve that innervates smooth muscle or sweat glands.

  3. Preganglionic fibers release acetylcholine; most sympathetic postganglionic neurons release norepinephrine.

 D. The parasympathetic system consists of nerves that emerge from the brain and from the sacral region of the spinal cord.

  1. The parasympathetic system acts to restore energy and is dominant during periods of relaxation.

  2. Parasympathetic preganglionic fibers synapse with postganglionic fibers in terminal ganglia located near or within the walls of the organs they innervate.

  3. Both preganglionic and postganglionic fibers release acetylcholine.

 E. Acetylcholine activates muscarinic and nicotinic receptors. There are two types of adrenergic receptors—alpha and beta.

 F. Many organs are innervated by both sympathetic and parasympathetic nerves, for example, the heart is stimulated by sympathetic nerves and its pumping effectiveness is decreased by parasympathetic (vagus) nerves.

## POST TEST

1. The part of the PNS that keeps the body in adjustment with the external environment is the _____ system.
2. The second cranial nerve is the _____ nerve; the tenth cranial nerve is the _____ nerve.
3. The cranial nerve that innervates the muscles of facial expression is cranial nerve (number) _____, the _____ nerve.
4. Axons of the _____ nerve pass through the cribriform plate and terminate in the _____ _____.
5. The vestibulocochlear nerve transmits sensory information from the _____ _____ and from the _____.
6. There are _____ pairs of cervical spinal nerves and _____ pairs of thoracic spinal nerves.
7. The dorsal root of a spinal nerve consists of _____ _____.
8. The ventral rami of several spinal nerves may interconnect to form a _____.
9. The segment of skin supplied by a spinal nerve is called a _____.
10. The portion of the PNS that functions to maintain a steady state within the internal environment is the _____ system.

11. The paravertebral ganglion chain consists of cell bodies of _____ neurons.
12. Preganglionic sympathetic and parasympathetic neurons secrete the neurotransmitter _____.
13. Most postganglionic sympathetic neurons release _____.
14. The rate and force of contraction of the heart are increased by its _____ nerves.
15. The digestive system is stimulated by _____ nerves.
16. Label the diagram below.

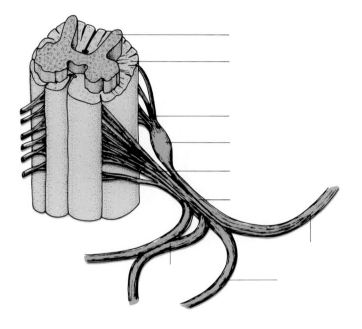

## REVIEW QUESTIONS

1. Contrast the somatic and autonomic nervous systems.
2. List the cranial nerves and their principal functions.
3. Identify the cell bodies found in each of the following: (a) paravertebral chain ganglion (b) collateral ganglion (c) terminal ganglion.
4. Identify the neurotransmitter released by (a) preganglionic autonomic fibers (b) postganglionic sympathetic neurons (c) postganglionic parasympathetic neurons.
5. Give several examples of how the sympathetic and parasympathetic systems work together to maintain homeostasis.
6. How might it be clinically important to know about the various types of receptors (for example, muscarinic, alpha, and beta) of the autonomic system and their effectors?

# Sense Organs

LEARNING OBJECTIVES

**After you study this chapter you should be able to**
1. Describe the structures and functions of the eye.
2. Give the functions of the rods and cones.
3. Describe the physiology of vision, including accommodation.
4. Describe the structures and functions of the three major parts of the ear.
5. Trace the transmission of sound through the ear.
6. Describe the receptors of taste and smell.
7. Describe tactile sensation and proprioception.

The sense organs maintain contact with the environment around us, establishing a sense of awareness that enriches our existence and that protects us from potentially dangerous situations. Traditionally the senses have been referred to as sight, hearing, taste, smell, and touch. In addition to these five senses, the body has many internal sensors that maintain homeostatic balance. As an example, certain blood vessels have receptors that maintain a normal balance of oxygen and carbon dioxide. Thus, how we respond to changes in our environment depends not only on our **exteroceptors** (ek″-stur-oh-**sep′**-tors) that sense changes in the outside world (cold versus hot, bitterness versus sweetness, pain versus pleasure, and so on), but also on the intricate internal operations of our **interoceptors** (in″-tur-oh-**sep′**-tors) that sense changes inside the body. To help us maintain balance and body position, we have interoceptors called **proprioceptors** (pro″-pree-oh-**sep′**-tors) (see Proprioception below).

# THE EYE

We live in a visual world that gives us a great deal of input about our environment. We see and interpret the images transmitted to the brain. The eye, an extremely delicate organ, is protected by its position in the body and by accessory structures. The eye and its musculature are set in the **orbit** formed by the skeletal bones of the face and are cushioned by layers of fat. The eyelashes and eyelids help to protect the eye anteriorly from foreign objects. The lids reflexively close if danger is perceived and frequent blinking lubricates and clears debris. Even though we are not aware of the process, tears flow at all times from the **lacrimal** (**lak′**-rih-mal) **glands**. They pass out through the **lacrimal ducts** to keep the eye moist and free from dust and minute objects.

Six extrinsic muscles extend from the bony structure of the orbit to the covering of the eyeball. These muscles work in a coordinated, precise fashion, enabling the two eyes to move together and focus on a single object in the visual field.

The eyeball is formed by three layers of tissue: the fibrous sclera and cornea, the vascular choroid layer, and the retina. A lens, ciliary muscle, iris, and inner fluid-filled cavities make up the remainder of the structure. The **sclera** (**sklay′**-rah), the white of the eye, is opaque and white. It is a tough, fibrous tissue, generously supplied with nerve endings. It covers the entire eyeball except the anterior colored portion. The sclera joins the **cornea** (**kor′**-nee-ah), the transparent layer that covers the iris and the pupil at the front of the eye. The cornea is frequently referred to as the window of the eye. The sclera is covered by the **conjunctiva** (kon-junk-**tie′**-vah), a moist mucous membrane that extends as a continuous lining of the inner layer of the eyelids.

The **choroid** (**ko′**-royd) layer is made of black pigment cells that absorb light rays so that they are not reflected back out of the eye. Blood vessels of the choroid nourish the retina.

The **iris**, the colored part of the eye, appears as blue, green, or brown. Its color is determined by the amount of pigment present. Composed of smooth muscle tissue, the iris regulates the amount of light entering the eye. The black spot, or opening in the center of the circular muscles of the iris, is the **pupil** of the eye. When the eye is stimulated by bright light, the circular muscle of the iris contracts, decreasing the size of the pupil. In dim light the iris increases the size of the pupil. Certain medications and levels of consciousness may also affect the size of the pupil.

The **lens** of the eye lies at the rear of the anterior cavity of the eyeball (Fig. 9–1). This cavity is filled with **aqueous humor**, a watery fluid, which helps to maintain an appropriate pressure within the eye. The lens is a clear, crystalline body that refracts (bends) light so that it can be focused on the retina. The lens is attached by tiny fibers, the **suspensory ligaments**, to the **ciliary muscle**.

Directly behind the lens is the posterior cavity of the eyeball, which contains a jellylike substance, the **vitreous humor**. The vitreous humor helps to maintain the ball-like shape of the eye and also aids in refracting images.

## Retina

The vitreous humor abuts the **retina** (**ret′**-ih-nah), the innermost layer of the eye. The retina contains specialized sensory cells, the **rods** and **cones**, that transmit signals through the retina to the optic nerve fibers. Because of these specialized microscopic cells the retina is the light-sensitive area of the eye. The cones are primarily responsible for color vision and vision during the daytime; the rods are mainly responsible for vision in dim light or darkness. Cones are most concentrated in the **fovea** (**foe′**-vee-ah), a small depression in the center of the posterior portion of the retina. The fovea is the region of sharpest vision.

The image of the object is carried from the retina to the brain through the **optic nerve** (cranial nerve II). The optic nerve is formed by the union of individual axons of sensory neurons of the retina. In

***Figure 9–1.*** *Structure of the eye. The eye has been partly dissected to show internal structure.*

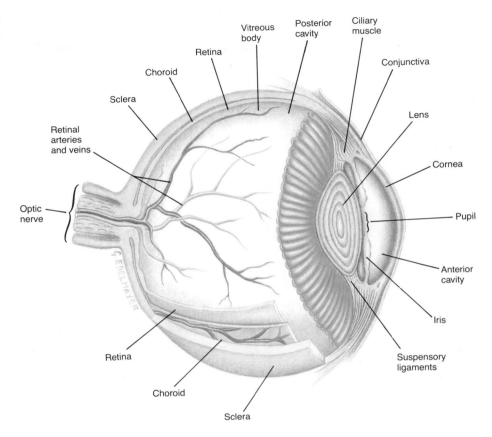

the area where the optic nerve forms there are no rods or cones. This area is known as the **optic disk**, or blind spot. Impulses of touch, pain, and temperature from the eye are transmitted to the brain by the trigeminal nerve (cranial nerve V).

## The Eye Compared to a Camera

The eye can be compared to a camera in many ways. It has an adjustable lens and a variable aperture system (pupil). The retina can be compared to the light-sensitive film used in a camera. Because of the ability of the eye to accommodate to different distances, the image is clearly focused on the retina unless there is some error in accommodation. The choroid layer absorbs light rays like the interior dark surface of a camera.

## The Physiology of Vision

For vision to occur light must pass through the eye and form an image on the retina. Light passes through the transparent cornea, the aqueous humor, the lens, and the vitreous body before reaching the retina. After an image is formed on the retina, nerve impulses must be transmitted to the visual areas of the cerebral cortex. Several processes are involved in focusing light rays on the retina. They include refraction (bending) of light rays by the cornea and lens, accommodation of the lens (see below), adjustment of the size of the pupil, and positioning the two eyeballs so that they are both directed toward the object. Positioning the eyeballs is the function of the six extrinsic eye muscles that control the movement of each eye.

The shape of the lens must be adjusted as we shift our focus on an object near or far from our position of viewing. Thus, the lens must be elastic so that the ciliary muscles can control its shape as we change our focus on objects. **Accommodation** is an automatic process in which the curvature of the lens is increased to permit focusing on close objects (Fig. 9–2). As we grow older the lens loses some of its elasticity and can no longer adjust to bring objects into focus. This age-related change is called **presbyopia** (prez-bi-**oh'**-pee-ah).

# FOCUS ON
## Cataract, A Case Study

As Mrs. West neared her seventy-third birthday she noticed that she had major visual changes with some cloudiness and some difficulty adjusting to images. When she looked at lights at night she saw circles and spectacular shapes around the point of brightness. Her crystal chandelier was a mass of colored prisms. This change in vision began to hamper her treasured independence. Finally, she asked her daughter to take her to the ophthalmologist to have her eyes checked. Much to her surprise she had a well-formed cataract in her right eye and the beginning of one in her left eye. Mrs. West and her physician discussed whether she wanted to go into the hospital for a 36-hour stay or have the surgery at a 1-day facility.

Her physician usually performed the surgical procedure called an *intracapsular extraction*. The entire lens is removed, including the capsule and its gelatinlike contents, through an incision made along the top edge of the cornea of the eye. The lens is emulsified with an instrument that works ultrasonically (see figure *a*) and is then aspirated from the eye. A transplant may be inserted at this point (see figure *b*). The incision is closed with minute sutures that do not have to be removed. It takes up to 3 months for the eye to heal completely.

After surgery, Mrs. West arrived home to carry on her usual activities. She was able to see well after the lens transplant with regular glasses for reading. As the cataract in the left eye progresses, the ophthalmologist will keep a check on the visual acuity and at the appropriate time Mrs. West will have surgery on that eye performed.

Many ophthalmologists today use intraocular lens implants as the most effective way to restore normal vision. Another alternative for Mrs. West was contact lenses. The hard lens is sometimes difficult for the elderly to handle on a daily basis. The extended wear soft lens is preferable but is not suitable for all people.

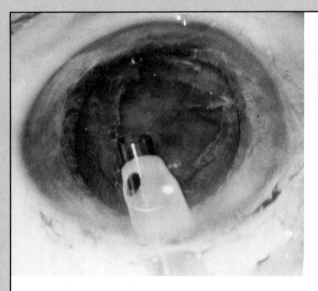 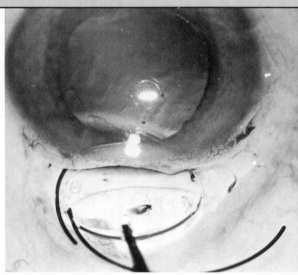

(a) *Ultrasonic emulsifying tip in operation. Instrument has been inserted under cornea through a 3-mm incision and is ultrasonically emulsifying the lens. (b) Implanting a posterior chamber intraocular lens. Lens is being slid underneath the cornea.*

*Haptics (dark half circles) hold intraocular lens in place within the eye. (Both photos by David A. Silva; courtesy of Wills Eye Hospital, Philadelphia, PA.)*

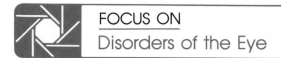

## FOCUS ON
## Disorders of the Eye

**Cataract:** an opaque area of the lens resulting in partial or total blindness; frequently seen in the elderly

**Glaucoma:** an increase in intraocular pressure due to a blockage of the aqueous humor between the lens and the root of the iris; may lead to blindness if untreated

**Emmetropia:** normal refraction of an image focusing directly on the retina

**Hyperopia:** focus of the image behind the retina; the eyeball may be short or the refractive power of the lens is weak; also called *farsightedness*

**Myopia:** focus of the image falls in front of the retina; only near objects can be seen clearly; also called *nearsightedness*

**Presbyopia:** decrease in accommodation power owing to loss of elasticity of the lens

**Strabismus:** one eye is not able to focus in synchrony with the other; one eye may deviate outward or toward the nose

**Astigmatism:** imperfection of the curvature of the cornea that causes faulty vision due to separate light rays not focusing on a single point

**Conjunctivitis:** inflammation of the conjunctiva

## THE EAR

As small children we learned to identify our facial structures, the eye, nose, mouth, and ear, but little did we know that these were only a part of the total organs. The external portion of the ear is viewed as an appendage on the head but the portion of the sense organ dealing with hearing and equilibrium lies internally hidden from sight. The ear actually has three parts.

1. The external ear includes the part we see and a canal connecting with the middle ear.
2. The middle ear contains three small bones that conduct sound waves.
3. The inner ear contains sensory receptors for sound waves and for maintaining the equilibrium of the body (Fig. 9–3).

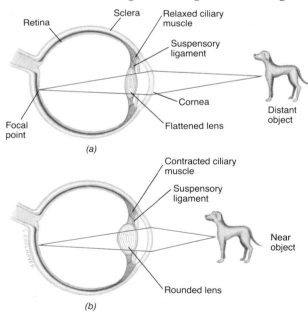

**Figure 9–2.** *Accommodation. How the lens changes in distant and near vision. (a) Relaxation of the ciliary muscles causes the suspensory ligament to draw the lens into a flattened shape suitable for distant vision. (b) Contraction of the ciliary muscle relieves the tension on the suspensory ligaments, allowing the lens to shorten and thicken for greater focusing power in near vision.*

### External Ear

The **pinna** (**pin′**-ah), the part of the ear that projects from the side of the head, primarily functions to collect sound waves and funnel them into the canal. This structure is composed mainly of cartilage and fat (which give individual shape to our ears) and is covered with skin that continues into the ear canal. This canal, known as the **external auditory meatus** (mee-**ay′**-tus), leads to the middle ear. In the lining of the canal are **ceruminous** (se-**roo′**-mih-nus) **glands**, which secrete a cerumen (earwax). Cerumen helps protect the epithelial lining of the canal from infection.

Separating the middle and external ear is a membrane, the **tympanic** (tim-**pan′**-ik) **membrane**, or eardrum. This flexible membrane vibrates as incoming sound waves move through the canal, transmitting the waves to the middle ear. Under normal circumstances the air pressure is equalized on the two sides of the tympanic membrane by the **eustachian** (u-**stay′**-kee-an) **tube**. This tube connects the middle ear and the external environment through the throat. Bacteria in the throat can pass

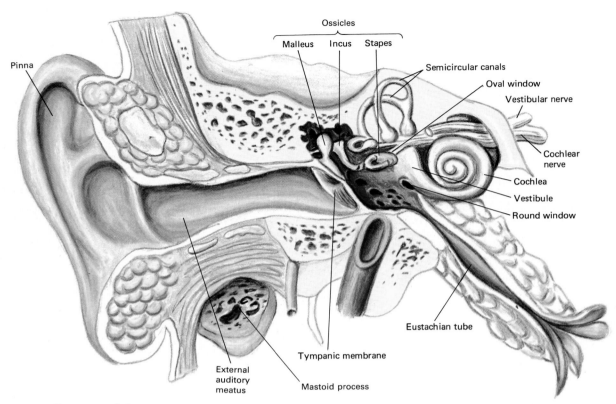

***Figure 9–3.*** *Structure of the ear.*

through the eustachian tube, leading to painful middle ear infection with swelling of the tympanic membrane.

## Middle Ear

The **middle ear** is a small moist cavity in the temporal bone containing air and three small **ossicles** (bones). At the rear of the cavity the middle ear opens into the mastoid process of the temporal bone. This area is filled with air spaces, which communicate with the middle ear and help equalize pressure. The three ossicles, **malleus**, **incus**, and **stapes**, are a chain of small bones that are attached from the tympanic membrane, to one another, and to the **oval window**, a small opening leading from the middle to the inner ear. Sound waves are amplified by vibrations of the ossicles during conduction from the tympanic membrane to the inner ear, where they are converted to nerve impulses.

## Inner Ear

The most important part of the ear, the **inner ear**, contains the mechanism for converting sound

waves to nerve impulses for transmission to the brain and also sends impulses to the brain that enable us to maintain our equilibrium. This inner structure inside the temporal bone is a **bony labyrinth** (**lab′**-ih-rinth) composed of the **vestibule** (which lies next to the oval window), the **cochlea** (**kok′**-lee-ah), and the vestibular apparatus. The bony labyrinth contains a fluid known as **perilymph**. The perilymph surrounds the **membranous labyrinth**, a group of ducts and sacs that lie within the bony labyrinth. The membranous labyrinth contains a fluid called **endolymph**. The two fluids are separated anatomically and have different chemical compositions but both carry vibrations through the system of canals within the inner ear.

The cochlea is a snail-shaped portion of the inner ear that contains the **organ of Corti**, the sound receptor. Within the organ of Corti are sensitive **hair cells**, which respond to sound waves by stimulating the **cochlear nerve**. The cochlear nerve then transmits the message to the brain.

## The Physiology of Hearing

We can summarize the steps in the physiology of hearing as follows. Sound waves enter the external auditory meatus, stimulating vibration of the tympanic membrane. These waves, in turn, stimulate the ossicles, which amplify the intensity of the sound waves. These vibrations are conducted through the perilymph to the endolymph inside the membranous portion of the inner ear. Vibrations of the endolymph stimulate the hair cells in the cochlea. Movement of the hair cells leads to transmission of neural impulses by the cochlear nerve to the brain.

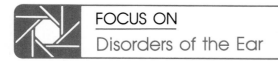

## FOCUS ON
## Disorders of the Ear

**Otitis media:** inflammation (usually infection) of the middle ear
**Otitis externa:** inflammation of the external ear canal
**Myringotomy:** small incision in the tympanic membrane to relieve pressure from infection in middle ear
**Presbycusis:** loss of the ability to discern high-pitched sounds in the elderly

**Otosclerosis:** changes in the composition of the bones in the middle ear, immobilizing the stapes and causing reduction in the transmission of sound waves
**Conduction deafness:** interference of the transmission of sound waves resulting from damage to ossicles or the tympanic membrane
**Nerve deafness:** due to damage of the cochlear nerve

## Equilibrium

The **vestibular** (ves-tib'-u-lar) **apparatus** detects sensations regarding body position and equilibrium. It includes the three semicircular canals and two small chambers, the saccule and utricle, which connect them to the vestibule. Within the vestibular apparatus are sensory hair cells that transmit information about the position of the body, mainly the head. The response of the hair cells is produced by the flow of endolymph within the semicircular canals as the position of one's head is changed. These responses in turn are transmitted to the vestibular nerve, which joins the cochlear nerve to form the vestibulocochlear nerve (cranial nerve VIII).

## TASTE

The sense of taste is perceived through the **taste buds** on the tongue and in various parts of the mouth. There are an average of 10,000 taste buds in the normal adult mouth. As an individual gets older the number of taste buds gradually decreases. It is of interest to note that taste buds respond only if the material to be tasted is in solution. The taste buds are able to discriminate among four primary tastes: sweet, sour, salty, and bitter (Fig. 9–4). However, they are not nerve structures and are constantly being replaced by new cells. Both the facial (cranial nerve VII) and the glossopharyngeal (cranial nerve IX) nerves transmit the sensory input to the brain.

## SMELL

**Olfactory** information is transmitted by receptor cells in the olfactory epithelium at the upper part of the nasal cavity (Fig. 9–5). In contrast to the taste buds, it is estimated that the olfactory epithelium may be able to discriminate among as many as 50 different smells. The smells discerned by the olfactory epithelium are transmitted to the olfactory center in the brain through the olfactory nerve (cranial nerve I). Olfactory cells are not replaced as are taste buds, therefore when they are damaged, our sense of smell is impaired. Both smell and taste are important in stimulating appetite and digestive juices. A bad head cold will decrease appetite, as the efficiency of the receptors is diminished because of inflammation.

## TACTILE SENSATION

There are several types of similar receptors referred to as *tactile receptors* that respond to pressure, touch, and vibration. They are located in various layers of the skin, in the fingertips and toes, and in the tip of the tongue. The **pacinian corpuscle** is the largest and most widely studied in regard to neural response and adaptability.

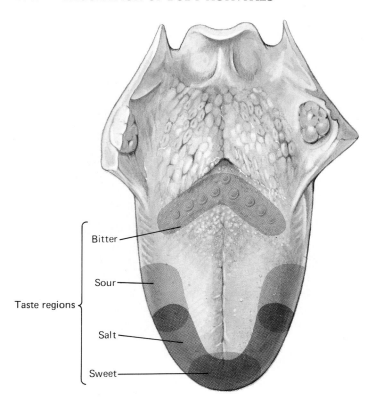

Taste regions {
Bitter
Sour
Salt
Sweet

*Figure 9–4. The sense of taste. Taste buds are most numerous on the tongue. Certain regions of the tongue respond more strongly than other regions to specific tastes.*

## PAIN

Pain is discussed in Chapter 7. However, it is worth noting here that pain is a sensory mechanism that is protective for the body. *Pain receptors* are sensory nerve endings found in the skin and certain internal tissues. An interesting feature in experiencing pain is that it may be felt in an area considerably distant from the primary area of pain. Because pain is frequently not a self-limiting sensation, it warns the body to attend to its source of stimulation.

## PROPRIOCEPTION

**Proprioception**, or position sense, helps us maintain the position of the body and its parts. The receptors performing this function are widely spread sensory organs known as **proprioceptors**. They are located within muscles, tendons, and joints. The brain coordinates the information from the proprioceptors with the information from the vestibular apparatus in the inner ear to maintain equilibrium and coordination of muscular activities. Signals are carried rapidly to the brain so that the central nervous system is aware of the location of the different parts of the body at all times.

## SUMMARY

   I. Through the sense organs we maintain contact with the environment, helping us to maintain a state of homeostasis.
  II. Sense organs are either exteroceptors or interoceptors. Proprioceptors are a form of interoceptor.
 III. The structure of the eye enables us to focus on objects so we visualize our environment in perspective.
   A. The eye is protected by its anatomical position in the orbit and by eyelids, lashes, and lacrimal ducts. The cornea keeps dust and other foreign matter out. The cornea is continuous with the sclera, a tough membrane that envelops the rest of the eyeball.
   B. The iris regulates the amount of light entering the eye. In bright light it contracts, narrowing its opening, the pupil; in weak light it dilates the pupil, permitting more light to enter.
   C. The internal surface of the eye is covered by a black coat, the choroid, which prevents light rays from scattering.
   D. Light passes through the lens and is received by light receptors in the retina.

**Figure 9–5.** *Location and structure of the olfactory epithelium. Note that the receptor cells are located within the epithelium.*

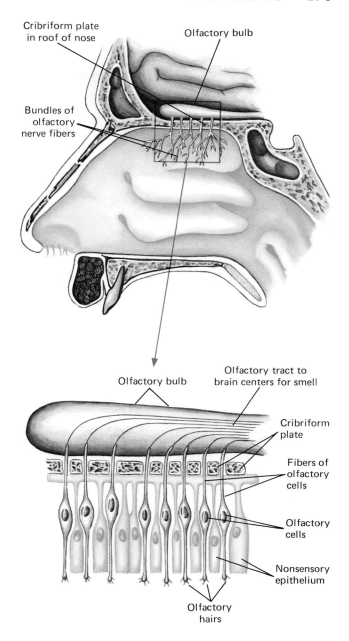

Cribriform plate in roof of nose

Olfactory bulb

Bundles of olfactory nerve fibers

Olfactory bulb

Olfactory tract to brain centers for smell

Cribriform plate

Fibers of olfactory cells

Olfactory cells

Nonsensory epithelium

Olfactory hairs

1. Rods are sensory cells in the retina sensitive to weak light but not to color.
2. Cones are sensory cells in the retina sensitive to color.

IV. Accommodation is an automatic process in which the curvature of the lens is increased to clearly focus on a close object.

V. In vision the image is focused on the retina. Then, the image is conducted from the retina to the brain by the optic nerve.

VI. The ear is a major exteroceptor dealing with hearing and equilibrium.
   A. The external ear serves as a tunnel collecting sound waves.
   B. The middle ear contains three small bones—malleus, incus, and stapes—that amplify sound waves from the tympanic membrane to the oval window leading to the inner ear.
   C. The inner ear contains the cochlea and vestibular apparatus.
      1. The cochlea contains the organ of Corti, which converts sound waves to nerve impulses for transmission to the brain.
      2. The vestibular apparatus contains three semicircular canals and two small chambers that transmit information about the body's position; they

play a major role in equilibrium.
VII. Taste is an important sense perceived through the taste buds on the tongue and transmitted through the facial and glossopharyngeal nerves.
VIII. Smell is perceived by the olfactory receptors, which transmit impulses to the brain through the olfactory nerve (cranial nerve I).
IX. Tactile sensations involve touch, pressure, and vibrations perceived through tactile receptors located in various parts of the skin.
X. Proprioception, or position sense, helps us maintain the position of the body and its parts.
XI. Pain serves as a protective mechanism for the body.

## POST TEST

*Select the most appropriate answer from Column B for each item in Column A.*
*You may use an answer once, more than once, or not at all.*

### Eye

**Column A**
1. _____ Loss of elasticity of the lens with age
2. _____ Colored part of the eye
3. _____ Area of clearest vision in retina
4. _____ Nearsightedness
5. _____ Senses color vision
6. _____ Window of the eye
7. _____ Crystalline body that adjusts for accommodation
8. _____ Sense(s) vision in dim light

**Column B**
a. fovea
b. cornea
c. ciliary body
d. iris
e. myopia
f. lens
g. rods
h. presbyopia
i. cones

### Ear

**Column A**
9. _____ Between middle and inner ear
10. _____ Porous bone that connects with middle ear
11. _____ Surrounds membranous labyrinth
12. _____ Outer portion of ear
13. _____ Inflammation of middle ear
14. _____ Bones in middle ear
15. _____ Connects middle ear with throat
16. _____ Transmits neural impulses from organ of Corti to brain

**Column B**
a. pinna
b. malleus, incus, stapes
c. eustachian tube
d. mastoid bone
e. bony labyrinth
f. otitis media
g. oval window
h. cochlear nerve

17. Label the diagrams on the opposite page.

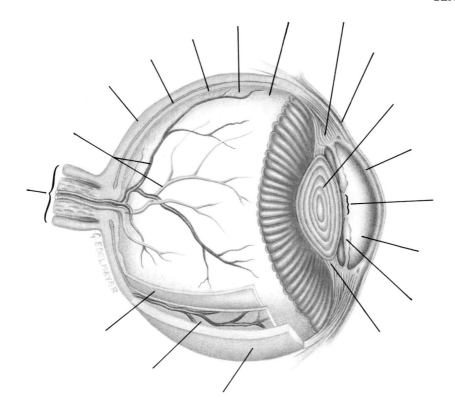

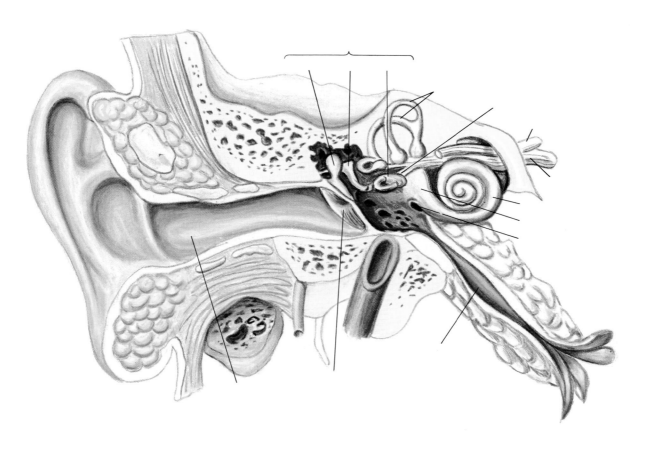

# REVIEW QUESTIONS

1. Distinguish among exteroceptors, interoceptors, and proprioceptors.
2. What are the layers of the eyeball?
3. What are the functions of (a) the pupil (b) the iris (c) the lens (d) rods and cones?
4. Summarize the steps in the physiology of hearing.
5. What are the functions of (a) malleus, incus, and stapes (b) cochlea (c) organ of Corti (d) eustachian tube?
6. What is the function of the vestibular apparatus?
7. Compare the function of the auditory and vestibular branches of cranial nerve VIII.
8. What are the four tastes recognized by the taste buds and how are these transmitted to the brain?
9. Where are the proprioceptors located?

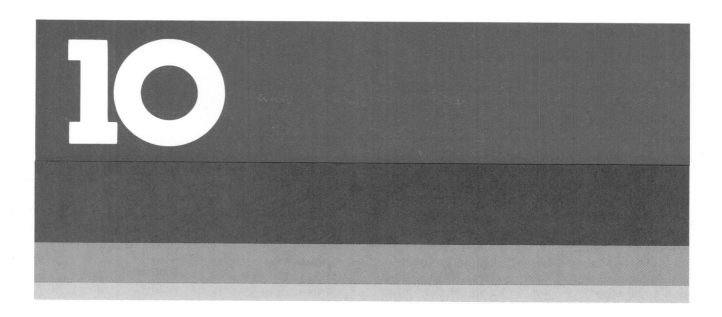

# The Endocrine System

## LEARNING OBJECTIVES

**After you study this chapter you should be able to**
1. Define the terms endocrine gland and hormone and describe how the endocrine system works to maintain homeostasis.
2. Locate the principal endocrine glands in the body, identify their principal hormones, and describe the functions of each hormone.
3. Describe how hormones are transported and how they affect their target tissues.
4. Draw a diagram illustrating how endocrine glands are regulated by negative feedback mechanisms.
5. Describe the mechanisms by which the hypothalamus links the nervous and endocrine systems.
6. Identify the hormones secreted by the anterior and posterior lobes of the pituitary gland and describe their actions; describe the effects of hyposecretion or hypersecretion of growth hormone.
7. State the actions of the thyroid hormones and describe the effects of their hyposecretion or hypersecretion.
8. Describe the mechanisms by which parathyroid hormone and calcitonin regulate calcium metabolism.
9. Contrast the actions of insulin and glucagon in maintaining blood-glucose homeostasis and

describe the homeostatic imbalances that occur in a diabetic.

10. Compare the effects of the adrenal medullary and adrenal cortical hormones in helping the body to cope with stress.

---

The **endocrine system** works with the nervous system in maintaining the steady state of the body. This system consists of endocrine glands and certain tissues that secrete chemical messengers called **hormones**. Recall from Chapter 3 that endocrine glands lack ducts and so release their hormones into the surrounding tissue fluid. Endocrine glands are vascular so that hormones diffuse into capillaries and are transported by the blood. Hormones affect specific tissues, their **target tissues**, generally by stimulating some change in metabolic activity. The principal endocrine glands and their hormones are listed in Table 10–1 and illustrated in Figure 10–1.

TABLE 10–1
**Principal Endocrine Glands and Their Hormones[1]**

| Endocrine Gland and Hormone | Target Tissue | Principal Actions |
| --- | --- | --- |
| **Hypothalamus** | | |
| Releasing and inhibiting hormones | Anterior lobe of pituitary gland | Stimulates or inhibits secretion of specific hormones |
| **Hypothalamus (Production) and Posterior lobe of Pituitary (Storage and release)** | | |
| Oxytocin | Uterus | Stimulates contraction |
| | Mammary glands | Stimulated ejection of milk into ducts |
| Antidiuretic hormone (ADH) | Kidneys (collecting ducts) | Stimulates reabsorption of water; conserves water |
| **Anterior Lobe of Pituitary** | | |
| Growth hormone (GH) | General | Stimulates growth by promoting protein synthesis |
| Prolactin | Mammary gland | Stimulates milk secretion |
| Thyroid-stimulating hormone (TSH) | Thyroid gland | Stimulates secretion of thyroid hormones; stimulates increase in size of thyroid gland |
| Adrenocorticotropic hormone (ACTH) | Adrenal cortex | Stimulates secretion of adrenocortical hormones |
| Gonadotropic hormones (FSH, LH) | Gonads | Stimulate gonad function |
| **Thyroid Gland** | | |
| Thyroxine ($T_4$) and triiodothyronine ($T_3$) | General | Stimulate metabolic rate; essential to normal growth and development |
| Calcitonin | Bone | Lowers blood-calcium level by inhibiting removal of calcium from bone |
| **Parathyroid Glands** | | |
| Parathyroid hormone (PTH) | Bone, kidneys, digestive tract | Increases blood-calcium level by stimulating bone breakdown; stimulates calcium reabsorption in kidneys; activates vitamin D |
| **Islets of Pancreas** | | |
| Insulin | General | Lowers blood-glucose level by facilitating glucose uptake and utilization by cells; stimulates glycogen production; stimulates fat storage and protein synthesis |
| Glucagon | Liver, adipose tissue | Raises blood-glucose level by stimulating manufacture of glucose from glycogen and noncarbohydrate nutrients; mobilizes fat |
| **Adrenal Medulla** | | |
| Epinephrine and norepinephrine | Skeletal muscle, cardiac muscle, blood vessels, liver, adipose tissue | Help body cope with stress; increase heart rate, blood pressure, metabolic rate; reroute blood; mobilize fat; raise blood-sugar level |
| **Adrenal Cortex** | | |
| Mineralocorticoids (aldosterone) | Kidney tubules | Maintain sodium and phosphate balance |
| Glucocorticoids (cortisol) | General | Help body adapt to long-term stress; raise blood-glucose level; mobilize fat |

TABLE 10–1
**Principal Endocrine Glands and Their Hormones** *Continued*

| Endocrine Gland and Hormone | Target Tissue | Principal Actions |
|---|---|---|
| **Ovary**[2] | | |
| Estrogens | General | Stimulate development of secondary sex characteristics |
| | Reproductive structures | Stimulate growth of sex organs at puberty; prompt monthly preparation of uterus for pregnancy |
| Progesterone | Uterus | Completes preparation of uterus for pregnancy |
| | Breasts | Stimulates development |
| **Testis** | | |
| Testosterone | General | Stimulates development of secondary sex characteristics and growth spurt at puberty |
| | Reproductive structures | Stimulates development of sex organs; stimulates spermatogenesis |
| **Pineal Gland** | | |
| Melatonin | Gonads, pigment cells, other tissues | Influences reproductive processes in hamsters and other animals; pigmentation in some vertebrates; may control biorhythms in some animals; may help control onset of puberty in humans |

[1]The digestive hormones are described in Chapter 16.
[2]The reproductive hormones will be discussed in Chapter 20.

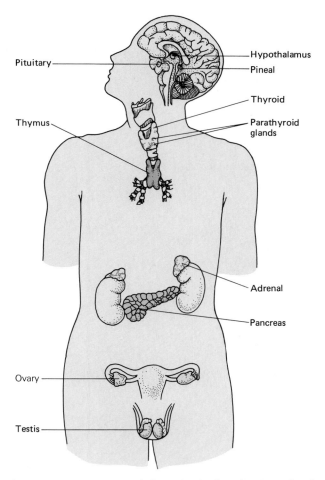

**Figure 10–1.** *Location of the principal endocrine glands. Both male and female gonads are shown.*

## HOW HORMONES WORK

A hormone may pass through many tissues seemingly "unnoticed" until it reaches its target tissue. How does the target tissue recognize its hormone? Specialized proteins in the cell membrane or cytoplasm of the target tissue act as *receptors* and bind with the hormone. This is a very specific process. The receptor is like a lock and the hormones like different keys. Only the hormone that fits the lock can influence the metabolic machinery of the cell. However, a cell can have receptors for several types of hormones.

Protein-type hormones combine with receptors in the cell membrane of a target cell. This results in a message being relayed into the cell by way of a second messenger. One second messenger that has been extensively studied is **cyclic AMP** (adenosine monophosphate). This compound triggers the chain of reactions that leads to the metabolic effect in the cell.

Steroid hormones are relatively small, lipid-soluble molecules that easily pass through the cell membrane into the cytoplasm. They combine with receptors within the cytoplasm, and the receptor-hormone complex then moves into the nucleus and activates a specific gene.

## REGULATION OF HORMONE SECRETION

Hormone secretion is self-regulated by **negative feedback** control mechanisms. Information regarding the hormone level or its effect is fed back to the gland, which then responds homeostatically. For example, the parathyroid glands release parathyroid hormone, which causes the level of calcium in the blood to rise. A low level of calcium in the blood signals the parathyroid glands to release more hormone (Fig. 10–2). However, when the calcium level rises above normal limits, the parathyroid glands are inhibited and slow their output of hormone. Both responses are negative feedback mechanisms because in both cases the effects are opposite (negative) to the stimulus.

## ENDOCRINE MALFUNCTIONS

An endocrine disorder may cause **hyposecretion**, a decrease in hormone output, or **hyperse-**

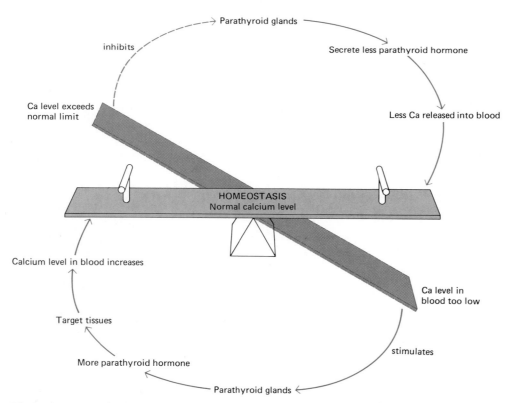

***Figure 10–2.*** *Endocrine glands are regulated by negative feedback mechanisms. When calcium level decreases below normal limits, the parathyroid glands secrete more parathyroid hormone. This hormone activates mechanisms that increase calcium level, thus restoring homeostasis. An abnormally high calcium level inhibits the parathyroid hormones so that less hormone is secreted.*

TABLE 10–2
**Consequences of Endocrine Malfunction**

| Hormone | Hyposecretion | Hypersecretion |
| --- | --- | --- |
| Growth hormone | Pituitary dwarf | Gigantism if malfunction occurs in childhood; acromegaly in adult |
| Thyroid hormones | Cretinism (in children); myxedema, a condition of pronounced adult hypothyroidism (BMR is reduced by about 40%; patient feels tired all of the time and may be mentally slow); goiter, enlargement of the thyroid gland | Hyperthyroidism; increased metabolic rate, nervous, irritable |
| Parathyroid hormone | Spontaneous discharge of nerves; spasms; tetany; death | Weak, brittle bones; kidney stones |
| Insulin | Diabetes mellitus | Hypoglycemia |
| Adrenocortical hormones | Addison's disease (body cannot synthesize sufficient glucose; patient is unable to cope with stress; sodium loss in urine may lead to shock) | Cushing's disease (edema gives face a full-moon appearance; fat is deposited about trunk; blood glucose level rises; immune responses are depressed) |

**cretion**, an abnormal increase in hormone output. Either condition results in homeostatic imbalance, leading to predictable clinical symptoms (Table 10–2). Some of these hormonal disorders will be described as specific endocrine glands are discussed.

## HYPOTHALAMUS AND PITUITARY GLAND

Nervous and endocrine systems are linked by the hypothalamus, which regulates the activity of the **pituitary** (pih-**too'**-ih-tar-ee) **gland**. Because it secretes at least nine distinct hormones that regulate the activities of several other endocrine glands and influence a wide range of physiological processes, the pituitary gland is referred to as the master gland of the body. This remarkable gland is about the size of a pea and weighs approximately 0.5 g (0.02 ounces).

Connected to the hypothalamus by a stalk of nervous tissue, the infundibulum, the pituitary gland lies within the sella turcica, a bony depression of the sphenoid bone. The pituitary gland consists of two main lobes, the anterior and posterior lobes.

### Posterior Lobe of the Pituitary Gland

Two peptide hormones, oxytocin and antidiuretic hormone, are secreted by the **posterior lobe** of the pituitary gland (Fig. 10–3). These hormones are actually produced by special cells in the hypothalamus. Enclosed within little vacuoles, the hormones pass slowly down the axons of these cells. These axons extend through the pituitary stalk into the posterior lobe. Hormone accumulates in the axon endings until the neuron is stimulated and then is released and diffuses into surrounding capillaries. Such production of hormones by neurons is called *neurosecretion*.

**Oxytocin** (ox''-se-**tow'**-sin) stimulates the uterus to contract and promotes release of milk from the breast. Toward the end of pregnancy, oxytocin levels rise, stimulating the strong contractions of the uterus needed to expel the baby. Oxytocin is sometimes administered clinically (under the name Pitocin) to initiate or speed labor. Males have about the same amount of oxytocin circulating in their blood as females, but its function in them is unknown.

**Antidiuretic hormone (ADH)** (an''-ti-die'-u-ret'-ik) helps the body to conserve water by increasing water reabsorption from the kidneys. This decreases the volume of fluid lost in the urine. ADH secretion is regulated by the volume and osmotic pressure of the blood.

Hyposecretion of ADH leads to the condition called **diabetes insipidus**, in which urine volume cannot be regulated effectively. Enormous quantities of urine, up to 30 l/day, may be excreted. Of course, this fluid loss must be replaced or serious dehydration will rapidly develop. Diabetes insipidus may now be treated by injection of ADH or with an ADH nasal spray.

### Anterior Lobe of the Pituitary Gland

The **anterior lobe** of the pituitary gland secretes six important hormones, including growth hormone, prolactin, and several tropic hormones. The anterior lobe also secretes a peptide called beta-lipotropin, which is now thought to be the precursor of endorphins and enkephalins (the morphine-

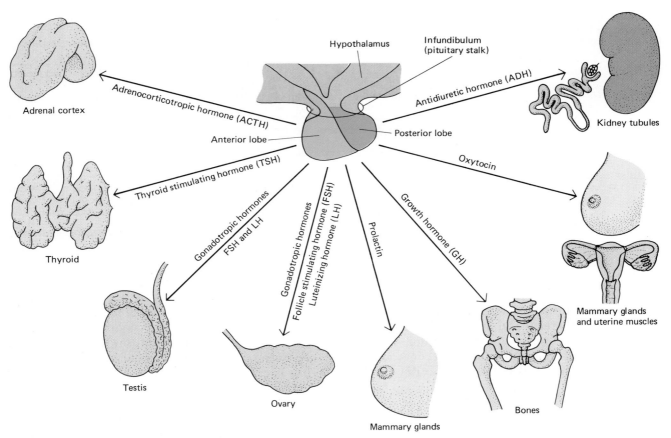

**Figure 10–3.** *The pituitary gland is suspended from the hypothalamus by a stalk of neural tissue, the infundibulum. The hormones secreted by the pituitary gland and the target tissues they act on are shown.*

like substances produced by the body that function in pain perception; see Chapter 7).

During lactation (milk production) **prolactin** (pro-**lak'**-tin) stimulates the cells of the mammary glands to secrete milk. As long as the infant continues to suckle, milk production continues, even for years. Once the mother stops nursing the baby, however, milk production ceases within a few days. The function of prolactin in males is not known.

The anterior lobe of the pituitary gland secretes four **tropic** (**trow'**-pik) **hormones**, that is, hormones that stimulate the activity of other endocrine glands. The tropic hormones are thyroid-stimulating hormone (TSH), which acts on the thyroid gland; adrenocorticotropic hormone (ACTH), which stimulates the adrenal cortex; and the gonadotropins, follicle-stimulating hormone (FSH) and luteinizing hormone (LH), which control the activities of the gonads (sex glands).

## Human Growth Hormone

**Human growth hormone** (HGH) (also called **somatotropin**) stimulates body growth mainly by increasing uptake of amino acids by the cells and by stimulating protein synthesis. The effects of growth hormone on growth of the skeleton is indirect. The hormone stimulates the liver (and perhaps certain other tissues) to produce peptides (called somatomedins), which are essential for growth of cartilage and bone. Growth hormone also affects fat and carbohydrate metabolism. It promotes mobilization of fat from adipose tissues, so that fat components become available for cells to use as fuel, a protein-sparing action.

Remember your parents telling you to get plenty of sleep and exercise to grow properly? These age-old notions are supported by recent studies. Growth hormone secretion increases during sleep and also during exercise. Children who get lots of loving also have an advantage in this regard. Cuddling, playing, and other forms of nurture are apparently essential to normal development. Growth is retarded in children who are deprived of emotional attention and support, even when their physical needs (food and shelter) are amply met. In extreme cases, childhood stress can produce actual dwarfism (psychosocial dwarfism). Some emotionally deprived children exhibit abnormal sleep patterns, which may be the basis for decreased secretion of growth hormone.

Have you ever wondered why circus midgets failed to grow normally? They are probably **pituitary dwarfs**, individuals whose pituitary gland did not produce sufficient growth hormone during childhood. Though miniature, a pituitary dwarf has normal intelligence and is usually well-proportioned. If the growth centers in the long bones are still open when this condition is initially diagnosed, it can be treated clinically by injection with growth hormone, which can now be synthesized commercially.

Abnormally tall individuals develop when the anterior pituitary secretes excessive amounts of growth hormone during childhood. This condition is referred to as **gigantism**. If hypersecretion of growth hormone (or somatomedin) occurs during adulthood, the individual cannot grow taller. However, a condition known as **acromegaly** (ak″-row-meg′-ah-lee) (large extremities) results in which the bones, especially those in the hands, feet, and face, increase in diameter. A patient may first become aware of the symptoms of acromegaly when his or her feet widen, requiring a larger shoe size, or when rings no longer fit his or her thickened fingers. Increase in the diameter of the mandible causes the lower jaw to protude.

### Control by the Hypothalamus

Each of the anterior pituitary hormones is regulated in some way by a **releasing hormone** and in some cases also by an **inhibiting hormone** produced in the hypothalamus. When released by the hypothalamus, these hormones diffuse into capillaries and circulate with the blood through portal veins to the hypothalamus. (A portal vein does not deliver blood to a large vein or directly to the heart but connects two sets of capillaries.) Within the anterior lobe of the pituitary the portal veins connect with a second set of capillaries from which the hormone diffuses into the tissue of the anterior pituitary gland.

## THYROID GLAND

Shaped somewhat like a shield, the **thyroid gland** is located in the neck, anterior to the trachea and just inferior to the larynx (Adam's apple) (Fig. 10–1). Its two lobes of dark red glandular tissue are connected by a bridge of tissue, the thyroid isthmus. The thyroid gland secretes two thyroid hormones and a hormone called calcitonin (which will be discussed in conjunction with the parathyroid glands).

### Thyroid Hormones

The principal **thyroid hormone** is **thyroxine**, or $T_4$ (because this compound has four iodine atoms).

The other thyroid hormone is **triiodothyronine**, or $T_3$ (because it has three iodine atoms). The thyroid hormones have widespread effects in the body. Their two principal actions are to stimulate metabolic rate and to promote growth. These hormones are thought to increase the rate of cellular respiration. Fuel is "burned" more quickly so oxygen consumption increases, as does heat production. Thyroid hormones are essential to normal growth and development. They promote protein synthesis and enhance the effect of growth hormone.

The regulation of thyroid hormone secretion depends mainly on a feedback system between the anterior lobe of the pituitary and the thyroid gland (Fig. 10–4). The pituitary gland secretes **thyroid-stimulating hormone (TSH)**, which acts by way of cyclic AMP to increase iodine uptake, promote synthesis and secretion of thyroid hormones, and increase the size of the gland itself. When the normal concentration of thyroid hormones in the blood falls, the anterior pituitary secretes more thyroid-stimulating hormone. When the level of thyroid hormones in the blood rises above normal, the anterior pituitary is inhibited and slows its release of thyroid-stimulating hormone.

Too much thyroid hormone in the blood may also affect the hypothalamus, inhibiting secretion of TSH-releasing hormone. However, the hypothalamus is thought to exert its regulatory effects primarily in certain stressful situations, such as extreme weather change.

### Disorders of the Thyroid Gland

Extreme **hypothyroidism** during infancy and childhood results in low metabolic rate and retarded mental and physical development, a condition called **cretinism** (kree′-tin-ism) (Fig. 10–5). When diagnosed and treated early enough, the effects of cretinism can be prevented.

An adult who feels like sleeping all the time, who is devoid of energy, and who is mentally slow or even confused may also be suffering from hypothyroidism. When there is almost no thyroid function, the basal metabolic rate (BMR) is reduced by about 40% and the patient develops the condition called **myxedema** (mik″-se-dee′-muh). Hypothyroidism, like cretinism, can be treated by using thyroid pills to replace the missing hormones.

**Hyperthyroidism** does not cause abnormal growth but does increase metabolic rate by 60% or even more. This increase in metabolism results in swift utilization of nutrients, causing the individual to be hungry and to increase food intake. However, this is not sufficient to meet the demands of the rapidly metabolizing cells, so these patients often lose weight. They also tend to be nervous, irritable, and emotionally unstable. In some forms of hyperthyroidism the thyroid gland and eyes are prominent.

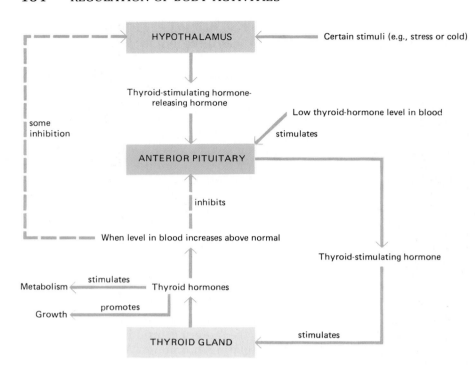

Figure 10–4. Regulation of thyroid hormone secretion. Dotted arrows indicate inhibition.

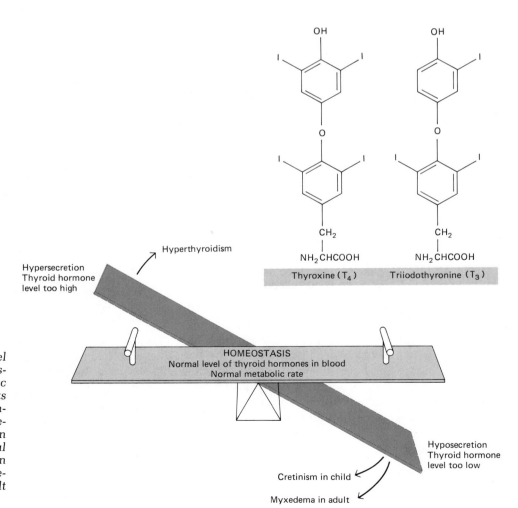

Figure 10–5. A normal level of thyroid hormone is necessary for a normal metabolic rate. Hypersecretion results in irritability and other clinical symptoms. Hyposecretion in children results in stunted physical and mental development, a condition known as cretinism. Hyposecretion in adults may result in myxedema.

Hyperthyroidism is often the result of **Graves' disease** (toxic goiter), in which the thyroid gland increases in both size and activity. Graves' disease can be treated with drugs, by surgery, or sometimes by injecting large amounts of radioactive iodine, which destroys some of the thyroid tissue.

Any abnormal enlargement of the thyroid gland is termed a **goiter** (goy'-ter) and may be associated with either hypo- or hypersecretion (Fig. 10–6). One cause is Graves' disease; another is **endemic goiter** caused by dietary iodine deficiency. Without iodine the gland cannot make thyroid hormones, so their concentrations in the blood decrease. In compensation, the anterior pituitary secretes large amounts of TSH and the thyroid gland enlarges, sometimes to gigantic proportions. Because the problem is lack of iodine, enlargement of the gland cannot increase production of the hormones, for the needed ingredient is still missing. Thanks to iodized salt, such simple goiter is no longer common in the United States. In other parts of the world, however, an estimated 200 million persons still suffer from this easily preventable disorder.

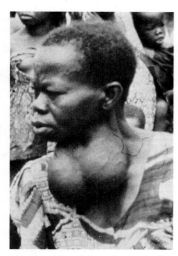

*Figure 10–6. Goiter resulting from iodine deficiency. (Courtesy of United Nations Food and Agricultural Organization.)*

## PARATHYROID GLANDS

The **parathyroid** (par"-uh-**thy'**-royd) **glands** are embedded in the connective tissue that surrounds the posterior surfaces of the lateral lobes of the thyroid gland. Usually there are four glands but the number may vary from 2 to 10. These glands secrete **parathyroid hormone (PTH)**, a small protein that regulates the calcium level of the blood and tissue fluid.

Appropriate concentrations of calcium are essential for normal nerve and muscle function, bone metabolism, cell-membrane permeability, and blood clotting. Parathyroid hormone stimulates release of calcium from the bones (Fig. 10–7). It also stimulates calcium reabsorption by the kidney tubules, raising the blood-calcium level while preventing loss by excretion. PTH activates vitamin D, which then increases the amount of calcium absorbed from the intestine. Vitamin D also

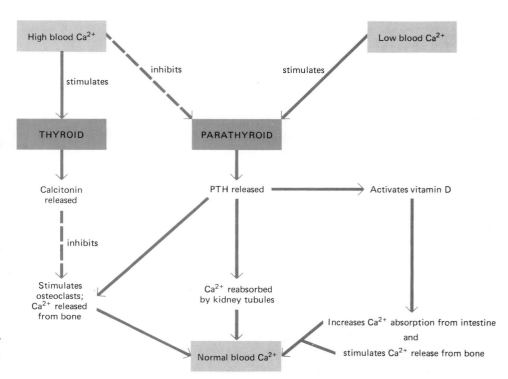

*Figure 10–7. Regulation of calcium metabolism. Dotted lines indicate inhibition.*

acts independently of PTH to stimulate calcium release from bone.

**Calcitonin** (kal″-si-**tow′**-nin), secreted by the thyroid gland, works antagonistically to parathyroid hormone. When calcium levels become excessive (about 20% above normal), calcitonin is released and inhibits removal of calcium from bone. Calcitonin acts rapidly to regulate calcium level.

Insufficient secretion of PTH results in a fall in calcium level in blood tissue fluid. Nerve fibers become more excitable and may discharge spontaneously, causing muscles to twitch and to go into spasms or even tetany. Spasm of the muscles of the larynx interferes with respiration and may lead to death. The symptoms of hypoparathyroidism can be relieved by injection of calcium or parathyroid hormone.

> Hyperparathyroidism is often caused by small benign tumors called **adenomas**, which cause overproduction of parathyroid hormone. So much calcium may be removed from the bones that they are weakened and may be easily fractured. The kidneys attempt to excrete the excess calcium mobilized from the bones. Crystals of calcium may precipitate in the urine and aggregate, forming kidney stones.

## ISLETS OF LANGERHANS

Usually thought of as a digestive organ, the pancreas is an elongated gland that lies in the abdomen posterior to the stomach and partially surrounded by a loop of the small intestine (Fig. 10–1). The pancreas has both exocrine and endocrine components.

More than a million small clusters of cells known as the **islets of Langerhans** (**eye′**-lits of **lahng′**-er-hanz) are scattered throughout the pancreas. About 70% of the islet cells are **beta** (B) **cells** that produce the hormone insulin. **Alpha** (or A) **cells** secrete the hormone glucagon.

## Actions of Insulin

**Insulin** (**in′**-suh-lin) is a protein hormone that exerts widespread influence on metabolism. Its principal action is to facilitate diffusion and storage of glucose into most cells, especially muscle and fat cells. By stimulating cells to take up glucose from the blood, insulin *lowers* the blood-sugar level. Insulin reduces the use of fatty acids as fuel and instead stimulates their storage in adipose tissue. It affects protein metabolism by increasing active transport of amino acids into cells and by stimulating protein synthesis.

## Actions of Glucagon

**Glucagon** (**gloo′**-kuh-gon), also a protein, acts antagonistically to insulin. It stimulates the mobilization of glucose, fatty acids, and amino acids from storage depots into the blood. Glucagon's principal action is to *raise* the blood-sugar level. It does this by stimulating liver cells to convert glycogen to glucose, and by stimulating the liver cells to make glucose from noncarbohydrates. Glucagon also promotes release of fat stores from adipose tissue, thereby raising fatty acid levels in the blood and providing nutrients for glucose production. Note that all these actions are opposite to those of insulin.

## Regulation of Insulin and Glucagon Secretion

Secretion of insulin and glucagon is directly controlled by the blood-sugar level (Fig. 10–8). After a meal, when the blood-glucose level rises as a result of absorption of nutrients from the intestine, the beta cells are stimulated to increase insulin secretion. Then, as the cells remove glucose from the blood, decreasing its concentration, insulin secretion decreases accordingly.

When one has not eaten for several hours, the blood-sugar level begins to fall from its normal fasting level of about 90 mg/100 ml. When it decreases to about 70 mg/100 ml, the alpha cells of the islets secrete large amounts of glucagon. Glucose is mobilized from the liver stores and the blood-sugar level returns to normal. The alpha cells respond to the glucose concentration within their own cytoplasm, which reflects the blood-sugar level. When the blood-sugar level is high, there is normally a high level of glucose within the alpha cells and glucagon secretion is inhibited.

Insulin and glucagon work together but in opposite ways to keep the blood-sugar level within normal limits. When glucose level rises, insulin release brings it back to normal; when it falls, glucagon acts to raise it again. The insulin-glucagon system is a powerful, fast-acting mechanism for keeping the blood-sugar level normal. Can you think of reasons why it is important to maintain a constant blood-sugar level? Perhaps the most important one is that brain cells are completely dependent on a continuous supply of glucose as they are normally unable to utilize any other nutrient as fuel.

## Diabetes Mellitus

The principal disorder associated with pancreatic hormones is **diabetes mellitus**. Although many of the symptoms of diabetes can be controlled, the long-term complications of this disorder reduce life expectancy by as much as one-third. There are an estimated 10 million diabetics in the United States alone and almost 40,000 persons die annually as a result of this disorder, making it the third most common cause of death.

Diabetes should be considered a group of diseases rather than a single disorder. Although there is an inherited tendency to diabetes, it is thought that certain environmental factors trigger its actual development. Two distinct clinical varieties of diabetes mellitus have been identified. More than 90% of all cases are **maturity onset diabetes**, which develops gradually, usually in overweight persons over age 40. In many cases of maturity onset diabetes, sufficient insulin is released by the islets of Langerhans. The problem is that the target cells are not able to take up the insulin and use it.

**Juvenile onset diabetes** usually develops before age 20. This disorder is marked by a dramatic decrease in the number of beta cells in the pancreas, resulting in insulin deficiency. Juvenile onset diabetes is insulin dependent, which means that insulin injections are necessary to relieve the carbohydrate imbalance.

## Metabolic Effects

Similar metabolic disturbances occur in all cases of diabetes mellitus. Three major metabolic effects of diabetes are (1) decreased utilization of glucose, (2) increased fat mobilization, and (3) increased protein utilization.

**Decreased Utilization of Glucose.** In diabetics, cells dependent on insulin can take in only about 25% of the glucose they require for fuel. Glucose remains in the blood and the blood-glucose level rises (*hyperglycemia*). Instead of the normal fasting level of about 90 mg/100 ml, the diabetic may have from 300 to more than 1000 mg/100 ml.

Whereas glucose does not appear in the urine of nondiabetics, the blood-glucose concentration is so high in the diabetic that sugar spills out into the urine (**glycosuria**). Although not completely reliable, a simple test for glucose in the urine is useful in screening for diabetes and for elevating control of glucose metabolism in known diabetics.

**Increased Fat Mobilization.** Despite the large quantities of glucose present in the blood of diabetics, the cells cannot utilize it and must turn to other sources of fuel. The absence of insulin promotes mobilization of fat stores, so that the blood–fatty acid level rises, providing nutrients for cellular respiration. Unfortunately, the blood-lipid level may reach five times the normal level, leading to development of atherosclerosis ("hardening of the arteries"). In addition, the increased fat metabolism by the cells increases formation of **ketone bodies** (acetone and other breakdown products of fat metabolism). Ketone bodies build up in the blood, causing **ketosis**, a condition in which the blood and body fluids become too acidic. If sufficiently marked, acidosis can lead to coma and death.

When the ketone level rises in the blood, ketones appear in the urine, providing another useful clinical indication of diabetes. Because of osmotic pressure, when ketone bodies and glucose are excreted in the urine, they take water with them, so that urine volume increases (**polyuria**). The resulting dehydration causes the diabetic to feel thirsty.

**Increased Protein Mobilization.** Lack of insulin also results in increased protein breakdown relative to protein synthesis. As a result the untreated diabetic becomes thin and emaciated, despite (usually) a voracious appetite.

## Treatment of Diabetes

Maturity-onset diabetes is generally a mild disorder and can be treated by maintaining an appropriate body weight and by carefully managing the diet. In more serious cases, tolbutamide and related drugs may be taken orally to stimulate the islets to produce insulin. However, it has been shown that these drugs have undesirable side effects, such as heart disease, and there has been a shift away from their use. In serious cases daily injections of insulin are used to regulate carbohydrate metabolism. Insulin is a protein so it cannot be taken orally because it would be digested by enzymes in the digestive tract.

## Hypoglycemia

**Hypoglycemia** (low blood-sugar level) is sometimes seen in people who later develop diabetes. It may be an overreaction by the islets to glucose challenge. Too much insulin is secreted in response to carbohydrate ingestion. About 3 hours after a meal the blood-sugar level falls below normal, making the individual feel drowsy. If this reaction is severe enough the patient may become incoordinated or even unconscious.

Serious hypoglycemia may develop if diabetics inject themselves with too much insulin or if too much is secreted by the islets because of a tumor. The blood-sugar level may fall drastically, depriving the brain cells of their needed supply of fuel. **Insulin shock** may result, a condition in which the patient may appear to be drunk or may become unconscious, experience convulsions or brain damage, or even die.

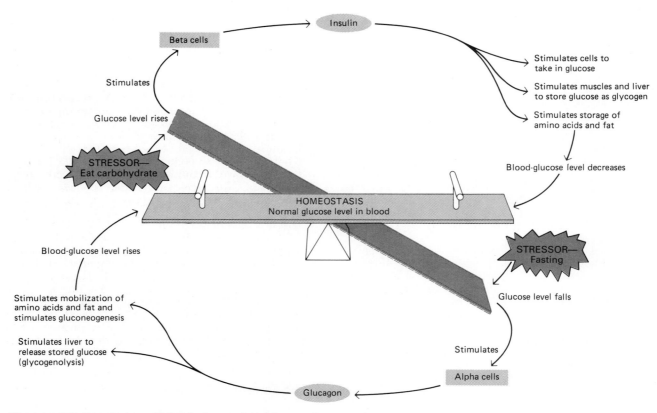

**Figure 10–8.** *Regulation of blood-glucose level by insulin and glucagon.*

## ADRENAL GLANDS

The paired **adrenal glands** are small yellow masses of tissue that lie in contact with the upper ends of the kidneys (Fig. 10–9). Each gland consists of a central portion, the **adrenal medulla**, and a larger outer section, the **adrenal cortex**. Although wedded anatomically, the adrenal medulla and cortex develop from different types of tissue in the embryo and function as distinct glands. Both secrete hormones that help to regulate metabolism, and both help the body deal effectively with stress.

### Adrenal Medulla

The adrenal medulla develops from neural tissue and its secretion is controlled by sympathetic nerves. Two hormones, epinephrine (sometimes called adrenaline) and norepinephrine (noradrenaline), are secreted by the adrenal medulla.

Often referred to as the emergency gland of the body, the adrenal medulla prepares an individual physiologically to deal with threatening situations. If a monster were suddenly to appear before you,

hormone secretion from this gland would initiate an alarm reaction enabling you to think quickly, then fight harder or run much faster than usual. Metabolic rate would increase as much as 100%.

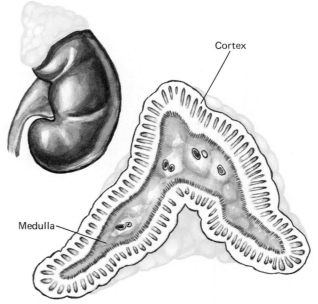

**Figure 10–9.** *The paired adrenal glands are small yellow masses of tissues that lie in contact with the upper ends of the kidneys. Each gland consists of a central medulla and an outer cortex.*

## Actions of Epinephrine and Norepinephrine

**Norepinephrine** is the same substance secreted as a neurotransmitter by sympathetic neurons and by some neurons in the central nervous system. Its effects on the body are similar but last about 10 times longer because the hormone is removed from the blood more slowly than it is removed from synapses. About 80% of the hormone output of the adrenal medulla is **epinephrine**.

The adrenal medullary hormones cause blood to be rerouted in favor of those organs essential for emergency action. Blood vessels to the skin and kidneys are constricted, whereas those to the brain, muscles, and heart are dilated. Constriction of the blood vessels to the skin has the added advantage of decreasing blood loss in case of hemorrhage. (It also explains the sudden paling that comes with fear or rage.) The heart beats faster and thresholds in the reticular activating system (RAS) of the brain are lowered, increasing alertness. Both glucose and fatty acid levels in the blood rise, assuring needed fuel for extra energy. Strength of muscle contraction increases. Virtually all of the airways enlarge so that one breathes more effectively. In fact, epinephrine and related drugs are used clinically to relieve nasal congestion and asthma.

Many of the effects of epinephrine and norepinephrine are similar but their effects on the cardiovascular system are somewhat different. Norepinephrine constricts the blood vessels, thereby increasing blood pressure. Epinephrine increases blood pressure by increasing cardiac output (the volume of blood pumped each minute).

Both epinephrine and norepinephrine are secreted continuously in small amounts. Their secretion is under nervous control. When anxiety is aroused, messages are sent from the brain through sympathetic nerves to the adrenal medulla. Acetylcholine released by these neurons triggers release of the hormones.

## Adrenal Cortex

All the hormones of the **adrenal cortex** are steroids. (Recall that steroids are a chemical group classified with the lipids.) Three different types of hormones are produced by the adrenal cortex: (1) sex hormones, (2) mineralocorticoids, and (3) glucocorticoids.

Small amounts of both **androgens** (hormones that have masculinizing effects) and **estrogens** (female hormones) are secreted by the adrenal cortex in both sexes. Normally the amounts of these hormones released are so small that they have little physiological effect. However, adrenal tumors may secrete large quantities, especially of the androgens, resulting in the "bearded ladies" of circus sideshows.

**Mineralocorticoids** (min″-er-al-o-**kor′**-ti-koids) help regulate salt balance. The principal mineralocorticoid is **aldosterone** (**al′**-do-ste-rone), a hormone that increases the rate at which sodium is reabsorbed by kidney tubules, thereby helping to maintain sodium balance in the body and an appropriate blood pressure. Aldosterone also helps to regulate potassium concentrations in the body. When the adrenal glands do not function, large amounts of sodium are excreted in the urine. Water leaves the body with the sodium (because of osmotic pressure) and the blood volume may be so markedly reduced that the patient dies of low blood pressure.

Aldosterone secretion depends on changes in blood pressure. When blood pressure decreases, the hypothalamus secretes a releasing hormone that stimulates the anterior pituitary to release **adrenocorticotropic hormone** (ACTH). ACTH, in turn, stimulates release of aldosterone, which increases sodium reabsorption. Water is reabsorbed with the sodium, so that blood volume and pressure increase. Decrease in blood pressure also stimulates release of the hormone **renin** from the kidneys. Renin catalyzes the production of a chemical group known as the **angiotensins** (an-jee-o-**ten′**-sins) in the blood. One of the angiotensins stimulates the adrenal cortex to release more aldosterone. By these mechanisms the adrenal glands help to keep the blood pressure constant and to maintain homeostasis.

**Cortisol** (**kor′**-ti-sol) also called hydrocortisone, accounts for about 95% of the **glucocorticoid** (gloo″-ko-**kor′**-ti-koid) activity of the adrenal cortex. The principal action of cortisol is to promote production of glucose from other nutrients in the liver. Cortisol stimulates transport of amino acids into liver cells and promotes fat mobilization so that these nutrients are available for glucose production. Large amounts of glucose and glycogen are produced in the liver and the blood-glucose level rises. Through these actions cortisol helps to ensure adequate fuel supplies for the cells when the body is under stress. Thus the adrenal cortex provides an important back-up system for the adrenal medulla.

Glucocorticoids are used clinically to reduce inflammation in allergic reactions, infections, arthritis, and certain types of cancer. These hormones help to stabilize lysosome membranes so that they do not destroy tissues with their potent enzymes. Glucocorticoids also reduce inflammation by decreasing the permeablility of capillary membranes, thereby reducing swelling. They also reduce the effects of histamine.

When used in large amounts over long periods of time, glucocorticoids can cause serious side effects. They decrease the number of lymphocytes (a type of white blood cell) in the body and can cause atrophy of lymph tissue, reducing the patient's ability to fight infections. Other side effects include ulcers, hypertension, diabetes mellitus, and atherosclerosis.

Glucocorticoid secretion is regulated by ACTH from the pituitary. In turn, ACTH secretion is controlled by a releasing hormone from the hypothalamus. Almost any type of stress is reported to the hypothalamus, which activates the system so that large amounts of cortisol are rapidly released. When the body is not under stress, high levels of cortisol in the blood inhibit both the hypothalamus and the pituitary.

Abnormally large amounts of glucocorticoids, whether due to disease or clinical administration, result in the condition called **Cushing's syndrome** (Fig. 10–10). Fat is mobilized from the lower part of the body and deposited about the trunk. Edema gives the patient's face a full-moon appearance. Blood-sugar level rises to as much as 50% above normal, causing adrenal diabetes. If this condition persists for several months it can cause the beta cells in the pancreas to "burn out" from secreting excessive insulin. This can result in permanent diabetes mellitus. Reduction in protein synthesis causes weakness and decreases immune responses, so that the patient often dies of infection.

Destruction of the adrenal cortex and the resulting decrease in aldosterone and cortisol secretion causes **Addison's disease**. Reduction in cortisol prevents the body from regulating blood-sugar levels because it cannot manufacture enough glucose. The patient also loses the ability to cope with stress. If cortisol levels are significantly depressed, even the stress of mild infections can cause death.

## The Adrenal Glands and Stress

**Stressors**, whether in the form of noise, disease, infection, or even the anxiety of taking a test for which one is not fully prepared, arouse the adrenal glands to action. The brain signals the adrenal medulla rapidly via neural connections to release epinephrine and norepinephrine, hormones that prepare the body for fight or flight. The hypothalamus also signals the anterior pituitary hormonally to secrete ACTH, which increases cortisol secretion, thereby adjusting metabolism to meet the increased demands of the stressful situation (Fig. 10–11).

Some forms of stress are short-lived. One reacts to the situation and quickly resolves it. Other stressors may last for days, weeks, or even years—a chronic disease, for example, or an unhappy marriage or job situation. General anxiety and tension are examples of nonspecific stress.

Physiologist Hans Selye introduced the term **general-adaptation syndrome (GAS)** to describe the body's response to stress. Selye suggested that chronic stress is harmful because of the side effects of long-term elevated levels of cortisol. Though glucocorticoids are helpful in reducing inflammation, they can also interfere with normal immune responses, so that infection spreads. Chronic high blood pressure may contribute to

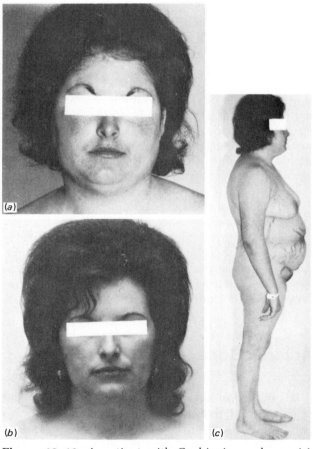

***Figure 10–10.*** *A patient with Cushing's syndrome (a) and (c) before treatment and (b) 1 year after treatment (removal of an adrenal adenoma). (From Cecil Textbook of Medicine, 17th ed. Philadelphia, W.B. Saunders Co., 1985, p. 1314.)*

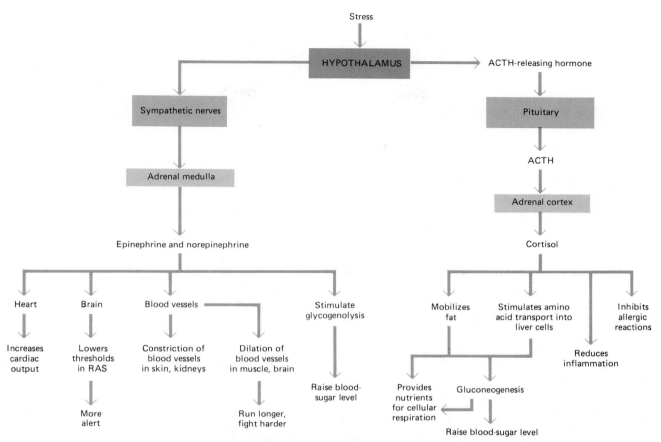

**Figure 10–11.** *The adrenal medulla and the adrenal cortex both play important roles in helping the body cope with stress. Some of the diverse effects of their hormones are shown here.*

heart disease, and increased levels of fat in the blood may promote atherosclerosis. When experimental animals are injected with large amounts of glucocorticoids, such disease states are induced, and similar effects are seen when large doses are administered clinically to patients. Among the diseases linked to excessive amounts of adrenocortical hormones are ulcers, high blood pressure, atherosclerosis, and arthritis.

## OTHER HORMONES

Many other tissues of the body secrete hormones. The digestive tract secretes hormones that stimulate digestion. The **thymus gland** releases a hormone (thymosin) that plays a role in immune responses and the kidneys release hormones, one of which (renin) helps to regulate blood pressure. The **pineal gland**, located in the brain, produces a hormone called **melatonin**, which may affect reproduction. In Chapter 20 we will discuss the principal reproductive hormones.

**Prostaglandins** are a group of local hormones released by many different tissues in the body, including the lungs, liver, and digestive tract. Prostaglandins influence a wide variety of metabolic activities and may help regulate other hormones. They dilate the bronchial passageways, inhibit gastric secretion, stimulate contraction of the uterus, affect nerve function, affect blood pressure, and influence metabolism. Those synthesized in the temperature-regulating center of the hypothalamus can cause fever, and it is now known that the ability of aspirin to reduce fever (long a mystery) depends on inhibiting prostaglandin synthesis. Prostaglandins are used clinically to initiate labor and induce abortion and their use as a birth control drug is being investigated.

## SUMMARY

I. The endocrine system regulates homeostasis of many metabolic processes; it consists of endocrine glands that release hormones.

A. Endocrine glands are ductless glands that secrete hormones into the surrounding tissue fluid.

B. Hormones are chemical messengers secreted by endocrine glands that are transported to target tissues by the blood and that stimulate the target tissue to change some metabolic activity.

II. Several mechanisms of hormone action are known.

A. Many nonsteroid hormones bind to receptors on the cell membrane of target cells. This activates a second messenger, such as cyclic AMP, which triggers the chain of events leading to the actual response.

B. Steroid hormones enter target cells and combine with receptors within the cytoplasm. The steroid-receptor complex moves into the nucleus and activates specific genes.

III. Endocrine glands are self-regulated by systems of negative feedback controls.

IV. The hypothalamus is the link between the nervous and endocrine systems.

A. Cells of the hypothalamus secrete several types of releasing and inhibiting hormones that regulate the secretion of hormones by the anterior pituitary gland.

B. Cells of the hypothalamus also produce the hormones oxytocin and ADH, which are released by the posterior lobe of the pituitary gland.

V. The posterior lobe of the pituitary gland releases the hormones oxytocin and ADH.

A. Oxytocin stimulates the uterus to contract and stimulates release of milk from the lactating breast.

B. ADH acts on the kidney ducts to promote reabsorption of water; this results in a small urine volume and thus conserves water.

VI. The anterior pituitary gland releases growth hormone, prolactin, and several tropic hormones.

A. Growth hormone promotes growth by promoting protein synthesis.
   1. Hyposecretion of growth hormone during childhood stunts growth.
   2. Hypersecretion causes gigantism; hypersecretion during adulthood may result in acromegaly.

B. Prolactin stimulates milk production in the lactating breast.

C. The tropic hormones include thyroid-stimulating hormone (TSH), ACTH, and the gonadotropic hormones.

VII. The thyroid hormones stimulate the rate of metabolism.

A. A rise in thyroid hormone level in the blood inhibits secretion of thyroid-stimulating hormone by the pituitary; a decrease stimulates TSH secretion.

B. Extreme hypothyroidism in childhood may result in cretinism; hypothyroidism in an adult leads to myxedema.

VIII. The parathyroid glands secrete parathyroid hormone (PTH), which increases calcium levels in the blood and tissue fluid.

A. PTH stimulates release of calcium from bones, stimulates calcium conservation by the kidneys, and helps activate vitamin D.

B. An increase in calcium level inhibits parathyroid hormone secretion; a decrease in calcium level stimulates secretion.

IX. The islets of Langerhans secrete insulin and glucagon, hormones that regulate the glucose level in the blood.

A. Insulin lowers the blood-sugar level by stimulating uptake and storage of glucose by the cells.

B. Glucagon raises the blood-sugar level by stimulating manufacture of glucose from glycogen and from noncarbohydrate nutrients.

X. The adrenal glands consist of the adrenal medulla and the adrenal cortex; both release hormones that help the body to cope with stress.

A. The adrenal medulla releases epinephrine and norepinephrine, hormones that increase heart rate, metabolic rate, and strength of muscle contraction and reroute the blood to organs that need more blood in times of stress.

B. The adrenal cortex releases cortisol, which promotes manufactured glucose in the liver, thereby raising the blood-sugar level; this hormone provides back-up to the adrenal medullary hormones.

C. The adrenal cortex also releases aldosterone, which helps maintain sodium and potassium balance.

XI. In response to stress the adrenal medulla initiates an alarm reaction that prepares the body physiologically to cope; secretion of cortisol by the adrenal cortex ensures a steady supply of needed nutrients for the rapidly metabolizing cells.

## POST TEST

1. Endocrine glands lack _____ and release _____.
2. A hormone may be defined as a _____ _____.
3. A second messenger important in the mechanism of action of many hormones is _____ _____.
4. The _____ serves as the link between nervous and endocrine systems.
5. The hormone _____ stimulates contraction of the uterus.
6. The hormone _____ stimulates milk production in the lactating breast.
7. Growth hormone is produced by the _____.
8. Oxytocin is produced by the _____.
9. Oxytocin is stored and released by the _____ when needed.
10. Hyoposecretion of growth hormone during childhood may result in a _____.
11. The main action of thyroid hormones is to stimulate _____.
12. The main action of glucagon is to _____.
13. Beta cells in the islets of Langerhans produce _____.
14. The appearance of glucose and ketone bodies in the urine is a symptom of _____ _____.
15. The principal glucocorticoid released by the adrenal cortex is _____.
16. Parathyroid hormone helps regulate _____ metabolism.
17. The master gland of the body is the _____; the emergency gland is the _____.

## REVIEW QUESTIONS

1. How does the hypothalamus serve as the link between the nervous and endocrine systems?
2. Contrast the functions of the anterior and posterior lobes of the pituitary gland.
3. Draw a diagram to illustrate how thyroid gland secretion is regulated by negative feedback.
4. What disorders are associated with impaired growth hormone and thyroid hormone secretion? Explain.
5. How do insulin and glucagon work together to maintain homeostasis?
6. What are the homeostatic imbalances associated with diabetes mellitus?
7. In what ways do the parathyroid glands regulate calcium balance? Which other gland secretes a hormone important in calcium balance?
8. How do the adrenal medulla and adrenal cortex work together in helping the body to cope with stress?

# IV

# INTERNAL TRANSPORT AND DEFENSE

# Blood

## OUTLINE

CHARACTERISTICS OF BLOOD
PLASMA
RED BLOOD CELLS
Life Cycle of a Red Blood Cell
Anemia
Polycythemia
WHITE BLOOD CELLS
FOCUS ON ROUTINE BLOOD TESTS
White Blood Cell Counts
Leukemia
PLATELETS
BLOOD CLOTTING
BLOOD GROUPS
Blood Transfusions
Rh Incompatibility

## LEARNING OBJECTIVES

**After you study this chapter you should be able to**
1. List six functions of the circulatory system.
2. Give the composition of blood plasma and describe the functions of plasma proteins.
4. Describe the structure and function of red blood cells.
5. Describe the structure and function of white blood cells.
6. Describe the following blood disorders: the anemias, leukemia, and polycythemia.
7. Give the origin and describe the structure and functions of a platelet.
8. Describe the formation of a platelet plug and summarize the chemical events of blood clotting.
9. Identify the antigen and antibody associated with each blood type in the ABO and Rh blood groups.
10. Explain why blood types must be carefully matched in transfusion therapy and identify the cause of erythroblastosis fetalis.

The **circulatory system** is the transportation system of the body. it delivers nutrients from the digestive system and oxygen from the lungs to all of the cells of the body. It transports wastes from the cells to the excretory organs and carries hormones from the endocrine glands to target tissues. The circulatory system also helps to regulate body temperature and fluid balance.

The circulatory system consists of two subsystems—the cardiovascular system and the lymphatic system. In the cardiovascular system the heart pumps blood through a vast system of blood vessels. The lymphatic system helps preserve fluid balance and protects the body against disease. In this chapter we will focus on the blood.

## CHARACTERISTICS OF BLOOD

Blood consists of red blood cells, white blood cells, and cell fragments called platelets, all suspended in a pale yellowish fluid called plasma (Fig. 11–1). In an adult weighing about 70 kg (154 pounds), blood volume (the amount of blood in the body) is normally about 5.6 l (about 6 quarts). The normal pH of blood is slightly alkaline, ranging between 7.35 and 7.45 (see Chapter 2 for discussion of pH).

## PLASMA

**Plasma** consists of 92% water, about 7% protein, a sprinkling of salts, and many materials being transported, including oxygen, various nutrients,

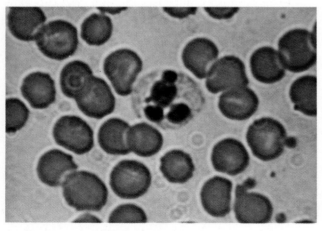

*Figure 11–1. Photomicrograph of blood. All the cells shown are red blood cells except for a single white blood cell (approximately ×1200).*

TABLE  11–1
**Some Important Components of Plasma**

| Component | Normal Range | Description |
|---|---|---|
| Water | 92% of plasma | |
| Total protein | 6–8 g/100 ml | |
| Albumins | 4–5 g/100 ml | Help maintain osmotic pressure; contribute to viscosity; transport fatty acids |
| Globulins | 2–3 g/100 ml | Some are antibodies |
| Fibrinogen | 0.3 g/100 ml | Important in clotting |
| Glucose | 70–100 mg/100 ml[1] | Nutrient in transport |
| Calcium | 8.5–10.5 mg/100 ml | |
| Urea nitrogen (BUN) | 8–25 mg/100 ml | Measurement of urea wastes in transport |
| Nonprotein nitrogen | 25–40 mg/100 ml | Nitrogen from urea and other nitrogen wastes and also from amino acids |
| Total lipids | 450–1000 mg/100 ml | |
| Cholesterol | 150–280 mg/100 ml | |
| Neutral fat | 80–240 mg/100 ml | |

[1]Also expressed as mg% or mg/dl (deciliter).

metabolic wastes, and hormones (Table 11–1). When the proteins involved in clotting have been removed, the remaining liquid is called **serum.**

Plasma proteins may be divided into three groups, or fractions: **albumins, globulins,** and **fibrinogen.** One of their homeostatic functions is to maintain blood volume. As blood flows through the tiny blood vessels called capillaries, some of the plasma seeps through the capillary walls and passes into the tissues. However, large protein molecules have difficulty passing through the capillary walls, so most of them remain in the blood. There they exert an osmotic force called **colloid osmotic pressure,** which helps pull plasma back into the blood.

Aside from their general functions some plasma proteins perform specific jobs. One group of the globulins, the **gamma globulins,** serves as **antibodies,** substances that provide immunity against disease. Fibrinogen and several other plasma proteins are involved in the clotting process. Certain albumins transport fatty acids; other albumins carry specific hormones, keeping them bound in the blood until needed and preventing their loss in urine. With the exception of the gamma globulins, which are produced in the lymph tissues, the plasma proteins are manufactured in the liver.

## RED BLOOD CELLS

**Red blood cells (RBCs),** or **erythrocytes** (ee-rith'-row-sites), are the most numerous and one of the most specialized cell types in the body. They are exquisitely adapted for the production and packaging of hemoglobin, the red pigment that transports oxygen. An adult male has about $3 \times 10^{13}$ (30 trillion) red blood cells circulating in his blood, or about 5,200,000 per cubic millimeter (mm³). A female has slightly fewer—about 4,700,00/mm³. About 3000 red blood cells lined up end to end would span only about 1 inch!

A mature red blood cell is a tiny, flexible, biconcave disc. (Biconcave means thinner in the center than around the edge.) When viewed under an ordinary light microscope the center portion of the red blood cell appears relatively clear because the cytoplasm is thinnest there. A mature red blood cell lacks a nucleus as well as most other organelles.

As blood circulates through the lungs, oxygen diffuses into the blood and into the red blood cells, where it combines weakly with hemoglobin to form oxyhemoglobin. When blood circulates through the brain or some other tissue where cells are low in oxygen, the reverse reaction occurs. The oxygen then diffuses out of the capillaries and into the cells.

Oxyhemoglobin is bright red and is responsible for the color of blood as it flows through arteries, which contain oxygen-rich blood. Reduced hemoglobin is not combined with oxygen; it is bluish in color and accounts for the darker appearance of venous blood.

## Life Cycle of a Red Blood Cell

Each second about 2.4 million red blood cells must be manufactured to replace a similar number that wear out and are destroyed. In adults the manufacture of red blood cells takes place in the red bone marrow of vertebrae, sternum, skull, and certain other bones. **Stem cells** multiply, giving rise to the blood cells. After a 3- to 5-day maturation period red blood cells squeeze through the walls of capillaries within the bone marrow and enter the circulation.

Without a nucleus and other organelles, a red blood cell is unable to synthesize proteins. When enzymes within a red blood cell break down they are not replaced. The cell becomes fragile and may rupture as it squeezes through a tight channel in the circulation. Old or damaged cells are phagocytized in the liver, spleen, or bone marrow by macrophages that are closely associated with blood vessels in these regions. The average circulating life span of a red blood cell is about 120 days.

## Anemia

A deficiency of hemoglobin, usually accompanied by a reduction in the number of red blood cells, is termed **anemia** (see Focus on Routine Blood Tests). With decreased amounts of hemoglobin, oxygen transport is reduced and cells do not receive enough oxygen. An anemic patient complains of feeling excessively tired and devoid of energy.

Three general causes of anemia are (1) loss of blood due to hemorrhage or internal bleeding, (2) decreased production of hemoglobin or red blood cells as in iron deficiency anemia, and (3) increased rate of red blood cell destruction (the **hemolytic anemias**, such as sickle cell anemia).

Two causes of decreased production of red blood cells are nutritional anemia and failure of the bone marrow to function normally (aplastic anemia). **Iron deficiency anemia** is the most common type of anemia. The body cannot synthesize hemoglobin without iron. That would be like trying to make a chocolate cake without chocolate; an essential ingredient would be missing.

**Pernicious** (per-**nish'**-us) **anemia** occurs when there is a vitamin $B_{12}$ deficiency. When this vitamin is inadequately present in the diet, or when sufficient amounts are not absorbed from the stomach, red blood cells do not mature normally. Great numbers of large, immature red blood cells pass into the circulation. These cells are fragile and rupture easily, leaving the patient deficient in oxygen-carrying capacity.

In **aplastic anemia** the bone marrow does not produce blood cells owing to injury by ionizing radiation or certain chemical substances. Benzene, arsenic, nitrogen mustard, and sometimes certain antibiotics (for example, chloramphenicol) or drugs used in cancer therapy (chemotherapy) can cause aplastic anemia.

**Sickle cell anemia** is a common type of hemolytic anemia. It is an inherited disorder caused by a mutation in the gene containing the "recipe" for making hemoglobin. The abnormal hemoglobin produced deforms the red blood cell so that it assumes a sickle shape (Fig. 11–2). These abnormal cells are fragile and are destroyed in great numbers. Sickle cell anemia is found mainly in persons of African descent. About 1% of American blacks have two genes for sickle cell anemia and exhibit symptoms of the disease. Another 8% of American blacks have one gene for sickle cell anemia and are described as having the sickle cell trait. In Africa, malaria was for centuries a major cause of death. Those with sickle cell trait are protected against the malaria parasite that lives in the blood. The spread of this mutant gene is thought to have been an advantage to natives of malaria-ridden areas.

## Polycythemia

Production of an excessive number of red blood cells is known as **polycythemia**. Secondary polycythemia may develop as a homeostatic compensation when insufficient oxygen is reaching the tissues. For example, when people move to a place with a high altitude, the decreased atmospheric pressure makes it more difficult for their hemoglobin to become saturated with oxygen. Their bodies compensate by manufacturing abnormally large numbers of red blood cells. Polycythemia also develops sometimes to compensate for the poor oxygenation typical of certain cardiovascular diseases. In **polycythemia vera**, a serious disorder of unknown origin, the number of red blood cells may double. This increases the viscosity (friction among the components) of the blood, causing it to flow sluggishly.

## WHITE BLOOD CELLS

**White blood cells (WBCs)**, or **leukocytes (loo'-koe-sites)**, defend the body against invading bacteria, viruses, and cancer cells. White blood cells develop from stem cells in the red bone marrow but some types complete their maturation elsewhere in the body. Whereas red blood cells function within the blood, many white cells leave the circulation and perform their duties in various tissues. They move through the tissues by ameboid motion, flowing along like amebas. As they wander through the body, the white blood cells phagocytize bacteria, dead cells, and foreign matter.

White blood cells may be classified in two groups, the granular leukocytes and nongranular leukocytes. **Granular leukocytes** have distinctive granules in their cytoplasm. These granules contain potent enzymes that destroy ingested bacteria.

Three types of granular leukocytes, distinguished by the staining properties of their granules, are neutrophils (**noo'**-troe-fils), basophils (**bay'**-so-fils), and eosinophils (ee-o-**sin'**-o-fils). They are illustrated in Figure 11–3 and their functions are summarized in Table 11–2. **Nongranular leukocytes** lack specific granules in their cytoplasm. This group includes the lymphocytes (**lim'**-foe-sites) and monocytes.

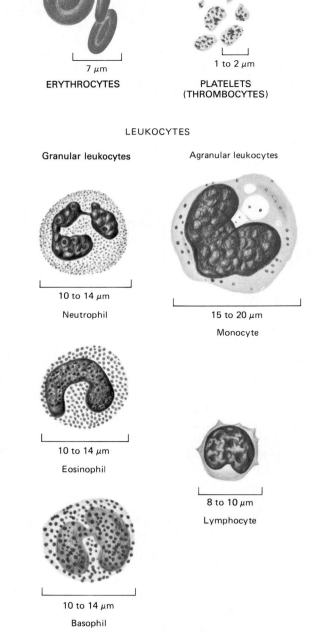

*Figure 11–3. Main types of blood cells in the circulating blood.*

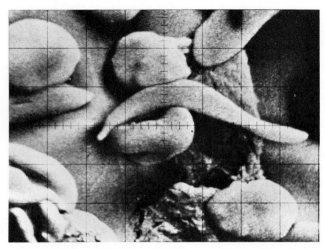

*Figure 11–2. Blood from a patient with sickle cell anemia. Note the abnormal shape of some of the red blood cells (approximately ×4000). (Courtesy of Irene Piscipe-Rodgers, Philips Electronic Instruments.)*

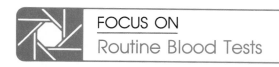
| Test | Description |
|------|-------------|
| **Complete blood count (CBC)** | Consists of four separate tests: (1) measurement of hemoglobin, (2) hematocrit, (3) white blood cell count and differential (percentage of each white cell type), (4) examination of red blood cells and platelets. (Sometimes a red blood cell count is also made.) |
| **Hemoglobin** | Hemoglobin and hematocrit tests are used to check for anemia and polycythemia and to follow the progress of an anemic patient. Normal adult value: 12–15 g/100 ml for women; 14–17 g/100 ml for men. Whole blood is treated chemically so that the hemoglobin forms a stable pigment (cyanmethemoglobin); then the optical density of the solution is measured in a photometer. (Optical density is directly proportional to concentration of hemoglobin.) |
| **Hematocrit** | Hematocrit is an indication of percentage of red cells per unit of blood volume. Normal adult values: 36–46% for women; 42–52% for men. Blood is centrifuged. Then the volume of red cells is read off a scale on the tube (see figure); expressed as percentage of whole blood volume. |
| **White blood cell count (WBC)** | Used in diagnosis of bacterial infection and in certain diseases such as leukemia. Used to monitor the effects of radiation or drug therapy that may depress WBC to dangerous levels. Whole blood is mixed with a weak acid solution for the purpose of diluting the blood and hemolyzing the red cells. The diluted blood is placed in a counting chamber (hemocytometer: a microscope slide with a well and a grid marking off tiny squares) and the white cells are counted. Then the number per cubic millimeter can be calculated. |
| **Red blood cell count (RBC)** | May be counted manually as in WBC, or an electronic cell counter may be used. |
| **Differential cell count** | Used to determine the relative number of each type of white cell in the blood. The differential cell count can be made by analysis of a stained blood smear. |
| **Platelet count** | Used in diagnosis of bleeding disorders. Blood is diluted and stained; then platelets are counted in a counting chamber. |
| **Prothrombin time (PT)** | Used when clotting disorder is suspected. Plasma is isolated from drawn blood. Calcium is added to plasma in the presence of tissue thromboplastin. Time elapsed between Ca addition and clot formation is prothrombin time (normal plasma clotting time is 12 seconds). |

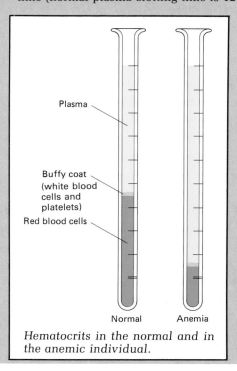

*Hematocrits in the normal and in the anemic individual.*

TABLE 11–2
**Cellular Components of Blood**

| Component | Normal Range | Function | Pathology |
|---|---|---|---|
| Red blood cells | Male: 4.2–5.4 million/$\mu$l<br>Female: 3.6–5.0 million/$\mu$l | Oxygen transport; carbon dioxide transport | Too few: anemia<br>Too many: polycythemia |
| Platelets | 150,000–400,000/$\mu$l | Essential for clotting | Clotting malfunctions; bleeding; easy bruising |
| White blood cells (WBC) (total) | 5000–10,000/$\mu$l | | |
| Neutrophils | About 60% of WBC | Phagocytosis | Too many may be due to bacterial infection, inflammation, leukemia (myelogenous) |
| Eosinophils | 1–3% of WBC | Some role in allergic response | Too many may result from allergic reaction, parasitic infection |
| Basophils | 1% of WBC | May play role in prevention of clotting in body | |
| Lymphocytes | 25–35% of WBC | Produce antibodies; destroy foreign cells | Atypical lymphocytes present in infectious mononucleosis; too many may be due to leukemia (lymphocytic), certain viral infections |
| Monocytes | 6% of WBC | Differentiate in tissues to form macrophages | May increase in monocytic leukemia, tuberculosis, fungal infections |

## White Blood Cell Counts

White blood cells are far less numerous than red blood cells, which outnumber them almost 700 to 1. Normally, an adult has about 7000 white blood cells per microliter of blood. A white blood cell count elevated above 10,000/$\mu$l, a condition called **leukocytosis** (loo″-koe-cy-**toe**′-sis), may indicate the presence of bacterial infection.

Viral infections can cause depressed white blood cell counts, a condition called **leukopenia** (loo-koe-**pee**′-nee-ah). Rheumatoid arthritis, cirrhosis of the liver, and certain other disorders are generally accompanied by leukopenia. Exposure to radiation and certain drugs, including those used in cancer chemotherapy, may also severely depress white blood cell production.

Because bacterial infections tend to increase the white blood cell count, whereas viral infections tend to decrease the white blood cell count, physicians often consider the results of blood tests before prescribing antibiotics. Such drugs (for exam-

Exposure to environmental factors such as radiation (especially during childhood) and certain chemicals have been linked to leukemia. Although no cure for leukemia has been found, radiation treatment and therapy with antimitotic drugs (drugs that inhibit cellular reproduction) can induce partial or complete remissions, lasting for months or years in some patients.

ple, penicillin and streptomycin) are effective against bacteria but do not kill viruses.

## PLATELETS

**Platelets**, or **thrombocytes**, are tiny fragments of cytoplasm that become detached from giant cells called **megakaryocytes** in the bone marrow. Platelets number about 300,000/$\mu$l of circulating blood—more than a quarter of a billion per cubic millimeter. These cell fragments function in **hemostasis** (he-mow-**stay**′-sis), prevention of blood loss. They physically plug breaks in blood vessel walls and they release chemicals that promote clotting.

## BLOOD CLOTTING

Within 2 seconds after a blood vessel is cut, the wall of the vessel contracts, slowing the flow of blood through the injured region. During this time platelets adhere to collagen fibers exposed when the blood vessel lining is damaged. These platelets release the compound ADP (adenosine diphosphate), which causes platelets to become sticky and activates other platelets. Great numbers of platelets accumulate at the injured site, forming a

## Leukemia

**Leukemia** is a form of cancer in which white blood cells multiply wildly within the bone marrow. They crowd out developing red blood cells and platelets, leading to anemia and impaired blood clotting. A common cause of death from leukemia is internal hemorrhaging, especially in the brain. Although there may be a dramatic rise in the white blood cell count, many of the white blood cells are immature or abnormal and are unable to protect the body against disease. Thus, death in leukemia patients often results from bacterial infection.

**platelet plug**, which can stop blood loss completely if the tear in the blood vessel wall is sufficiently small.

A more permanent blood clot begins to form within 20 seconds of a serious injury, or within 2 minutes of a minor wound. The process of blood clotting, called **coagulation**, leads to the formation of a blood clot, a gel consisting of insoluble fibers and trapped blood cells and platelets. More than 30 different substances that affect clotting have been found in the blood.

Although the process of blood clotting is quite complex, we can summarize its three main steps.

1. In response to damaged tissue, a series of reactions takes place involving certain proteins in the blood called **clotting factors**. This results in formation of a complex of substances known as **prothrombin activator**.
2. The prothrombin activator catalyzes the conversion of a plasma globulin called **prothrombin** to its active form, **thrombin**. Calcium ions must be present for this reaction to take place. Prothrombin is manufactured in the liver with the help of vitamin K.
3. The thrombin acts as an enzyme to convert the plasma protein fibrinogen to **fibrin**, a fibrous protein that forms long fibrin threads. These threads form the webbing of the clot. They trap blood cells, platelets, and plasma, which help to strengthen the clot.

Within a few minutes after clot formation the clot begins to contract and squeezes out serum, that is, plasma containing neither fibrinogen nor clotting factors. As the clot contracts, the ends of the damaged blood vessel are pulled closer together and the clot itself becomes smaller and harder. The clotting process is summarized in Figure 11–4 (also see Fig. 11–5).

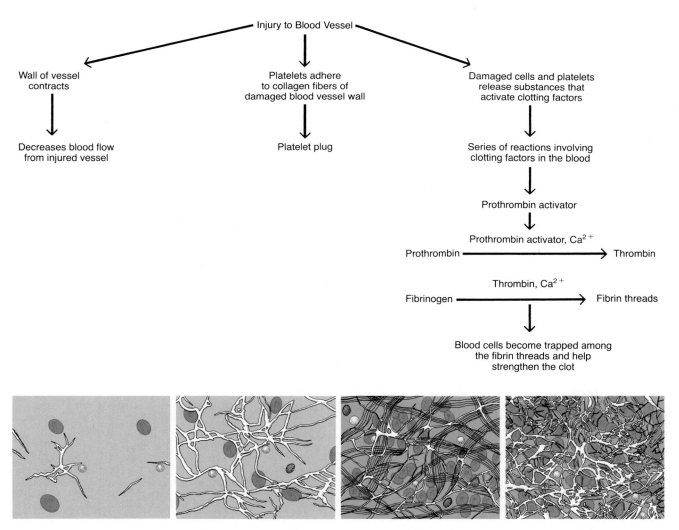

***Figure 11–4.*** *Overview of blood clotting. Fibrin threads form the webbing of the clot. Blood cells, platelets, and plasma become trapped among the fibrin threads and help to strengthen the clot.*

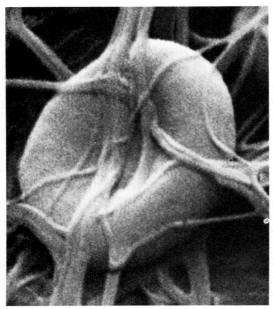

**Figure 11–5.** *Scanning electron micrograph of a red blood cell enmeshed in fibrin (approximately ×14,000). (From Emil Bernstein: Science, 173: cover photo, August 27, 1971. Copyright 1971 by the American Association for the Advancement of Science.)*

In persons with **hemophilia** ("bleeder's disease"), one of the clotting factors is absent owing to a genetic mutation. Transfusion of the appropriate purified clotting factor (or of normal fresh plasma) into a hemophiliac relieves the tendency to bleed for a few days.

Clots do not usually form in intact blood vessels because the lining is smooth and is coated with a layer of negatively charged proteins that repel the platelets and clotting factors. When injured or diseased, however, the lining becomes rough and loses its negative charge. Platelets are then attracted to the roughened blood vessel lining, where they may be damaged, and initiate a clotting reaction. A clot that forms within a blood vessel is called a **thrombus** (throm′-bus). A thrombus may become so large that the flow of blood through the vessel is impeded. Anticoagulants in the blood usually help to prevent abnormal clotting.

## BLOOD GROUPS

Red blood cells have specific proteins known as **antigens** (an′-tih-jins) on their surfaces. These antigens are different in persons with different blood types. Specific types of antibodies found in the plasma are associated with some blood types. Although there are several blood typing systems, the most important clinically are the ABO and Rh systems.

Based on the **ABO system**, each of us has type A, B, AB, or O blood. Those with type A blood have type A antigen on the surface of their red blood cells (Fig. 11–6). They also have anti-B antibodies, which circulate in the plasma and act against type B antigens. Individuals with type B blood have red blood cells coated with type B antigen and have type A antibody. Those with type AB have both types of antigen and neither type of antibody. Persons with type O blood have neither A nor B antigens but they have antibodies against both A and B (Table 11–3).

Named in honor of the rhesus monkeys in which it was originally worked out, the **Rh system** consists of at least eight different kinds of Rh antibodies, each referred to as an *Rh factor*. By far the most important is antigen D. Most persons of western European descent are Rh-positive, which means that they have antigen D on the surfaces of their red blood cells (as well as the antigens of the ABO system appropriate to their blood type). The 15% or so of the population who are Rh-negative have no antigen D and will produce antibodies against that antigen when exposed to Rh-positive blood. Unlike the antibodies of the ABO system, antibody D does not occur in the blood of Rh-negative persons unless they have been exposed to the D antigen. However, once antibodies to Rh blood have been produced, they remain in the blood.

## Blood Transfusions

Transfusing blood from a healthy person to a patient is a routine, life-saving procedure. During surgery or after hemorrhage whole blood can be transfused to restore an adequate volume of circulating blood. Blood components can be separated by centrifuging (spinning the blood at high speed so that the heavier components settle at the bottom of a tube) (see figure in Focus on Routine Blood Tests). Then, plasma itself can be used to expand blood volume in patients who are in circulatory shock (discussed in Chapter 13). Plasma is also sometimes used to supply needed clotting factors. Packed red blood cells are given to patients with severe anemia or those whose blood is otherwise deficient in oxygen-carrying capacity. Similarly, white blood cells or platelets can be transfused in patients whose bone marrow is not producing these blood components adequately. Whole blood or blood components can be stored in blood banks and withdrawn as needed.

In transfusing blood, the blood of the donor must be carefully matched with the blood of the recipi-

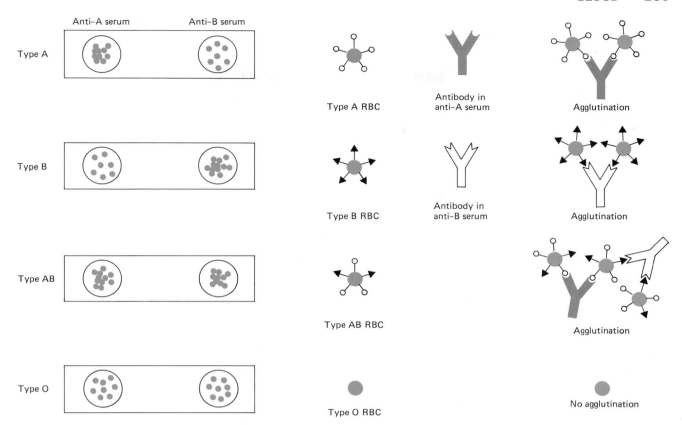

**Figure 11–6.** *Typing blood. Each blood type has a different combination of antigen and antibody. In typing blood, serum containing antibody to type A blood is placed on a slide and serum containing antibody to type B is placed on a separate area of the slide. A drop of blood is mixed with each type of serum. If the blood contains A antigen, it will agglutinate with the anti-A serum. If the blood contains B antigen, it will agglutinate with the anti-B serum.*

ent. If the blood is not compatible, a **transfusion reaction** will occur. This is a serious allergic reaction in which antibodies in the recipient's blood attack the foreign red blood cells in the transfused blood, causing them to **agglutinate** (clump). Red blood cells may break, releasing hemoglobin into the plasma, a process known as **hemolysis**. For example, if a patient with type A blood is accidentally given type B blood, her or his antibodies will combine with the type B antigens on the surfaces of the donated red blood cells, causing them to agglutinate and producing hemolysis. This could prove fatal. Blood typing is routinely carried out by mixing a sample of a person's blood with serum containing different types of antibodies to determine if agglutination occurs. (Fig. 11–6).

## Rh Incompatibility

Although several kinds of maternal-fetal blood type incompatibilities are known, Rh incompatibility is probably the most important. Rh incompatibility can cause serious problems when an Rh-negative woman and an Rh-positive man produce an Rh-positive baby. At the time of birth a small amount of the baby's blood may mix with the mother's, stimulating her body to produce antibodies against the Rh-positive blood. If she should carry an Rh-positive child in a subsequent pregnancy,* her antibodies can cross the placenta (the organ of exchange between mother and developing baby) and cause hemolysis of the baby's red blood cells (Fig. 11–7). Breakdown products of the hemoglobin released into the circulation damage many organs, including the brain. This type of hemolytic disease is known as **erythroblastosis** (ee-rith-row-blas-**toé**-sis) **fetalis**.

When Rh incompatibility problems are suspected, blood can be exchanged in utero, that is, while the child is still within the mother's uterus. An Rh-negative woman is now treated immediately after childbirth with an anti-Rh drug that clears the Rh-positive cells from her blood quickly, minimizing the change of her sensitizing her own white blood cells. As a result, her cells do not produce the anti-D that could harm her next baby.

---

*Rh incompatibility often develops slowly over a period of several pregnancies.

TABLE 11–3
**ABO Blood Types[1]**

| Blood Type | Antigen on RBC | Antibodies in Plasma |
|---|---|---|
| O | | Anti-A, anti-B |
| A | A | Anti-B |
| B | B | Anti-A |
| AB | A, B | |

[1]This table and the discussion of the ABO system have been simplified somewhat. Actually, some type A individuals have two type A antigens and are designated type $A_1$, whereas those with only one antigen are termed type $A_2$.

## SUMMARY

I. The circulatory system transports nutrients, oxygen, wastes, and hormones; helps regulate body temperature; and protects the body against disease.

II. Blood consists of red blood cells, white blood cells, and platelets suspended in plasma.

III. Blood plasma consists of about 92% water, about 7% plasma proteins, salts, nutrients, oxygen and other gases, hormones, and wastes. Three fractions of plasma proteins are albumins, globulins, and fibrinogen.

IV. Red blood cells, or erythrocytes, are tiny, biconcave discs that transport hemoglobin.

V. White blood cells, or leukocytes, defend the body against pathogens and other foreign substances.

A. Granular leukocytes include the neutrophils, basophils, and eosinophils.

B. Nongranular leukocytes include the lymphocytes and monocytes.

VI. Platelets are cell fragments formed from megakaryocytes in the bone marrow; they function in hemostasis.

VII. In hemostasis platelets patch tears in blood vessel walls by aggregating and forming a platelet plug. Platelets also release chemicals that promote blood clotting.

VIII. Blood is typed on the basis of specific antigens on the surfaces of red blood cells.

A. People with type A blood have type A antigen and type B antibodies.

B. People with type B blood have type B antigen and type A antibodies.

C. People with type AB blood have both

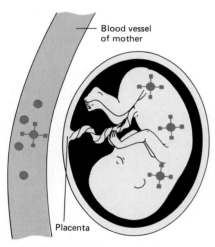

Blood vessel of mother

Placenta

A few Rh+ RBCs leak across the placenta from the fetus into the mother's blood

(a)

The mother produces anti-Rh antibodies in response to Rh antigen on Rh+ RBCs

(b)

Anti-Rh antibodies cross the placenta and enter the blood of the fetus. Hemolysis of Rh+ blood occurs. The fetus may develop erythroblastosis fetalis.

(c)

● Rh— RBC of mother

Rh+ RBC of fetus with Rh antigen on surface

Anti-Rh antibody made against Rh+ RBC

Hemolysis of Rh+ RBC

***Figure 11–7.*** *Rh incompatibility can cause serious problems when an Rh-negative woman and an Rh-positive man produce Rh-positive offspring. (a) Some $Rh^+$ red blood cells (RBCs) leak across the placenta from the fetus into the mother's blood. (b) The woman produces antibodies in response to the D antigen on the $Rh^+$ RBCs. (c) Some of the D antibodies cross the placenta and enter the blood of the fetus, causing hemolysis. The fetus may develop erythroblastosis fetalis.*

types of antigens and those with type O blood have neither type of antigen but both types of antibodies.

D. People with Rh-positive blood have antigen D on the surface of their red blood cells, as well as the antigens of the appropriate ABO type. Rh-negative individuals may produce antibody D when exposed to antigen D.

IX. In transfusion therapy blood types must be carefully matched to prevent transfusion reaction.

## POST TEST

1. The function of red blood cells is to transport _____.
2. The liquid portion of the blood is called _____.
3. Some of the gamma globulins serve as _____.
4. Fibrinogen functions in blood _____.
5. Red blood cells are produced in the _____ _____.
6. A deficiency of hemoglobin is called _____.
7. The function of white blood cells is to _____
8. Leukocytosis refers to an elevation of the _____ _____ _____ _____ count.
9. Platelets are formed from large cells in the _____ _____.
10. Fibrinogen is converted to _____ in the presence of a catalyst called _____.
11. A clot formed within a blood vessel is a _____.
12. A person with type B blood has _____ antigens on the surfaces of his or her red blood cells and _____ antibodies in his or her plasma.
13. Erythroblastosis fetalis may occur when there is _____ incompatibility. This may occur when a woman with _____ _____ type blood produces a baby with _____ type blood.

## REVIEW QUESTIONS

1. List five functions of the circulatory system and identify which specific blood components carry out each job.
2. What are the functions of the plasma proteins as a group? of globulins specifically?
3. In what ways are mature red blood cells specifically adapted to their function?
4. Give three general causes of anemia.
5. What are the functions of platelets? Explain.
6. Imagine that a patient with type AB blood is accidentally given type A blood in a transfusion. What, if any, ill effects might occur? What if a patient with type O blood is given type A blood?
7. Describe the physiological cause of the disease erythroblastosis fetalis.

# The Heart

LEARNING OBJECTIVES

**After you study this chapter you should be able to**
1. Locate the heart in the mediastinum.
2. Describe the structure of the pericardium and of the wall of the heart.
3. Identify the chambers of the heart and compare their structures.
4. Locate the atrioventricular and semilunar valves, compare their structures, and describe how they function.
5. Trace the path of an action potential through the conduction system of the heart.
6. Compare and contrast cardiac muscle with skeletal muscle.
7. Describe the events of the cardiac cycle, define systole and diastole, and correlate normal heart sounds with the events of the cardiac cycle.
8. Define cardiac output and identify the factors that determine it.
9. Explain how the nervous system regulates the heart rate and identify other factors that influence the heart rate.
10. Relate Starling's law of the heart to cardiac output.
11. Correlate the principal waves of a normal EKG with the events of the cardiac cycle. Describe common arrhythmias and other disorders that can be diagnosed with the help of the EKG.

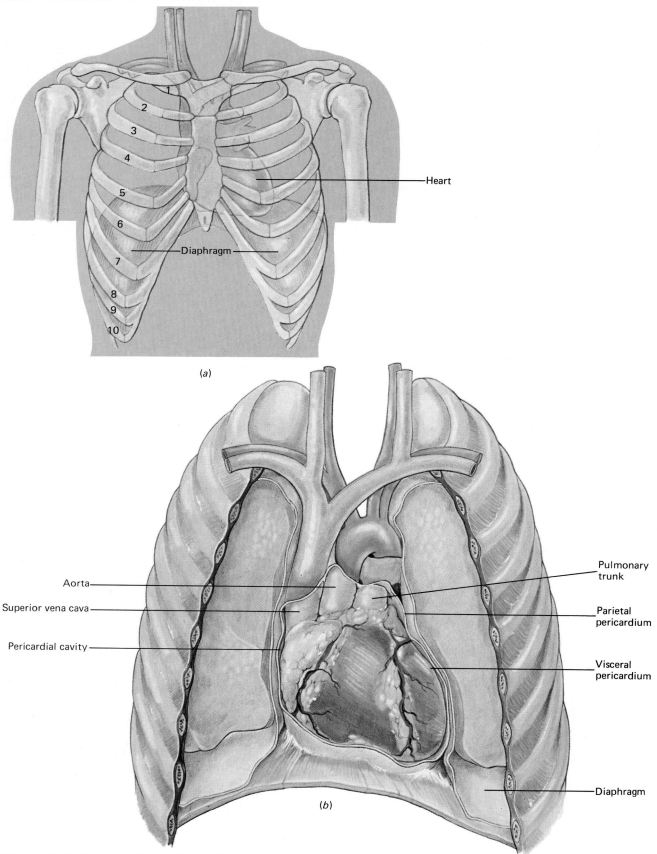

(a)

(b)

**Figure 12–1.** The heart lies in the mediastinum between the lungs. Its apex rests on the diaphragm. The heart and the roots of the great blood vessels are loosely enclosed by the pericardium.

In an average lifetime the heart pumps about 300 million l (80 million gallons) of blood through the vast complex of blood vessels that bring oxygen and nourishment to the cells of the body. This hollow, muscular organ is not much bigger than a fist and weighs less than a pound. Ever sensitive to the changing needs of the body, it can vary its output from 5 to 35 l of blood per minute.

## LOCATION OF THE HEART

The heart lies well protected in the mediastinum and is flanked by the lungs. About two-thirds of this cone-shaped organ lies to the left of the body's midline (Fig. 12–1). The base of the heart, its broad end, is its superior aspect and lies beneath the second rib. Its apex, or pointed end, points downward and to the left and rests on the diaphragm. When you place your fingers on the left side of the chest between the fifth and sixth ribs, you can feel the apical pulse each time the heart beats, bringing the apex in contact with the chest wall.

## COVERING OF THE HEART

The heart and the origins of the great blood vessels are enclosed in a loose-fitting sac called the **pericardium** (per-ih-**kar'**-dee-um). This protective covering consists of an outer layer called the **parietal pericardium** and an inner layer called the **visceral pericardium**. The parietal pericardium forms a strong sac for the heart and helps to anchor it within the mediastinum. The visceral portion of the pericardium forms the outer layer of the heart.

Between the visceral and parietal pericardia is a potential space, the **pericardial cavity** (Fig. 12–1). Normally, a thin film of lubricating fluid moistens the apposing surfaces, facilitating smooth movement of the heart as it contracts and relaxes.

> Inflammation of the pericardium, called **pericarditis**, may occur following some types of infections or may accompany certain diseases. In pericarditis, abnormal accumulation of pericardial fluid or fibrous adhesions between the layers of the pericardium may occur, interfering with normal heart function.

## THE HEART WALL

From the inside out, the layers of the heart are the endocardium, myocardium, and visceral pericardium. The **endocardium** (en"-doe-**kar'**-dee-um) consists of a smooth endothelial lining resting on connective tissue. By far the greatest bulk of the heart wall consists of **myocardium** (my"-o-**kar**-dee-um), the cardiac muscle that contracts to pump the blood. The outer layer of the heart is the visceral pericardium. The wall of the heart is richly supplied with nerves, blood vessels, and lymph vessels.

## CHAMBERS OF THE HEART

The heart consists of four chambers: right atrium, right ventricle, left atrium, and left ventricle (Figs. 12–2 and 12–3). The **atria** receive blood returning to the heart from the veins and act as reservoirs between contractions of the heart. The **ventricles** pump blood into the great arteries leaving the heart.

The heart is actually a double pump. The right side receives **deoxygenated blood** (blood somewhat depleted of its oxygen supply) returning from the tissues and organs and pumps it into the **pulmonary circulation**. **Pulmonary arteries** convey blood to the lungs, where gases are exchanged. **Pulmonary veins** then return oxygen-rich blood to the left side of the heart. This oxygenated blood is pumped into the **systemic circulation**, the network of blood vessels that serves all of the body systems.

Right and left sides of the heart are separated by walls or **septa** (Fig. 12–3). Between the atria is the **interatrial** (in"-ter-**a'**-tree-al) **septum**; between the ventricles is the **interventricular** (in"-ter-ven-**trik'**-u-lar) **septum**. On the interatrial septum a shallow depression, the **fossa ovalis**, marks the place where an opening called the **foramen ovale** existed in the fetus. Before birth this opening permitted blood to flow directly from right atrium to left atrium, diverting blood from the fetus's nonfunctioning lungs. A small, muscular pouch called an **auricle** increases the surface area of each atrium (Fig. 12–3).

The walls of the atria are thinner than those of the ventricles. This is probably because their job is to pump blood into the ventricles, which requires much less force than pumping blood into the blood vessels. The left ventricle has the thickest wall; it must create sufficient pressure to force blood into the **aorta** (ay-**or'**-ta) (the largest artery in the body) and on through the thousands of miles of blood vessels in the systemic circulation.

The right atrium, which receives blood returning from all parts of the systemic circulation, is slightly larger than the left. This blood is delivered

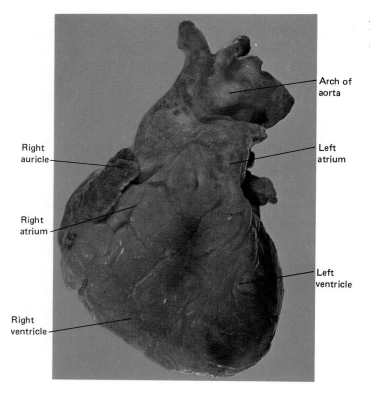

*Figure 12–2.* Photograph of human heart, anterior view. (Courtesy of Phil Horne, Stanford University School of Medicine.)

Arch of aorta

Right auricle

Left atrium

Right atrium

Left ventricle

Right ventricle

by two large veins, the **inferior vena cava** and the **superior vena cava**. The **coronary sinus**, which returns blood from the heart wall, also opens into the right atrium. The left atrium receives oxygenated blood from the four pulmonary veins.

The right ventricle pumps blood into the **pulmonary trunk**, the large common stem of the two pulmonary arteries. The thick-walled left ventricle, which pumps blood into the aorta, forms the apex of the heart.

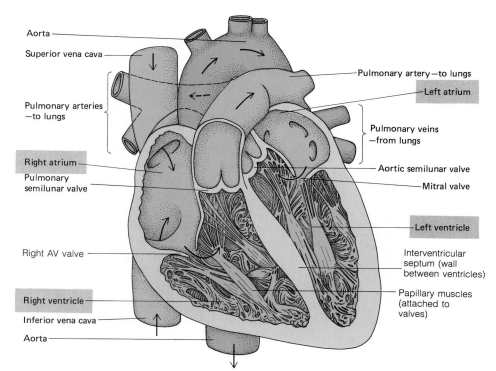

Aorta

Superior vena cava

Pulmonary arteries —to lungs

Right atrium

Pulmonary semilunar valve

Right AV valve

Right ventricle

Inferior vena cava

Aorta

Pulmonary artery—to lungs

Left atrium

Pulmonary veins —from lungs

Aortic semilunar valve

Mitral valve

Left ventricle

Interventricular septum (wall between ventricles)

Papillary muscles (attached to valves)

*Figure 12–3.* Internal view of the heart showing chambers, valves, and connecting blood vessels. Arrows indicate the direction of blood flow.

Irregular muscle columns project from the inner surface of both ventricles. One set of these, the **papillary (pap'-il-ler"-ee) muscles**, are continuous with the **chordae tendineae (kor'-dee ten'-di-nee)** ("heart strings"), cords of connective tissue attached to the edges of the valves between the atria and ventricles.

## VALVES

After blood is pumped from either atrium into the corresponding ventricle, pressure in the ventricle becomes greater than in the atrium. When the atrium relaxes, blood must be prevented from flowing back into it. To prevent such backflow of blood, an **atrioventricular (a"-tree-o-ven-trik'-u-lar) (AV) valve** guards the passageway between each atrium and ventricle (Fig. 12–3).

Each AV valve consists of flaps or **cusps** of fibrous tissues that project from the heart wall. The AV valve between the right atrium and the right ventricle has three cusps and is appropriately named the **tricuspid valve**. The left AV valve, with only two cusps, is called the **bicuspid valve** but is more frequently referred to as the **mitral valve**.

As stated previously, the cusps of the AV valves are anchored to papillary muscles by the chordae tendineae (Fig. 12–4). As blood fills the atria, the pressure on the AV valves increases, forcing them open into the ventricles. Then, as the ventricles contract, blood is forced back against the valves, pushing them closed. However, contraction of the papillary muscles and tensing of the chordae tendineae prevent these valves from opening backward into the atria. You might think of them as swinging doors that swing in only one direction.

**Semilunar (Sem"-ee-loo'-nar) valves**, so named because their three cusps are shaped like half moons, guard the exits from the ventricles. The semilunar valve between the left ventricle and the aorta is known as the **aortic valve** and the one between the right ventricle and the pulmonary trunk as the **pulmonary valve**.

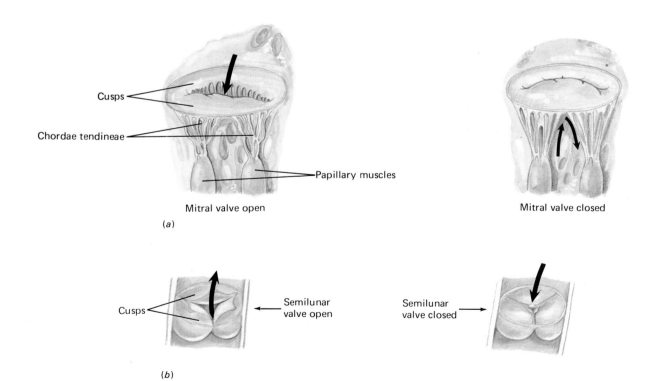

Cusps

Chordae tendineae

Papillary muscles

Mitral valve open

(a)

Mitral valve closed

Cusps

Semilunar valve open

Semilunar valve closed

(b)

*Figure 12–4. How the valves of the heart work. (a) The mitral valve in the open and closed positions. (b) A semilunar valve in the open and closed positions.*

Valve deformities sometimes occur as birth defects but more often develop following inflammation. Rheumatic fever and syphilis are two diseases that often lead to valve deformity. One of the more common valve deformities is **mitral stenosis**, a narrowing of the opening of the mitral valve. In this condition, the valve is thickened and thus impedes the flow of blood from the left atrium into the left ventricle. Mitral stenosis is almost always the result of rheumatic fever inflammation.

Another valve problem occurs when a valve cusp is shortened, preventing the valve from closing completely and allowing blood to be regurgitated in the wrong direction. This condition is known as **valvular insufficiency**. Mitral valve defects result in the accumulation of blood in the left atrium. In such cases blood backs up into the pulmonary circulation, increasing pulmonary blood pressure and possibly causing pulmonary edema. Diseased valves can sometimes be surgically removed and replaced with artificial valves.

## CONDUCTION SYSTEM

The horror film heart that beats spookily after being separated from the body of its owner is not totally a product of overactive imaginations; some script writers may have rooted their fantasies in a knowledge of cardiac physiology. When removed from the body the heart can continue to beat for many hours if it is perfused with appropriate nutrients and salts. This is possible because the heart has its own specialized conduction system and can beat independently of its nerve supply.

The heart's conduction system includes the sinoatrial node, the atrioventricular node, and the atrioventricular bundle (Fig. 12–5). These structures are composed of specialized types of cardiac muscle. The **sinoatrial (SA) node** is a small mass of specialized muscle in the posterior wall of the right atrium. Because automatic self-excitation of the SA node initiates each heartbeat, the SA node is known as the **pacemaker** of the heart. The ends of the fibers of the SA node fuse with surrounding ordinary atria muscle fibers so that the action potential spreads through the atria, producing atrial contraction.

One group of atrial muscle fibers conducts the action potential directly to the **atrioventricular (AV) node**, located in the right atrium along the lower part of the septum. Here transmission is delayed briefly, allowing time for the atria to complete their contractions before the ventricles begin to contract.

From the AV node the action potential spreads into specialized muscle fibers called **Purkinje fibers**, which form the **atrioventricular (AV) bundle**

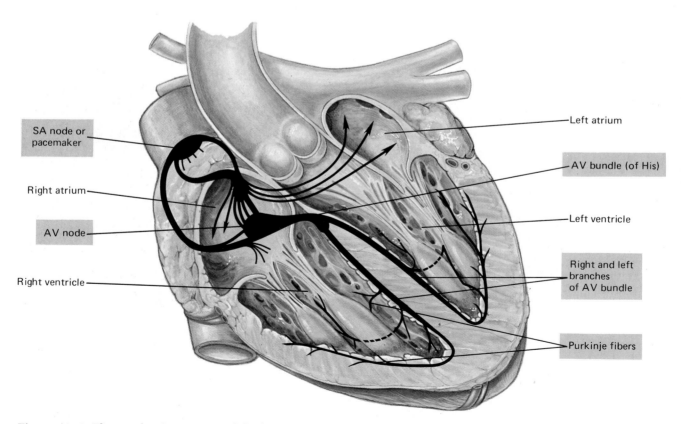

**Figure 12–5.** *The conduction system of the heart.*

(also called the **bundle of His**). The large Purkinje fibers conduct impulses about six times faster than ordinary cardiac muscle fibers. The AV bundle divides into right and left Purkinje bundles, which extend into the right and left ventricles just beneath the endocardium. Each bundle then divides into smaller branches. The terminal Purkinje fibers extend beneath the endocardium and penetrate about one-third of the way into the myocardium. Their fibers end on fibers of ordinary cardiac muscle within the myocardium, so that after an impulse reaches the ends of the Purkinje fibers, it spreads through the ordinary muscle fibers of the ventricles.

## CARDIAC MUSCLE

In some ways cardiac is similar to skeletal muscle. It is striated, has dark Z lines, and has myofibrils that contain actin and myosin filaments. During contraction these filaments slide over one another just as in skeletal muscle contraction.

In several ways, though, cardiac muscle is unique. It is capable of contracting without being triggered by a nerve impulse. Another feature of cardiac muscle is its characteristic branching (Fig. 12–6). Cardiac muscle cells are separated at their ends by dense bands called **intercalated** (in-**ter'**-kah-lay-ted) **discs**. These discs are specialized junctions between the cardiac muscle cells. Physi-

ologically, these junctions are of great significance because they offer little resistance to the passage of an action potential. Stimulation of a single muscle fiber results in contraction of all the muscle fibers.

## THE CARDIAC CYCLE

The sequence of events that occurs during one complete heartbeat is referred to as the **cardiac cycle**. Each complete cycle lasts for about 0.8 second and occurs about 72 times per minute. It consists of both a contraction, in which blood is forced out of the heart, and a subsequent relaxation, in which the heart fills with blood. The period of contraction is known as **systole** (**sis'**-toe-lee); the period of relaxation is **diastole** (die-**as'**-toe-lee).

Each cardiac cycle begins with the spontaneous generation of an action potential in the SA node that spreads throughout the myocardium, resulting in contraction of the atria. Blood is forced from the two atria into the two ventricles. As the atria contract, the AV valves are open, but the semilunar valves are closed (Fig. 12–7). As the atria relax, they are filled with blood from the veins. During this time the AV valves are closed and the ventricles are contracting, forcing blood through the semilunar valves into the aorta and pulmonary arteries. Then, as the ventricles begin to relax, the aortic and pulmonary valves close, the tricuspid

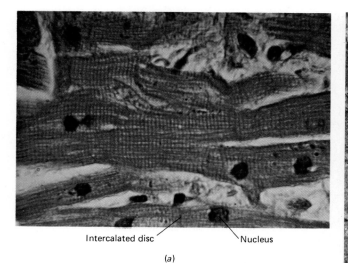

Intercalated disc      Nucleus

*(a)*

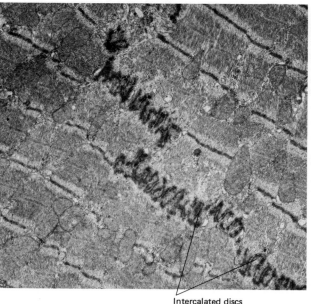

Intercalated discs

*(b)*

***Figure 12–6.*** *Cardiac muscle. (a) Cardiac muscle as seen with the light microscope (approximately ×400). (b) An electron micrograph of cardiac muscle. (Courtesy of Lyle C. Dearden.)*

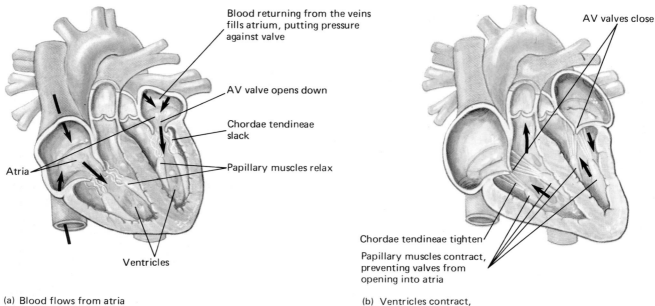

Blood returning from the veins
fills atrium, putting pressure
against valve

AV valve opens down

Chordae tendineae
slack

Papillary muscles relax

Atria

Ventricles

(a) Blood flows from atria
to ventricles

Atria contract
forcing additional
blood into ventricles

AV valves close

Chordae tendineae tighten

Papillary muscles contract,
preventing valves from
opening into atria

(b) Ventricles contract,
forcing blood against
valve cusps

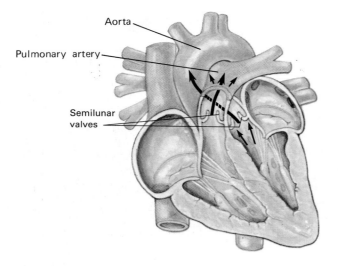

Aorta

Pulmonary artery

Semilunar
valves

(c) When ventricles
contract, blood is
pushed up against
semilunar valves,
forcing them open

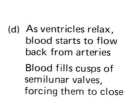

(d) As ventricles relax,
blood starts to flow
back from arteries

Blood fills cusps of
semilunar valves,
forcing them to close

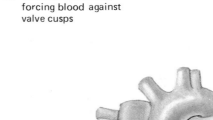

*Figure 12–7. Blood flow through the heart during the cardiac cycle.*

and mitral valves open, and blood flows into the
ventricles so that the cycle may begin again. At the
time the atria are contracting, the ventricles are relaxed. Then the atria relax during ventricular systole and remain relaxed during the first part of
ventricular diastole.

## HEART SOUNDS

When you listen to the heart through a stethoscope you can hear certain characteristic sounds,
usually described as a **"lub-dup."** These sounds
are produced each time the valves close. The first

sound, the "lub," marks the beginning of ventricular systole. Heard as a low-pitched, relatively long sound, it is caused by the closure of the mitral and tricuspid valves as the ventricles begin to contract.

The second sound marks the beginning of ventricular diastole and is caused by the closing of the aortic and pulmonary valves. Because these valves close rapidly, the "dup" sound is heard as a quick snap. Diastole is longer than systole, so when the heart is beating at a normal rate there is a slight pause after the second sound. Thus one hears, "lub-dup" pause, "lub-dup" pause. Sometimes a third normal sound can be heard, although it is faint and difficult to hear even with a stethoscope. This sound is caused by blood rushing into the partially filled ventricles.

> Abnormal heart sounds also occur commonly and some of them give the physician valuable diagnostic information. For instance, one common type of abnormal sound, a **heart murmur**, is the result of turbulence. The turbulence sets up vibrations that give rise to sound waves. Sometimes, as during strenuous exercise, a murmur may be heard even in a healthy heart as a result of blood flowing so fast that turbulence occurs. More often, though, a murmur indicates a valve disorder. When the valve does not close properly it allows blood to flow backward (regurgitation). When this occurs, a hiss may be heard.
>
> Characteristic murmurs may also be detected when a valve becomes narrowed and rough. In **aortic stenosis** (narrowing of the lumen of the aorta), passage of blood from the left ventricle into the aorta is impeded. During systole, therefore, the blood is forced through the narrowed opening in a small stream but at tremendous speed. This causes a great deal of turbulence within the aorta, resulting in intense vibration and a loud murmur.

## CARDIAC OUTPUT

The volume of blood pumped by one ventricle during one beat is called the **stroke volume**. By multiplying the stroke volume by the number of times the ventricles beat per minute (the **heart rate**), one can calculate the cardiac output. **Cardiac output** is the volume of blood pumped by one ventricle in 1 minute. In a resting adult the heart might beat about 72 times per minute and pump about 70 ml of blood with each contraction.

$$\text{Cardiac output} = \text{stroke volume} \times \text{heart rate}$$
$$= \frac{70 \text{ ml}}{\text{stroke}} \times \frac{72 \text{ strokes}}{\text{min}}$$
$$= 5040 \text{ ml/min} \ (5.04 \text{ l/min})$$

During stress, such as exercise, the normal heart can increase its cardiac output four to five times, so that up to 25 l of blood can be pumped per minute. An athlete's heart can increase its output up to seven times. From the equation above, it should be clear that cardiac output can be varied by a change in either the stroke volume or the heart rate (Fig. 12–8). How are these mechanisms regulated?

## Regulation of Heart Rate

Although the heart is capable of beating independently, it is able to adapt its rate to the changing needs of the body because it is carefully regulated by the nervous system. A number of other factors, including hormones, ion concentration, and change in body temperature, can influence the heart rate.

The heart is innervated by parasympathetic nerves that slow its rate and by sympathetic nerves that speed it up. Parasympathetic innervation originates in the cardiac centers in the medulla and passes to the heart by way of the vagus nerves. Vagus nerve fibers richly supply the SA and AV nodes. When stimulated, these parasympathetic nerves release acetycholine, which slows the heart. Normally, the parasympathetic nerves are the dominant neural influence of the heart.

Sympathetic nerves that serve the heart originate in the upper thoracic portion of the spinal cord and reach the myocardium by way of several nerves sometimes called **accelerator nerves**. These nerves supply the nodes and also the muscle fibers themselves. When stimulated, they release norepinephrine, which increases the heart rate, as well as the strength of ventricular contraction.

The cardiac centers in the medulla maintain a balance between the inhibitory effects of the parasympathetic nerves and the stimulating effects of the sympathetic nerves. Various parts of the circulatory system send messages (for example, regarding blood pressure) to the cardiac centers. These centers respond by sending messages via parasympathetic nerves to the heart. When parasympathetic messages decrease, the sympathetic nerves are able to dominate and increase the heart rate.

During stress, epinephrine and norepinephrine released from the adrenal medulla accelerate the heartbeat. An elevated body temperature can greatly increase heart rate. A heart rate of more than 100 beats per minute commonly occurs during fever. On the other hand, heart rate decreases when the body temperature is lowered. This is why a patient's temperature is sometimes deliberately lowered during heart surgery.

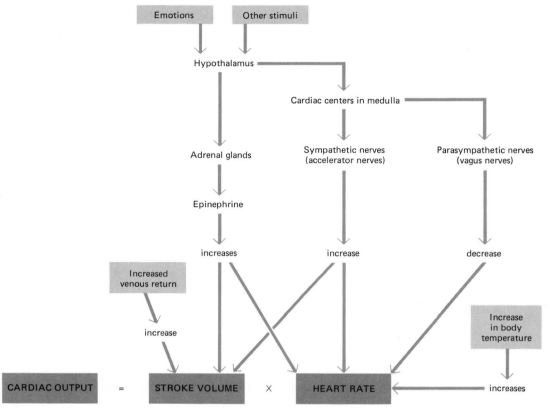

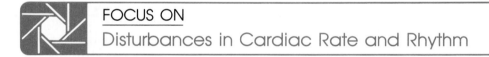

***Figure 12–8.*** *Some factors that influence cardiac output.*

## FOCUS ON
## Disturbances in Cardiac Rate and Rhythm

Although rapid or slow heart rates sometimes occur in individuals with normal hearts, these conditions can indicate cardiac disorders. **Tachycardia** (tak″-ee-**kar′**-dee-ah) (from *tachy*, "fast", and *cardia*, "heart") means fast heart rate, usually defined as more than 100 beats per minute. Tachycardia may be caused by fever, stimulation of the heart by its sympathetic nerves, certain hormones or drugs, or weakening of the heart muscle. When the myocardium cannot pump blood effectively, homeostatic reflexes are activated that increase the heart rate.

**Bradycardia** (brad″-ee-**kar′**-dee-ah) (from *brady*, meaning "slow") describes a heart rate of less than 60 beats per minute. This condition is common in athletes. Bradycardia may also result from decreased body temperature, certain drugs, or stimulation of the heart by its parasympathetic nerves. Bradycardia may occur in patients with atherosclerotic lesions in the carotid sinus region of the carotid artery. (The carotid sinus will be discussed in Chapter 13.)

Any variation from the normal *rhythm* of the heart beat is called an **arrhythmia** (ah-**rith′**-me-ah).

In **atrial flutter** the atria may contract about 300 times per minute, contracting two or three times for every one ventricular contraction. This arrhythmia is often due to dilation of the atria as a result of diseased valve.

In **fibrillation** the heart beats rapidly and its contractions are incoordinated. Numerous small waves of depolarization may spread in all directions through the myocardium so that the heart cannot contract as a whole and thus cannot pump blood. A patient can live for many years with **atrial fibrillation** because venous pressure continues to force blood into the ventricles. The effectiveness of the heart may be reduced up to 30% but this level of functioning is sufficient to sustain life. However, **ventricular fibrillation** can result in rapid death because in this conditon blood is not pumped into the arteries. About one out of every four persons dies in ventricular fibrillation. There are many causes of this condition, including electrical shock, inadequate oxygen to the heart muscle, heart attacks, injury, and effects of certain drugs. When a heart is in ventricular fibrillation, it cannot restore its normal rhythm by itself.

Clinically, the heart can be **defibrillated** by briefly applying a strong electrical current to the chest wall. This stimulates depolarization of all the cardiac muscle fibers simultaneously, so that all contractions momentarily cease. If the SA node then begins to function, normal cardiac rhythm may be reestablished.

In **heart block**, transmission of an action potential becomes delayed or blocked at some point in the conduction system. **Atrioventricular heart block** may occur when the AV bundle becomes damaged or when impulses through it are depressed for some reason, for instance, electrolyte imbalance. When conduction is not completely interrupted, the condition is called **incomplete heart block**.

In **complete AV heart block**, all the impulses are totally blocked between atria and ventricles. The atria may continue to beat at their normal rate but, although the ventricles also beat, they do so independently and at a slower rate (about 40 beats per minute). In such a case, ventricular beat is determined by the AV node acting independently. The ventricles are said to have "escaped" from control of the atria.

Artificial pacemakers are now implanted in patients with severe heart block syndromes. The **pacemaker** is implanted beneath the skin and its electrodes are connected to the heart. This device provides continuous rhythmic impulses that drive the heart.

Sometimes a heartbeat results from an impulse that originates at a region other than the SA node. Such an impulse initiates a premature **ectopic beat** that, owing to the refractory period that follows, delays the onset of the next beat. When the next contraction does occur, it may be unusually strong and startling, giving rise to a pounding sensation. Ectopic beats are not serious in themselves but can indicate heart damage. They can also result from the action of drugs such as caffeine or from stress.

## Regulation of Stroke Volume

Stroke volume, the volume of blood pumped by one ventricle during one contraction, also has a direct effect on cardiac output. The ventricles do not eject all the blood within them when they contract. The more forcefully they contract, the greater the volume of blood ejected. Furthermore, the volume of blood delivered to the heart varies from time to time. Stroke volume is regulated mainly by venous return and by sympathetic stimulation.

Perhaps the most important determinant of cardiac output is **venous return**, the amount of blood delivered to the heart by its veins. The greater the amount of blood delivered to the heart by the veins, the more blood the heart pumps. This relationship, known as **Starling's law of the heart**, explains that the heart pumps all the blood delivered to it within physiological limits. Because the cardiac muscle fibers are stretched to a greater extent when extra amounts of blood fill the heart chambers, these muscle fibers contract with greater force, pumping the greater volume of blood into the arteries. By increasing the stroke volume in this way the heart can increase its normal output of about 5 l/minute to a maximum of about 14 l/minute. At greater volumes the heart can keep pace with the tremendous venous return only if the nerves serving it increase the heart rate and the force of contraction.

## THE ELECTROCARDIOGRAM

The **electrocardiogram** (ee-lek″-trow-**kar′**-dee-o-gram) (**ECG** or **EKG**), is probably the single most useful indicator of cardiac function. EKG patterns are used to indicate various cardiac disorders, including heart damage during or following heart attacks.

As each wave of depolarization spreads through the heart, electrical currents spread into the tissues surrounding the heart and onto the body surface. Electrical potentials can be recorded by placing electrodes on the surface of the body on opposite sides of the heart. The **electrocardiograph** is used to amplify and record the electrical activity and the record produced is called the **electrocardiogram** (Fig. 12–9). When desired, the output of an

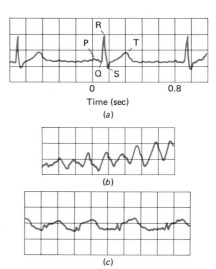

*Figure 12–9. Electrocardiograms. (a) Normal. (b) Ventricular fibrillation. (c) Some of the cardiac muscle has been damaged during a "heart attack" (myocardial infarction). Note the marked ST interval.*

electrocardiograph can also be tape recorded. In intensive care units and in operating rooms an instrument called an oscilloscope is used instead of an ink-writing electrocardiograph. The oscilloscope continuously monitors the heart, displaying a visual representation of electrical variations on a fluorescent screen. The pattern displayed reflects the difference in electrical potential between the electrodes (electrocardiographic leads) placed on various parts of the body.

An electrocardiogram begins with what is called the **P wave**. This is the graphic record of the spread of depolarization of a multitude of muscle cells over the atria just prior to atrial contraction. This is followed by the **QRS complex**, which reflects the spread of a similar collective impulse through the ventricles just before ventricular contraction. As the ventricles recover after contraction, that is, their cells repolarize, further currents are generated that are reflected on the graph as the **T wave**.

The shapes of the waves and the time intervals between them are important in evaluating an EKG. The **PR interval** is the duration of time between the beginning of a P wave and the beginning of a QRS wave. It represents the time between the beginning of the contraction of the atrium and the beginning of the contraction of the ventricle. In patients with heart disease, scarred or inflamed tissue may result in lengthening of the PR interval. This is because more time is required for the wave of depolarization to pass through the atrial myocardium and AV node. The **QRS duration**, the time required for the QRS wave, represents depolarization of the ventricles. The **QT interval** extends from the beginning of the Q wave to the end of the T wave. It represents the time of ventricular contraction and repolarization. The **ST interval** represents the time during which the ventricles repolarize; it extends from the S wave to the end of the T wave.

# SUMMARY

I. The heart is a hollow, muscular organ that lies in the mediastinum between the lungs. Its apex is directed toward the left and rests on the diaphragm.

II. The heart is enclosed by a tough sac called the pericardium.

III. The bulk of the heart wall consists of myocardium, the middle muscular layer. The inner layer of the heart wall is the endocardium and the outer layer is the visceral pericardium.

IV. The heart has four chambers—the right and left atria, which receive blood returning to the heart, and the right and left ventricles, which pump blood out into the great arteries.

V. Each atrium is separated from its ventricle by an atrioventricular (AV) valve, which prevents backflow of blood. The semilunar valves are located between each ventricle and the artery into which it pumps blood.
  A. The AV valve between the right atrium and right ventricle is the tricuspid valve.
  B. The AV valve between the left atrium and left ventricle is the mitral valve.
  C. The aortic valve is located between the left ventricle and the aorta.
  D. The pulmonary valve is located between the right ventricle and the pulmonary trunk.

VI. The heart has its own conduction system and can beat independently of its nerve supply. However, elaborate mechanisms exist to regulate the heartbeat so that its rate and strength of contraction adjust to the changing needs of the body.
  A. Each heartbeat begins in the SA node. The action potential spreads through the atria, causing atrial contraction. One group of fibers conducts the action potential to the AV node.
  B. From the AV node the action potential spreads through the Purkinje fibers and finally reaches the ordinary fibers of the ventricles.

VII. The sequence of events that occurs during one complete heartbeat is a cardiac cycle.
  A. Each cardiac cycle begins with the generation of an action potential in the SA node that produces atrial systole.
  B. As the atria contract, additional blood is forced into the ventricles.
  C. Ventricular systole occurs next, forcing blood through the semilunar valves into the systemic and pulmonary circulations. At the same time the atria have returned to diastole and are again filling with blood.

IX. When listening to the heart through a stethoscope, one can hear a "lub" sound when the mitral and tricuspid valves close, followed by a "dup" sound when the aortic and pulmonary valves snap shut.

X. Cardiac output is the amount of blood pumped by one ventricle in 1 minute. According to Starling's law of the heart, the more blood returned to the heart by the veins, the greater the volume of blood that will be pumped during the next systole.

XI. Cardiac output equals stroke volume multiplied by heart rate.

    A. Heart rate is regulated mainly by sympathetic and parasympathetic nerves but can be influenced by other factors such as hormones.

XII. Stroke volume depends on venous return and sympathetic stimulation.

XIII. An electrocardiogram (EKG) begins with a P wave, which represents the spread of an impulse over the atria just prior to atrial contraction. This is followed by the QRS complex, which indicates that the impulse is spreading over the ventricles just prior to ventricular contraction. As the ventricles recover, currents generated cause a T wave.

## POST TEST

1. The heart is enclosed by a tough sac called the _____.
2. The visceral pericardium is the _____ layer of the heart.
3. The bulk of the heart wall consists of _____.
4. The wall separating the ventricles of the heart is called the _____ _____.
5. The left AV valve is most often called the _____ valve.
6. Aortic and pulmonary valves are _____ valves.
7. The cusps of the AV valves are anchored to _____ muscles by the chordae tendineae.
8. The _____ is called the pacemaker of the heart.
9. From the AV node, the action potential spreads into specialized muscle fibers called _____ _____.
10. Cardiac muscle fibers are separated by specialized junctions known as _____ _____.
11. In the cardiac cycle the period of contraction is called _____ and the period of relaxation is called _____.
12. The volume of blood pumped by one ventricle during one beat is the _____ _____.
13. The volume of blood pumped by one ventricle in 1 minute is the _____ _____.
14. Heart rate is slowed by _____ nerves and speeded by _____ nerves.
15. The amount of blood delivered to the heart by the veins is called _____ _____.
16. Starling's law states that, within physiological limits, the heart will pump _____.
17. An electrocardiogram begins with a _____ wave, which represents the spread of an impulse over the _____.
18. Label the diagram on the following page.

## REVIEW QUESTIONS

1. Relate the structure of the heart wall to the heart's function. Distinguish between parietal and visceral pericardium.
2. How does cardiac muscle differ from skeletal muscle structurally and physiologically?
3. Trace a heartbeat through the conduction system of the heart.

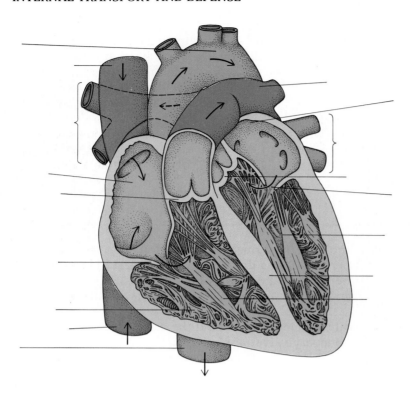

4. Trace blood through the heart chambers, describing the events of the cardiac cycle.
5. Define stroke volume and cardiac output and relate both to Starling's law of the heart.
6. Describe the regulation of heart rate by sympathetic and parasympathetic nerves.

# Circulation of Blood and Lymph

## LEARNING OBJECTIVES

**After you study this chapter you should be able to**

1. Compare the structure and functions of arteries, capillaries, sinusoids, and veins.
2. Trace a drop of blood through the pulmonary and systemic circulations, listing the principal vessels and heart chambers through which it must pass on its journey from one part of the body to another. (For example, trace a drop of blood from the inferior vena cava to an organ such as the brain and then back to the heart.)
3. Identify the main divisions of the aorta and its principal branches.
4. Trace a drop of blood through the hepatic portal system.
5. Give the physiological basis for arterial pulse and describe how pulse is measured.
6. Define blood pressure and give its relationship to blood flow and peripheral resistance.
7. Compare blood pressure in the different types of blood vessels of the systemic circulation.
8. Describe the homeostatic mechanisms that regulate blood pressure and explain how blood pressure is measured clinically.

Tonsils
The Spleen
The Thymus Gland

9. Give the physiological basis of circulatory shock.
10. Describe the progressive pathological changes in atherosclerosis, give its risk factors and common complications, and tell how it is treated.
11. Describe the following cardiovascular diseases: hypertension, angina, coronary occlusion, and myocardial infarction.

---

So extensive is the network of blood vessels in the body that blood flows within close proximity of almost every cell. The various types of blood vessels form pathways through the body, and complex physiological dynamics are involved in circulating the blood. The lymphatic system is composed of a second set of vessels that return fluid to the blood.

## THE BLOOD VESSELS

The principal types of blood vessels are the arteries, capillaries, and veins. As shown in Figure 13–1, the heart delivers blood into the arteries. These vessels and their smallest branches, the arterioles, carry blood to the various organs of the body. From the arterioles blood flows through capillaries, tiny vessels that form extensive networks within each tissue. Blood passes from the capillaries into venules and then is conducted back toward the heart by larger veins. These different types of blood vessels vary with respect to their length, diameter, thickness, and the composition of their walls.

### General Structure of the Blood Vessel Wall

The wall of an artery or vein has three layers, or **tunics**: an internal tunica intima, a middle tunica media, and an external tunica adventitia (Fig. 13–2). The **tunica intima** consists of a lining of endothelium (a simple squamous epithelium), which is in contact with the blood in the **lumen** (space inside) of the vessel, and an underlying thin layer of connective tissue.

**Tunica media** consists of connective tissue and smooth muscle cells. In large arteries tunica media is the thickest layer and contains several layers of elastic fibers.

**Tunica adventitia** (ad-ven-**tish**'-ee-ah) is a relatively thin layer in arteries but is the thickest layer in the walls of large veins. It consists of connective tissue rich in elastic and collagen fibers. Nerves,

lymphatic vessels, and even tiny blood vessels are found within the connective tissue of tunica adventitia. It may seem strange that blood vessels themselves must be supplied with blood and a system of blood vessels, but the walls of large arteries and veins are so thick that nutrients and ox-

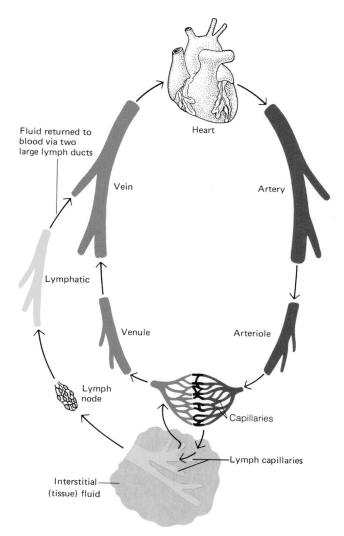

**Figure 13–1.** *Types of blood vessels and their relationship to one another. Lymphatic vessels return excess tissue fluid to the blood.*

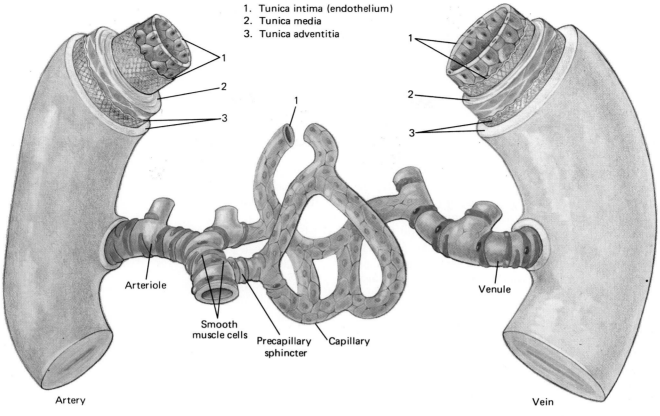

1. Tunica intima (endothelium)
2. Tunica media
3. Tunica adventitia

Arteriole

Smooth muscle cells

Precapillary sphincter

Capillary

Venule

Artery

Vein

***Figure 13–2.*** *Structure of blood vessel walls.*

ygen could not otherwise effectively reach all of their cells.

## Arteries

An **artery** is a blood vessel that conducts blood away from the heart to the organs and tissues of the body. All arteries except the pulmonary arteries carry oxygen-rich blood. Arteries are strong vessels adapted to carry blood under high pressure.

**Arterioles** are small arteries important in regulating blood pressure and in determining the amount of blood distributed to any tissue. The smooth muscle in the tunica media of arterioles is innervated by sympathetic nerves. Impulses from these nerves stimulate the smooth muscle to contract, reducing the diameter of the blood vessel. Such narrowing of the blood vessel is called **vaso-constriction** (vas-oh-kon-**strik'**-shun). When sympathetic impulses are inhibited, the muscle fibers relax and the diameter of the blood vessel increases. This is called **vasodilation** (vas-oh-die-**lay'**-shun).

Changes in blood vessel diameter depend on the metabolic needs of the tissue served, as well as the demands of the body as a whole. For example, arterioles may dilate in response to increased carbon dioxide or decreased oxygen in the tissues. During exercise, when skeletal muscle tissue is rapidly metabolizing, the blood supply to the muscles must be increased. The arterioles dilate, increasing the amount of blood flowing to the muscle cells by more than 10-fold.

It is important to understand that if all of the blood vessels in the body were dilated at the same time, there would not be enough blood to fill them completely. Blood is routed to the various tissues according to their needs at any particular moment. Normally the liver, kidneys, and brain receive the lion's share of the blood. However, in cases of sudden stress requiring rapid action, the blood is quickly rerouted in favor of the heart and skeletal muscles. At such times organs such as the kidneys and digestive organs can do with less blood.

## Capillaries

**Capillaries** are the organs of exchange in the cardiovascular system because their walls are so thin that oxygen and nutrients easily diffuse through them. The capillary wall is also somewhat porous, so plasma itself may leave the circulation through it. Blood enters the arterial end of a capillary network at rather high pressure, forcing some plasma out of the capillaries and into the tissues. Once out of the blood, this fluid is called **interstitial** (in-tur-**stish'**-ul) **fluid**, or tissue fluid. Rich in oxygen and nutrients, interstitial fluid bathes all the cells of the body. Most of the interstitial fluid is returned to the blood at the venous end of the capillary network where blood pressure is lower. Excess interstitial fluid enters the lymphatic system and is also eventually returned to the blood.

Each individual capillary is only about 1 mm (0.04 inch) long and many are so narrow that red blood cells must pass through them in single file (Fig. 13–3). Yet these vessels form complex networks so extensive that if they could be placed end to end they would span about 60,000 miles!

The capillary wall consists mainly of tunica intima, that is, of endothelium. At the point where a capillary branches from an arteriole a smooth muscle cell surrounds the vessel, forming a **precapillary sphincter.** By contracting or relaxing, precapillary sphincters regulate the flow of blood into the capillaries.

In the liver, spleen, and bone marrow, arterioles and venules are connected by vessels called **sinusoids** rather than by typical capillaries. The endothelial cells lining a sinusoid do not all come into contact with one another, leaving gaps in the wall. For this reason sinusoids are leaky. Macrophages lie along the outer walls of sinusoids and extend their pseudopods into the vessels to remove worn-out blood cells, debris, and foreign matter from the circulation.

## Veins

Blood from the capillaries is connected by the **venules** (**ven'**-yools), which join to form larger veins. A **vein**, you may recall, is a blood vessel that conducts blood from the tissues back toward the heart. In general, veins have thinner walls than arteries. Most veins larger than 2 mm in diameter have valves positioned so that they can conduct blood against the force of gravity. A vein valve usually consists of two cusps formed by inward extensions of the intima. These valves are arranged to permit blood to flow toward the heart, not backward in the opposite direction.

When one stands for a long period of time, blood accumulates in the veins of the legs. In persons engaged in occupations in which they must stand for long periods each day, such pooling of the blood can eventually stretch the veins. Then, because the cusps no longer meet, the competence of the valves is destroyed. This often leads to **varicose veins**, especially in those who have inherited weak vein walls and in obese individuals. A varicose vein is wider than the usual vein and is elongated and tortuous as well. Varicose veins occur mainly in the superficial veins of the legs because these veins are not well supported but must bear the weight of the blood within them. **Hemorrhoids** are varicosities of the veins in the anal region. They occur when venous pressure is constantly elevated, as in chronic constipation (because of straining) and during pregnancy (owing to pressure of the enlarged uterus on veins in the pelvic region).

## Anastomoses

The distal ends of blood vessels supplying a body structure may be joined by a **collateral chan-**

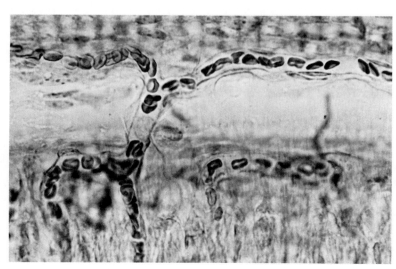

***Figure 13–3.*** *Red blood cells pass through capillaries in single file.*

**nel**, also called a **vascular anastomosis**. Anastomoses permit blood to flow between the joined vessels. Such junctions may occur between arteries, between veins at their origin, or between an arteriole and a venule. An anastomosis between an arteriole and a venule permits blood to bypass a capillary network.

An anastomosis provides an alternative channel of blood supply to a particular area. For example, anastomoses are commonly found around joints, where movement may temporarily impede blood flow through one channel. If an artery supplying a particular organ is slowly blocked by disease or is tied off during surgery, blood may flow through the alternate pathway provided by the anastomosis. Sometimes an entirely new capillary network develops from a collateral channel. This **collateral circulation** may be life preserving in certain cardiovascular disease states. For example, when normal circulation to an area, such as part of the heart wall, is impeded, blood can flow through the collateral circulation.

## THE PATTERN OF CIRCULATION

Blood flows through a continuous network of blood vessels that forms a double circuit connecting (1) heart and lungs and (2) heart and all tissues. The left ventricle pumps blood into the **systemic circulation**, which brings oxygen-rich blood to all the different organs and tissues. Blood returns to the right atrium of the heart somewhat deoxygenated but loaded with carbon dioxide wastes. It is pumped by the right ventricle into the **pulmonary circulation**. The pulmonary arteries carry blood to the lungs, where gases are exchanged. Then pulmonary veins return the blood, rich in oxygen once more, to the left atrium. Blood then passes into the left ventricle and is pumped into the systemic circulation again, repeating the double cycle. This general pattern of circulation is shown diagrammatically in Figure 13–4. A more detailed view is shown in Figure 13–5.

### Pulmonary Circulation

Deoxygenated blood returning to the heart from the systemic circulation passes into the right atrium and then into the right ventricle. From the right ventricle it is pumped into the **pulmonary trunk**, a large artery that divides almost immediately to form the **right** and **left pulmonary arteries**. These vessels deliver blood to the right and left lungs, respectively. On reaching the lung each pulmonary artery gives rise to branches that service all regions of the organ.

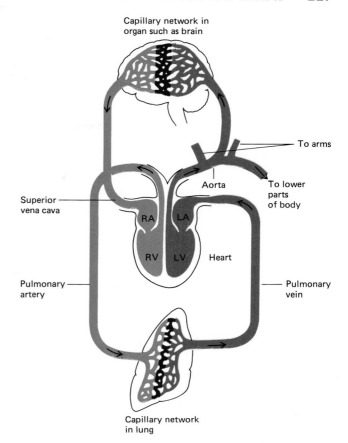

**Figure 13–4.** *Simplified diagram of circulation through the systemic and pulmonary circuits. Red represents oxygenated blood; blue represents deoxygenated blood.*

Eventually blood flows into the extensive capillary networks in the walls of the air sacs, where carbon dioxide diffuses out of the blood and oxygen diffuses into it. **Pulmonary capillaries** deliver the now oxygenated blood to pulmonary venules, which join to form larger veins. Two **pulmonary veins** exit from each lung and conduct oxygenated blood to the left atrium of the heart. Note that the pulmonary veins are the only veins that carry oxygen-rich blood and the pulmonary arteries are the only arteries that transport deoxygenated blood. (A few exceptions occur in the circulatory system of the fetus.)

In summary, blood flows through the vessels of the pulmonary circulation in the following sequence: right atrium→right ventricle→pulmonary trunk→pulmonary artery→pulmonary arterioles →pulmonary capillaries→pulmonary venules→ pulmonary veins→left atrium.

### Systemic Circulation

Blood returns from the pulmonary circulation, enters the left atrium, then passes into the left ven-

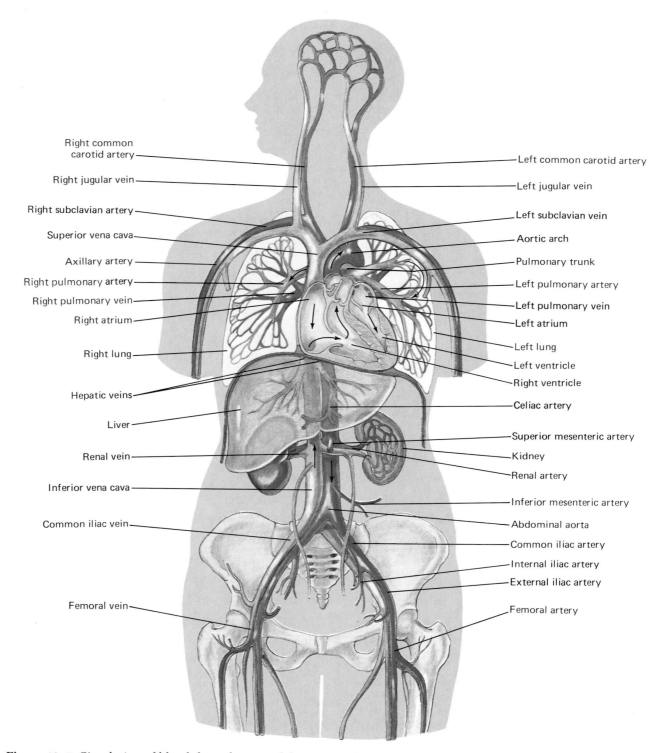

**Figure 13–5.** *Circulation of blood through some of the principal arteries and veins. Blood vessels carrying oxygen-rich blood are red; those carrying blood low in oxygen are blue.*

tricle. From there it is pumped into the largest artery in the body, the **aorta**.

The first portion of the aorta, which travels upward (anteriorly), is known as the **ascending aorta** (Fig. 13–6). Coronary arteries branch off from the

ascending aorta and enter the heart muscle (Table 13–1). After a short distance the aorta makes a U turn, the **aortic arch**. Three large arteries that branch off from the aortic arch are the (1) **brachiocephalic** (brak″-ee-o-se-**fal′**-ik) **(innominate) ar-**

CIRCULATION OF BLOOD AND LYMPH 229

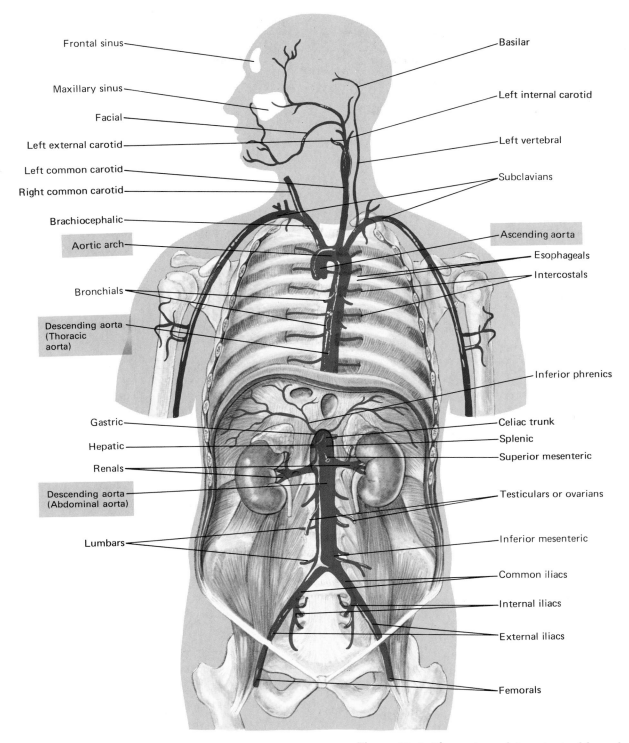

Frontal sinus

Maxillary sinus

Facial

Left external carotid

Left common carotid

Right common carotid

Brachiocephalic

Aortic arch

Bronchials

Descending aorta
(Thoracic
aorta)

Gastric

Hepatic

Renals

Descending aorta
(Abdominal aorta)

Lumbars

Basilar

Left internal carotid

Left vertebral

Subclavians

Ascending aorta

Esophageals

Intercostals

Inferior phrenics

Celiac trunk

Splenic

Superior mesenteric

Testiculars or ovarians

Inferior mesenteric

Common iliacs

Internal iliacs

External iliacs

Femorals

*Figure 13–6.* The aorta and its principal branches.

tery, which supplies the right upper portion of the body; (2) the **left common carotid artery**, which supplies the left side of the head and neck; and (3) the **left subclavian** (sub-**klay'**-vee-an) **artery**, which supplies the neck and left arm. As the aorta passes down through the thoracic and abdominal cavities it is called the **descending aorta**. The descending aorta is referred to as the **thoracic aorta** as it passes through the thorax. Below the diaphragm the descending aorta is called the **abdomi-**

TABLE 13–1
**The Aorta and its Principal Branches**

| Division of Aorta | Arterial Branch | Region Supplied |
|---|---|---|
| Ascending aorta | Coronary arteries | Wall of heart |
| Aortic arch | Brachiocephalic (innominate) | |
| | Right common carotid | Branches into external carotid (supplying head and neck) and internal carotid (supplying brain and head) |
| | Right subclavian | Sends branches to neck and right upper extremity |
| | Left common carotid | Branches into external carotid (supplying head and neck) and internal carotid (supplying brain and head) |
| | Left subclavian | Sends branches to neck and left upper extremity |
| Thoracic aorta | *Visceral Branches* | |
| | Bronchial | Bronchi of lungs |
| | Esophageal | Esophagus |
| | *Parietal Branches* | |
| | Several pairs of posterior inter-costal arteries | Intercostal and other chest muscles, and pleurae; join with other arteries that serve chest wall |
| | Subcostal | Last pair of arteries to branch from thoracic aorta; serve chest wall |
| Abdominal aorta | *Visceral Branches* | |
| | Celiac | Branches to supply the liver (hepatic artery), stomach (gastric artery), and spleen, pancreas, and stomach (splenic artery) |
| | Superior mesenteric | Small intestine and first part of large intestine |
| | Suprarenal | Adrenal glands |
| | Renal | Kidneys |
| | Ovarian (in female) | Ovaries |
| | Testicular (in male) | Testes |
| | Inferior mesenteric | Colon, rectum |
| | Common iliac | |
| | External | Lower extremities |
| | Internal | Branches supply gluteal muscles, urinary bladder, uterus, vagina |
| | *Parietal Branches* | |
| | Inferior phrenic | Diaphragm |
| | Lumbar | Spinal cord and lumbar region of back |
| | Middle sacral | Sacrum, coccyx, gluteus maximus, and rectum |

**nal aorta.** Branches are given off to all the major organs and tissues. For example, **renal arteries** branch off to the kidneys. In the lower abdominal cavity the aorta itself divides to form the left and right **common iliac arteries**, which deliver blood to the lower extremities and pelvic structures.

In the systemic circulation blood returns to the heart through two large veins, the **superior** and **inferior venae cavae.** The inferior vena cava receives blood returning from the portion of the body below the level of the diaphragm. Two **brachiocephalic (innominate) veins** receive blood from the upper portions of the body and empty it into the superior vena cava (Table 13–2). The brachiocephalic veins, in turn, receive blood from the **jugular veins,** which drain blood from the brain and from the **subclavian veins,** which drain blood from the upper extremities, as well as from several other

TABLE 13–2
**Veins Draining into the Venae Cavae**

| Vein | Formed From | Area(s) Drained |
|---|---|---|
| ***Into Superior Vena Cava*** | | |
| Internal jugular | Sinuses of dura mater | Brain, skull |
| External jugular | Veins of face | Muscles and skin of face and scalp |
| Subclavian | Axillary, cephalic, basilic and their tributaries, scapular, and thoracic veins | Upper appendages, chest, mammary glands |
| Brachiocephalic (innominate) | Internal jugular, external jugular, and subclavian | Brain, face, neck |
| Azygos | Lumbar and intercostal veins | Posterior aspect of thorax and abdominal cavities |
| ***Into Inferior Vena Cava*** | | |
| Hepatics | Sinusoids of liver | Liver |
| Renals | Veins of kidney | Kidney |
| Ovarians or testiculars | Veins of gonads | Ovaries or testes |
| Common iliac | External iliac (extension of the femoral vein) | Lower appendages |
| | Internal iliac | Organs of lower abdomen |

veins. In the following sections we will consider in more detail the circulation through the heart, brain, and liver.

### Coronary Circulation

The heart is a large, actively metabolizing organ that requires a continuous supply of nutrients and oxygen. Blood flowing through its chambers cannot serve these needs because the layers of the heart are far too thick to depend on diffusion. The heart requires its own system of blood vessels, the **coronary circulation**.

Two coronary arteries branch off from the ascending aorta just as it leaves the heart. The **right coronary artery** emerges from the aorta on the anterior surface of the heart. Its branches mainly supply the right atrium and ventricle. The right coronary artery passes to the inferior margin of the heart and gives off a branch (the marginal artery) before circling to the posterior surface of the heart.

The **left coronary artery** is markedly larger than the right. It passes under the left atrium and divides into branches that supply the left atrium and ventricle. (Among its main branches are the anterior interventricular (descending) artery and the circumflex artery.) Many anastomoses are present within the coronary circulation.

As blood passes through the extensive capillary networks of the coronary circulation, oxygen and nutrients are delivered to the heart muscle and wastes are removed. Blood from the capillaries drains into coronary veins that join to form a large vein, the **coronary sinus**. The coronary sinus lies in the posterior side of the heart and empties into the right atrium.

### Cerebral Circulation

Four arteries—the two **internal carotid arteries** and the two **vertebral arteries** (branches of the subclavian arteries)—supply the brain with blood (Fig. 13–7). The vertebral arteries pass through the foramen magnum and join on the ventral surface of the brain stem to form the **basilar artery**. The basilar artery branches into the right and left **posterior cerebral arteries**. The internal carotid arteries enter the cranial cavity in the midportion of the cranial floor. Their terminal branches are the **anterior cerebral arteries** and **middle cerebral arteries**. Small communicating arteries join the two anterior and the middle and posterior cerebral arteries, forming a circular anastomosis at the base of the brain. This anastomosis is known as the **circle of Willis**. Should one of the arteries serving the brain become blocked or impaired in some way,

this interconnecting arterial circuit helps ensure that the brain cells will continue to receive an adequate blood supply through other vessels.

From the brain capillaries, blood drains into large venous sinuses located in folds of the dura mater. These empty into the internal jugular veins at either side of the neck, and blood returns to the heart through the brachiocephalic veins and superior vena cava.

### Hepatic Portal System

As you have seen, blood generally flows from arteries to capillaries and then to veins, which conduct it back to the heart. However, there are a few exceptional veins that carry blood to a second set of exchange vessels—either capillaries or sinusoids. Such veins are called **portal veins**. One such system of veins, the **hepatic portal system**, transports blood from the organs of the digestive system to the liver (Fig. 13–8).

Blood reaches the intestines through the **mesenteric** (mes″-en-ter′-ik) **arteries** and enters the capillaries in the intestinal wall. Nutrients are absorbed into these capillaries and then pass into the **superior mesenteric vein**. This vein empties into the **hepatic portal vein**, which also receives blood returning from the lower portion of the intestine and from the spleen. The hepatic portal vein conducts blood to the liver, where it gives rise to an extensive network of hepatic sinusoids. As blood flows through these sinusoids liver cells remove nutrients whose concentrations in the blood are above homeostatic levels. Eventually the hepatic sinusoids deliver blood to the **hepatic veins**, which leave the liver and empty into the inferior vena cava.

## PHYSIOLOGY OF CIRCULATION

In Chapter 12 some of the factors that influence the flow of blood through the heart were discussed. Here we will turn our attention to the movement of blood through the blood vessels.

### Pulse

Each time the left ventricle pumps blood into the aorta, the elastic wall of the aorta stretches. This expansion moves down the aorta and its branches in a wave that is faster than the flow of the blood itself. As soon as the wave has passed, the elastic arterial wall snaps back to its normal size. This alternate expansion and recoil of an artery is the **arterial pulse**.

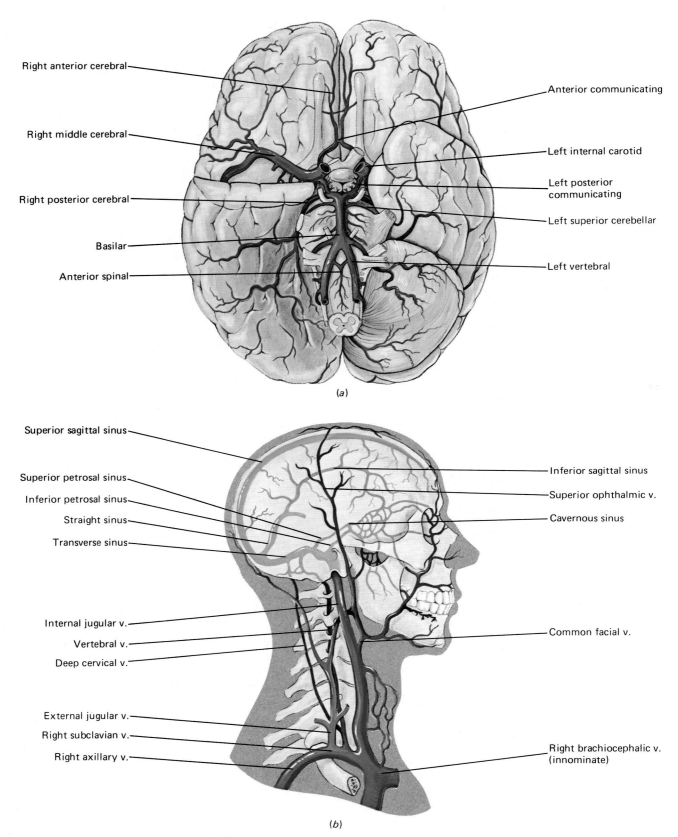

**Figure 13-7.** (a) Arterial circulation in the brain. Note the circle of Willis, which is made up of arterial anastomoses. It provides alternative circulatory pathways to ensure an adequate blood supply to the brain cells. (b) Venous drainage of the brain.

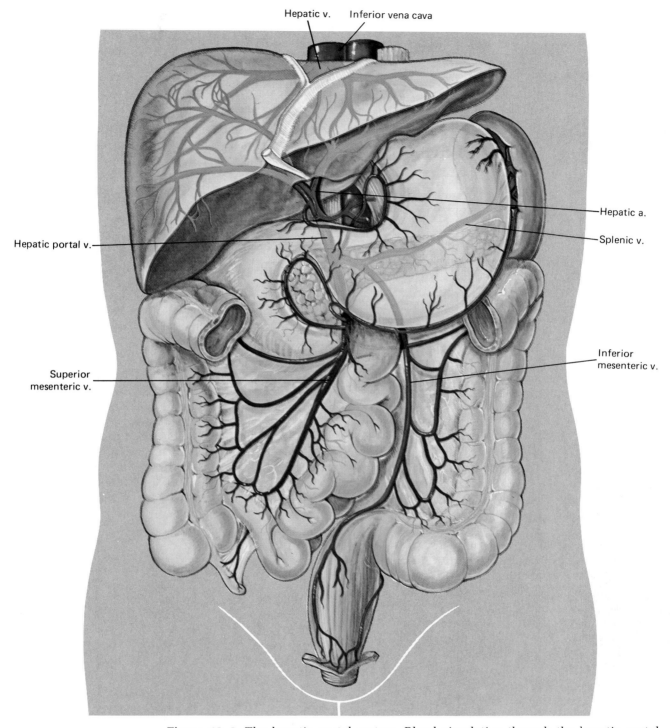

**Figure 13–8.** The hepatic portal system. Blood circulating through the hepatic portal vein has already passed through capillaries in the intestine and is partly depleted of its oxygen supply. Oxygen-rich blood is delivered to the liver by the hepatic arteries. Its branches deliver blood to the hepatic sinuses where it mixes with the venous blood from the hepatic portal vein.

The ability of the large arteries to expand and then snap back to their original diameters is important in maintaining a continuous flow of blood. As the left ventricle forces a large volume of blood into the aorta during systole, the aorta expands to accommodate it. During diastole, as the walls of the aorta recoil to normal size, the blood is kept flowing into the capillaries. Were it not for this mechanism, blood would rush through the arteries and into the arterioles and capillaries in enormous

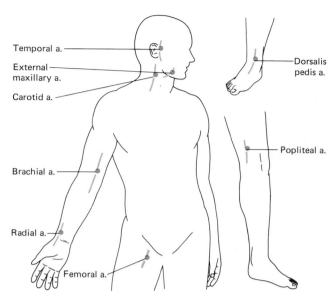

*Figure 13–9.* The pulse may be felt at any of the locations indicated in the diagram. All of the arteries indicated lie near the body surface over a bone or other firm structure.

gushes each time the ventricle contracted, and the delicate walls of the capillaries would soon be damaged.

When you place your finger over an artery near the skin surface, you can feel the pulse. The **radial artery** in the wrist is most frequently used to measure pulse, but the common carotid artery in the neck region or any other superficial artery that lies over a bone or other firm structure may be used (Fig. 13–9). These locations are sometimes referred to as *pressure points* because pressure applied directly on the vessel at these points may stop arterial bleeding if the wound is distal to the pressure point.

The number of pulsations counted per minute indicates the number of heartbeats per minute, because every time the heart contracts a pulse wave is initiated. Because it takes time for the pulse wave to pass from the ventricle to the artery, the pulse is felt just after ventricular contraction.

Large veins near the heart also develop a pulse owing to the contraction of the right atrium. The external jugular vein in the neck region is sometimes used to measure venous pulse.

## Blood Pressure

**Blood pressure** is the force exerted by the blood against the inner walls of the blood vessels. It is determined by the flow of blood and the resistance to that flow.

Blood pressure = blood flow × resistance

## Blood Flow

The flow of blood depends directly on the pumping action of the heart. When cardiac output increases, blood flow increases, causing a rise in blood pressure (Fig. 13–10). When cardiac output decreases, blood flow decreases, causing a fall in blood pressure. Recall from Chapter 12 that cardiac output depends on heart rate and stroke volume. Any change in either of these factors may result in a change in blood pressure.

Blood always flows from regions of high pressure to regions of lower pressure. If there were no pressure difference it would not flow at all. Blood pressure in arteries increases and decreases in a pattern that corresponds to the events of the cardiac cycle. Blood pressure in the arteries is at its highest during ventricular systole when blood is pumped into the aorta and pulmonary arteries. Blood pressure in the arteries is at its lowest at the end of ventricular diastole, after the arteries have recoiled, forcing blood to flow into the smaller blood vessels.

The volume of blood flowing through the system also affects blood pressure. As you have learned, the normal volume of blood in the body is about 5 l. If blood volume is reduced by hemorrhage or by chronic bleeding, the blood pressure drops. On the other hand, an increase in blood volume causes an increase in blood pressure. For example, a high dietary intake of salt causes retention of water. This may result in an increase in blood volume and lead ultimately to an increase in blood pressure.

## Peripheral Resistance

Blood flow is impeded by resistance and, as indicated by the previous equation, when the resistance to flow increases, blood pressure increases. **Peripheral resistance** is the impedence to blood flow caused by blood viscosity and by friction between the blood and the wall of the blood vessel.

Blood viscosity offers resistance to flow because there is friction between the blood cells and between the plasma proteins. In anemia or conditions of blood loss, blood viscosity decreases, causing a fall in blood pressure. However, in healthy blood viscosity remains fairly constant and is only a minor factor in changes in blood pressure.

More important is the friction between the blood and the wall of the blood vessel. The length and diameter of a blood vessel determine the surface area of the vessel that is in contact with the blood. The length of a blood vessel does not ordinarily change but the diameter, particularly of the arteri-

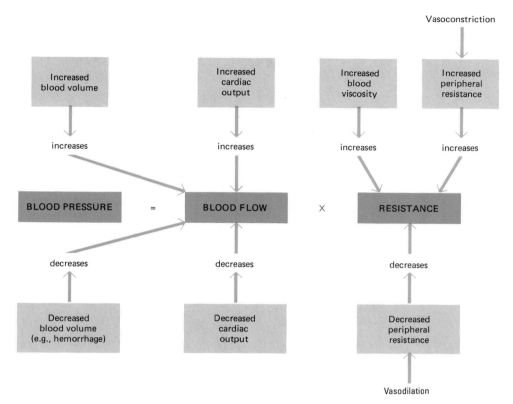

**Figure 13–10.** *Some factors that influence blood pressure. Any factor that increases either blood flow or resistance increases blood pressure. Any factor that decreases either blood flow or resistance decreases blood pressure.*

oles, does. *A small change in the diameter of a blood vessel causes a big change in blood pressure.*

### Pressure Changes As Blood Flows Through the Systemic Circulation

Because arteries are large, their walls offer little resistance to blood flow. Arterioles, though, have a much smaller diameter and so offer a great deal of resistance to blood flow. This permits relatively high pressures to build up behind them. More important, because arterioles can dilate and constrict, they can alter the amount of resistance to blood flow and thereby influence the blood pressure and the rate of flow. In fact, the amount of blood pressure within the arterial system as a whole is regulated mainly by the degree of vasoconstriction or vasodilation of the arterioles.

Because the diameter of a capillary is small, capillaries individually offer great resistance to blood flow. However, blood has so many capillary channels through which to pass that the total resistance, when all the capillaries are considered together, is far less than that of the arterioles.

As blood flows through capillaries, most of the

pressure caused by the action of the heart is spent. By the time the blood passes into the venules its pressure is only about 15 mm Hg compared with 120 mm Hg in the arteries (Fig. 13–11). This venous pressure falls steadily as blood passes into the larger veins but even this small pressure (perhaps 10 mm Hg) is usually sufficient to push blood through the veins to the heart. When the blood finally enters the right atrium its pressure is about 0 mm Hg.

It takes little pressure to force the blood through the veins because veins offer little resistance to blood flow. Their diameters are large and vein walls are so thin and distensible that they can hold large volumes of blood. Indeed, at any moment more than half of all the blood in the circulation may be found within the veins. Thus, veins serve as a blood reservoir. When blood is lost during hemorrhage, arterial pressure begins to fall. Special receptors (baroreceptors) respond, causing the veins to constrict and thereby releasing large amounts of blood into the heart. This response prevents the heart from failing and keeps the circulation going even when large amounts of blood are lost.

Veins are so arranged that when the body is in

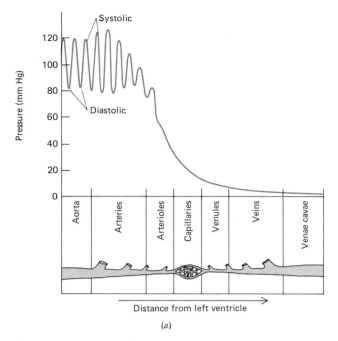

**Figure 13–11.** *Blood pressure in various parts of the systemic circulatory system.*

an upright position gravity offers a great deal of resistance to venous blood flow. It is really quite remarkable that blood in the feet manages to make its way back to the heart. How is this accomplished? Recall that a system of valves prevents backflow of blood within the veins. Blood is pushed along by the pressure of blood behind it and by compression of veins when skeletal muscle contracts.

During exercise increased muscle contraction results in increased flow of blood through the veins and into the heart, thereby increasing cardiac output. On the other hand, when one stands perfectly still for a long period of time, for example, when a soldier stands at attention, blood pools in the veins. Within a few moments, pressure also increases in the capillaries (veins are not accepting blood from them because they are dammed up with their own) and plasma is lost to the interstitial fluid. Arterial blood pressure falls and blood supply to the brain is diminished, sometimes resulting in fainting.

## Regulation of Blood Pressure

Whenever you change position blood pressure fluctuates. It is kept within normal limits by the interaction of several complex homeostatic mechanisms. Specialized receptors, called **baroreceptors**, present in the walls of certain arteries and in the heart wall, are sensitive to changes in blood pressure. When blood pressure increases, the walls of the baroreceptors stretch and messages are sent to the **vasomotor center** in the medulla. Then, parasympathetic nerves signal the heart to slow, thus lowering blood pressure. In addition, the vasomotor center lowers blood pressure by inhibiting sympathetic nerves that constrict arteries.

Low blood pressure stimulates the kidneys to release the hormone **renin**. Then, renin converts a plasma protein to **angiotensins** (an-gee-o-**ten′**-sins), a group of hormones that act as powerful vasoconstrictors. Their action raises blood pressure. The kidneys also act indirectly to maintain blood pressure by helping to regulate blood volume. Hormones signal the kidneys to excrete more or less water or salts, which, in turn, affects blood volume.

## Circulatory Shock

In **circulatory shock** blood pressure may fall so drastically that blood flow to the tissues is inadequate and tissue damage results. Shock can result from a number of conditions, including hemorrhage. In hemorrhage blood loss results in decreased venous return and therefore reduced cardiac output. **Traumatic shock**, which usually results from physical injury, can occur without hemorrhage because of actual damage to the capillaries. Fluid is lost from the blood and the person may "bleed to death" physiologically without actually losing a drop of blood. Venous return and cardiac output become too low to sustain life.

In fainting, peripheral blood vessels become dilated, so that blood pools in them and cardiac output falls. If a person who has fainted is kept in an upright position the shock may deepen, resulting in death. Luckily, when a person faints he or she generally falls into a horizontal position, which helps to restore normal cardiac output.

In **nonprogressive** (or compensated) **shock** sympathetic reflexes and other mechanisms are able to compensate for the decreased blood volume. By vasoconstriction and increased fluid conservation, cardiac output can be increased sufficiently to maintain life. In **progressive shock** blood flow is so reduced that the compensatory mechanisms are not successful. A vicious cycle develops involving positive feedback in which the heart weakens, brain activity decreases, and cardiac output progressively decreases. As shock continues to deepen, the heart, brain, blood vessels, and other organs become more damaged, further worsening the shock.

## Measuring Blood Pressure

In arteries, blood pressure rises during systole and falls during diastole. A blood pressure reading is expressed as systolic pressure over diastolic pressure. For example, normal blood pressure for a young adult would be about 120/80. (The numbers refer to millimeters of mercury.) Systolic pressure is represented by the numerator, diastolic by the denominator. Pulse pressure is the difference between the systolic and diastolic pressures. The systolic pressure may vary greatly with physical exertion and emotional stress.

Clinically, blood pressure is measured with a **sphygmomanometer** (sfig″-mow-mah-**nom**′-eh-ter) and stethoscope. The sphygmomanometer consists of a manometer (a column of mercury calibrated in millimeters) connected by a rubber tube to an inflatable rubber cuff. An air pump with a valve is attached to the cuff.

To measure the pressure, the cuff is wrapped around a patient's arm over the brachial artery. Air is pumped into the cuff until the air pressure is great enough to compress the artery so that no pulse is heard on the anterior surface of the elbow joint (using the stethoscope). Then the valve is opened slightly so that the pressure in the cuff begins to fall. Soon, a distinct sound is heard as blood spurts into the artery again. The pressure at that instant is read as the systolic pressure. The sound gets louder, then changes in quality, and finally becomes inaudible. Pressure at the instant the sound is no longer audible is read as the diastolic pressure.

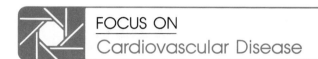

## FOCUS ON
## Cardiovascular Disease

Cardiovascular disease is the number one cause of death in the United States and in most other industrial societies. Most often death results from some complication of **atherosclerosis**\* (hardening of the arteries as a result of lipid deposition). Although atherosclerosis can affect almost any artery, the disease most often develops in the aorta and in the coronary and cerebral arteries. When it occurs in the cerebral arteries it can lead to a **cerebrovascular accident (CVA)**, commonly referred to as a *stroke*.

Although there is apparently no single cause of atherosclerosis, several major risk factors have been identified:

1. Elevated levels of cholesterol in the blood, often associated with diets rich in total calories, total fats, saturated fats, and cholesterol.
2. Hypertension. The higher the blood pressure, the greater the risk.
3. Cigarette smoking. The risk of developing atherosclerosis is two to six times greater in smokers than nonsmokers and is directly proportional to the number of cigarettes smoked daily.
4. Diabetes mellitus, an endocrine disorder in which glucose is not metabolized normally.

The risk of developing atherosclerosis also increases with age. Estrogen hormones are thought to offer some protection in women until after menopause, when the concentration of these hormones decreases. Other suggested risk factors that are currently being studied are obesity, hereditary predisposition, lack of exercise, stress and behavior patterns, and dietary factors such as excessive intake of salt or refined sugar.

In atherosclerosis, lipids are deposited in the smooth muscle cells of the arterial wall. Cells in the arterial wall proliferate and the inner lining thickens. More lipid, especially cholesterol from low-density lipoproteins, accumulates in the wall. Eventually calcium is deposited there, contributing to the slow formation of hard plaque. As the plaque develops, arteries lose their ability to stretch when they fill with blood, and they become progressively occluded (blocked), as shown in the figure. As the artery narrows, less blood can pass through to reach the tissues served by that vessel and the tissue may become **ischemic** (lacking in blood). Under these conditions the tissue is deprived of an adequate oxygen supply.

When a coronary artery becomes narrowed, **ischemic heart disease** can occur. Sufficient oxygen may reach the heart tissue during normal activity, but the increased need for oxygen during exercise or emotional stress results in the pain known as **angina pectoris**. Persons with this condition often carry nitroglycerin pills with them for use during an attack. This drug dilates veins so that venous return is reduced. Cardiac output is lowered so that the heart is not working so hard and requires less oxygen. Nitroglycerin also dilates the coronary arteries slightly, allowing more blood to reach the heart muscle.

---

\*Atherosclerosis is the most common form of arteriosclerosis, any disorder in which arteries lose their elasticity.

**Myocardial infarction (MI)** is the serious, often fatal, form of ischemic heart disease that often results from a sudden decrease in coronary blood supply. The portion of cardiac muscle deprived of oxygen dies within a few minutes and is then referred to as an **infarct**. The term myocardial infarction is used as a synonym for heart attack. MI is the leading cause of death and disability in the United States. Just what triggers the sudden decrease in blood supply that causes MI is a matter of some debate. It is thought that in some cases an episode of ischemia triggers a fatal arrhythmia, such as **ventricular fibrillation**, a condition in which the ventricles contract rapidly without actually pumping blood. In other cases, a **thrombus** (clot) may form in a diseased coronary artery. Because the arterial wall is roughened, platelets may adhere to it and initiate clotting. If the thrombus blocks a sizable branch of a coronary artery, blood flow to a portion of heart muscle is impeded or completely halted. This condition is referred to as a **coronary occlusion**. If the coronary occlusion prevents blood flow to a large region of cardiac muscle, the heart may stop beating, that is, **cardiac arrest** may occur, and death can follow within moments. If only a small region of the heart is affected, however, the heart may continue to function. Cells in the region deprived of oxygen die and are replaced by scar tissue.

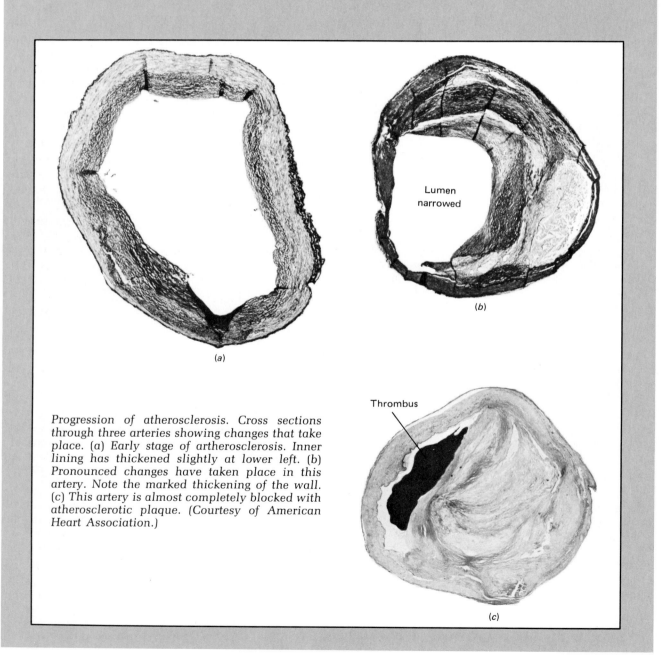

Lumen narrowed

(a)

(b)

Thrombus

(c)

*Progression of atherosclerosis. Cross sections through three arteries showing changes that take place. (a) Early stage of artherosclerosis. Inner lining has thickened slightly at lower left. (b) Pronounced changes have taken place in this artery. Note the marked thickening of the wall. (c) This artery is almost completely blocked with atherosclerotic plaque. (Courtesy of American Heart Association.)*

# THE LYMPHATIC SYSTEM

The **lymphatic system** is a subsystem of the circulatory system. Its three principal functions are (1) to collect and return interstitial fluid, including plasma proteins, to the blood and thus help maintain fluid balance; (2) to defend the body against disease by producing lymphocytes; and (3) to absorb lipids from the intestine and transport them to the blood.

The lymphatic system consists of the clear, watery **lymph** formed from interstitial fluid, the lymphatic vessels that conduct the lymph, lymph tissue organized in lymph nodules and nodes, the tonsils, spleen, and thymus. The lymph system has neither a heart nor arteries (Fig. 13–12). Its microscopic dead-end capillaries extend into most tissues, paralleling the blood capillaries. The lymph circulation is a drainage system. Its job is to collect excess interstitial fluid and to return it to the blood. The lymph capillaries conduct lymph to larger lymph vessels called **lymphatics**. At strategic locations, lymphatics enter lymph nodes. As the lymph flows slowly through the lymph sinuses within the tissue of the lymph node, it is filtered. Macrophages remove bacteria and other foreign matter as well as debris.

Lymphatics that leave the lymph nodes conduct lymph toward the shoulder region. Lymphatic vessels from all over the body except the upper right quadrant drain into the **thoracic duct**. This duct delivers the lymph into the base of the left subclavian vein. Lymph from the lymphatic vessels in the upper right quadrant of the body drains into the **right lymphatic duct**, which empties lymph into the base of the right subclavian vein. In this way lymph is continuously emptied into the blood, where it mixes with the plasma.

## Lymph Nodes

**Lymph nodes**, sometimes called lymph glands, are masses of lymph tissue surrounded by a connective tissue capsule. Their two main functions are (1) to filter the lymph and (2) to produce lymphocytes. Lymph nodes are distributed along the main lymphatic routes. As illustrated in Figure 13–12, they are most numerous in the axillary and groin regions and many are located in the thorax and abdomen.

By filtering and phagocytizing bacteria from the lymph, the lymph nodes help prevent the spread of infection. When bacteria are present, lymph nodes may increase in size and become tender. You may have experienced the swollen cervical lymph nodes that often accompany a sore throat. An infection in almost any part of the body may result in swelling and tenderness of the lymph nodes that drain that area.

## Tonsils

**Tonsils** are masses of lymph tissue located under the epithelial lining of the oral cavity and pharynx. The **lingual (ling′-gwal) tonsils** are located at the base of the tongue. The **pharyngeal tonsil** is located in the posterior wall of the nasal portion of the pharynx above the soft palate. When enlarged (usually owing to infection or allergy), the pharyngeal tonsil is called the *adenoids*.

Most prominent are the paired **palatine tonsils** on each side of the throat. These oval masses of lymphatic tissue are thickenings in the mucous membrane of the throat. The stratified squamous epithelium of the throat that overlies the tonsils dips down to form 10 to 20 pits, or **crypts**, in each tonsil. Bacteria often accumulate in these crypts and may invade the lymphatic tissue of the tonsil. This may cause an increase in the mass of the tonsil. Sometimes bacterial invasion of the tonsils becomes a chronic problem, and the tonsils are surgically removed by the well-known procedure called tonsillectomy. After about age 7 the lymphatic tissue of the tonsils begins to shrink in size.

## The Spleen

The **spleen** is the largest organ of the lymphatic system (Fig. 13–12). It lies in the abdominal cavity protected by the ribs, and posterior and lateral to the stomach. Because it holds a great deal of blood, the spleen has a distinctive rich purple color.

One of the main functions of the spleen is to bring blood into contact with lymphocytes. As blood flows slowly through the spleen, any disease organisms within it activate lymphocytes in the spleen tissue. The activated lymphocytes then attack the foreign invaders. As blood flows through the spleen, macrophages remove worn-out red and white blood cells and platelets. The spleen stores platelets and a large percentage of the body's platelets are normally found there.

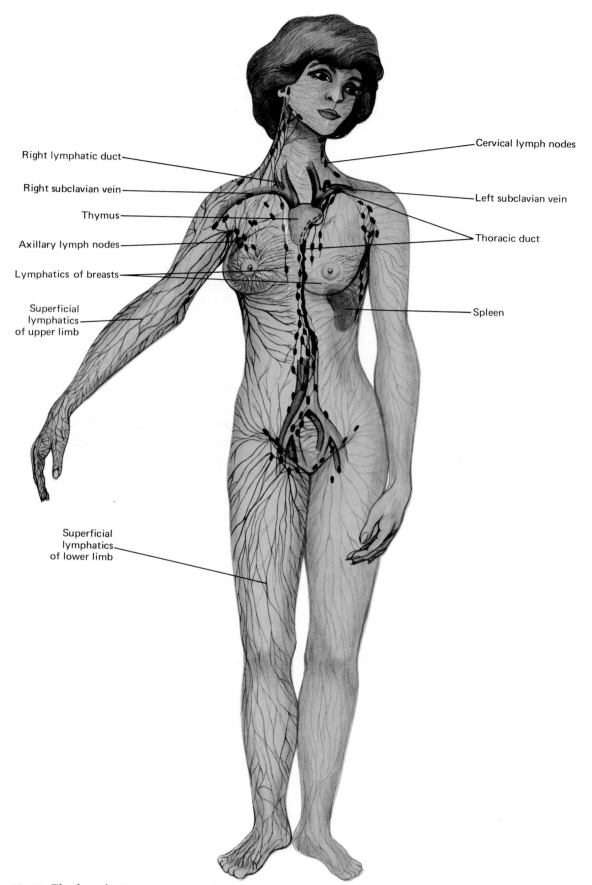

Right lymphatic duct

Right subclavian vein

Thymus

Axillary lymph nodes

Lymphatics of breasts

Superficial
lymphatics
of upper limb

Superficial
lymphatics
of lower limb

Cervical lymph nodes

Left subclavian vein

Thoracic duct

Spleen

***Figure 13–12.*** *The lymphatic system. Lymphatic vessels extend into most tissues of the body but lymph nodes are clustered in certain regions. The right lymphatic duct drains lymph from the upper right quadrant of the body. The thoracic duct drains lymph from other regions of the body.*

Although the spleen performs these important functions, it is not vital to life. Fortunately so, for of all the abdominal organs, the spleen is the one most easily and most frequently injured. A severe blow or crushing injury to the upper abdomen or lower left chest may fracture the ribs that protect the spleen and cause rupture of the spleen itself. When the spleen is ruptured, extensive, sometimes massive hemorrhage occurs. This condition is usually treated by prompt surgical removal of the spleen (splenectomy) to prevent death due to loss of blood and shock. (When surgery—either splenectomy or occasionally surgical repair—is not performed on an injured spleen, the mortality rate is about 90%.) When the spleen is surgically removed some of its functions are taken over by the bone marrow and liver; other functions are simply absent and the body does without them.

## The Thymus Gland

The **thymus** (**thy′**-mus) **gland** is a pinkish gray lymphatic organ located in the superior mediastinum anterior to the great vessels as they emerge from the heart and posterior to the sternum (Fig. 13–12). During fetal life and childhood it is quite large. It reaches its largest size at puberty and then begins to involute and become smaller with age. The thymus gland plays a key role in the body's immune processes.

## SUMMARY

I. Blood is conducted through two circulatory circuits by a system of blood vessels. In each circuit blood leaving the heart flows through arteries, arterioles, capillaries, venules, and veins.
   A. An artery conducts blood away from the heart and toward some organ or tissue.
   B. An arteriole is a small artery that can constrict or dilate, thereby changing the flow of blood into a tissue and affecting blood pressure.
   C. Capillaries are microscopic blood vessels with thin walls through which oxygen, nutrients, and other materials diffuse.
   D. A venule is a small vein that receives blood from the capillaries.
   E. A vein conducts blood away from the tissues and organs and back toward the heart.
II. The blood vessel wall consists of three layers: tunica intima, the innermost layer that lines the blood vessel; a middle layer, the tunica media; and an outer connective tissue layer, tunica adventitia.
III. Blood is pumped by the left ventricle into the systemic circulation, which brings oxygen-rich blood to all the tissues of the body. After circulating through the tissues, blood is conducted through veins back to the heart. Blood enters the right atrium and then passes into the right ventricle, which pumps it into the pulmonary circulation. In the lungs, carbon dioxide wastes diffuse out from the blood and oxygen diffuses into the blood. Blood recharged with oxygen returns to the left atrium of the heart and is pumped by the left ventricle back into the systemic circulation.
IV. The aorta is the largest artery in the body.
   A. The aorta receives blood from the left ventricle and gives off branches that deliver blood to all parts of the body.
   B. The main divisions of the aorta are ascending aorta, aortic arch, and descending aorta, subdivided into the thoracic and abdominal aortae.
   C. The main branches of each division of the aorta are listed in Table 13–1.
V. Two coronary arteries that branch from the ascending aorta bring blood to the wall of the heart. Blood circulates through a complex network of arteries and capillaries and then empties into the coronary veins. These join to form the coronary sinus, a large vein that empties into the right atrium (Table 13–2).
VI. Blood is conducted into the brain by the internal carotid arteries and the vertebral arteries. Branches of these arteries join to form the circle of Willis. From the brain capillaries, blood passes into venous sinuses in the dura mater and then into the internal jugular veins.
VII. Blood from the digestive system drains into the hepatic portal vein, which conducts it to the liver. Within the liver, blood flows into an extensive network of sinusoids from which the liver removes excess nutrients. Blood from the hepatic sinusoids passes into hepatic veins, which empty into the inferior vena cava. This hepatic portal system is characterized by an extra set of exchange vessels (sinusoids), so that instead of conducting blood into another vein, the hepatic portal vein empties into a set of sinusoids.
VIII. Pulse is caused by the elastic expansion and recoil of arteries as they fill with blood; it is measured with a sphygmomanometer and a stethoscope.

IX. Blood pressure is the force exerted by the blood against the inner walls of the blood vessels. Blood pressure = flow × resistance.
   A. A small change in the radius of a blood vessel causes a big change in resistance and thus in blood pressure.
   B. The amount of blood pressure within the arteries as a whole is regulated mainly by the degree of vasoconstriction or vasodilation of the arterioles.
   C. Blood pressure is greatest in the arteries, decreases in the arterioles, and continues to decrease as blood flows through capillaries, venules, and finally veins.
X. Blood pressure is regulated by neural and hormonal mechanisms. Arterial baroreceptors provide feedback to the cardiac centers in the medulla.
XI. Major cardiovascular diseases include hypertension, atherosclerosis, and ischemic heart disease.
   A. In atherosclerosis plaques develop within the arterial wall, eventually impeding the flow of blood. Atherosclerosis can lead to CVA, ischemic heart disease, or MI.
   B. Some patients with ischemic heart disease suffer from attacks of angina pectoris, especially during physical exertion or emotional excitement.
   C. Myocardial infarction (MI) usually results from a sudden decrease in blood supply to the myocardium.
XII. The lymphatic system collects and returns interstitial fluid to the blood, defends the body against disease, and absorbs lipids from the intestine.
   A. The lymph is formed from interstitial fluid.
   B. The lymph circulates through a system of lymph capillaries and veins; as it passes through lymph nodes it is filtered.
   C. The lymphatic system includes the tonsils, spleen, and thymus gland.

## POST TEST

1. Blood vessels that transport blood away from the heart and toward some organ or tissue are called _____.
2. Materials are exchanged between blood and tissues through the thin walls of _____.
3. By constricting and dilating, arterioles help determine the amount of _____ that enters a tissue and also help regulate blood _____.
4. The left ventricle pumps blood into the _____ circulation.
5. Blood from the right ventricle is pumped into the _____.
6. The pulmonary vein carries _____ (oxygen-rich or deoxygenated) blood.
7. The coronary arteries branch from the _____.
8. In the lower abdominal cavity, the aorta divides to form the _____ _____ arteries.
9. Blood returning to the heart from the tissues above the level of the diaphragm drains into a large vein, the _____ _____.
10. The brachiocephalic artery branches from the _____ and delivers blood to the right _____ carotid artery and the right _____ artery.
11. The coronary sinus drains blood from the _____ veins and delivers it to the _____ _____.
12. An important arterial circuit at the base of the brain is the _____ _____.
13. Blood is delivered to the brain by the _____ _____ _____ arteries and the _____ arteries.
14. Blood from the digestive tract passes from the superior mesenteric vein into the _____ _____ vein, which takes it to the _____.

15. Blood from the kidneys passes into the _____ veins, which deliver it to the _____ _____ _____.

16. The alternate expansion and recoil of an artery is arterial _____.

17. The force exerted by the blood against the inner walls of the blood vessels is called _____ _____.

18. A small change in the radius of a blood vessel causes a big change in resistance and _____ _____.

19. Three functions of the lymphatic system are _____, _____, and _____.

20. Tonsils are masses of _____ _____.

21. Two main functions of lymph nodes are to _____ _____ and to _____ _____.

22. Vessels that conduct lymph into a lymph node are called _____.

23. The spleen filters _____.

24. The _____ is a lymphatic organ that plays a key role in immunity.

25. When interstitial fluid enters a lymph capillary it is called _____.

26. Label the diagram below.

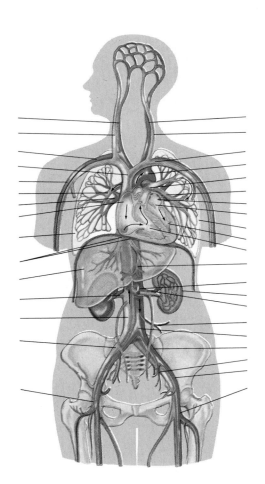

## REVIEW QUESTIONS

1. Compare the wall of an artery with that of a capillary.
2. Why is the ability of arterioles to dilate and constrict physiologically important?

3. Some veins have valves. Why is this useful?
4. Why are capillaries sometimes referred to as the "functional structures" of the circulatory system.
5. Name the divisions of the aorta and list the main arteries that branch from each division.
6. Trace a drop of blood from the inferior vena cava to the thoracic aorta by listing each blood vessel and each part of the heart through which it must pass in sequence.
7. What blood vessels bring blood to the brain? What is the significance of the circle of Willis?
8. Why does the heart, which is always full of blood, require a system of blood vessels to serve its wall? Trace the blood through the principal vessels that serve the heart.
9. Trace a drop of blood from the (a) subclavian vein to the coronary artery (b) right atrium to the renal vein (c) inferior vena cava to the superior vena cava (d) hepatic portal vein to the right common carotid artery.
10. Trace a drop of blood from the (a) coronary vein to a pulmonary capillary (b) iliac vein to the brain (c) kidney to the liver (d) inferior vena cava to the arm (e) heart to the celiac artery.
11. How does blood manage to travel against gravity through veins in the legs on its way back to the heart?
12. How do the angiotensins influence blood pressure?
13. What is ischemic heart disease and what are some of its consequences?
14. Describe the progression of atherosclerosis, list its risk factors, and relate this disease to various types of heart disease.
15. How does the lymphatic system help maintain homeostasis?
16. What are the functions of (a) lymph nodes (b) tonsils (c) spleen (d) thymus?

# 14

# The Body's Defense Mechanisms

## LEARNING OBJECTIVES

**After you study this chapter you should be able to**
1. Distinguish between specific and nonspecific defense mechanisms and identify several nonspecific defense mechanisms.
2. Describe the process of inflammation and tell how inflammation works in the defense of the body.
3. Compare the functions of B lymphocytes with those of T lymphocytes.
4. Define the terms antigen and antibody.
5. Describe the mechanism of cell-mediated immunity, including development of memory cells.
6. Describe the mechanism of antibody-mediated immunity, including the effects of antigen-antibody combination on pathogens both directly and through the complement system.
7. Describe the role of the thymus in immune mechanisms.
8. Contrast active and passive immunity and give examples of each.
9. Explain the theory of immunosurveillance and what happens when immunosurveillance fails.

245

10. Describe the problem of graft rejection and how physicians minimize its effects in transplant patients.
11. Define hypersensitivity and give the immunological basis of allergy.
12. Briefly describe a common allergic response such as hayfever and tell what happens in systemic anaphylaxis.

---

The body has remarkable defense mechanisms that provide protection against **pathogens** (disease organisms). Defense mechanisms can be nonspecific or highly specific (Fig. 14–1).

## NONSPECIFIC DEFENSE MECHANISMS

Nonspecific defense mechanisms prevent pathogens from entering the body and destroy them quickly when they do penetrate the skin. The skin is the body's first line of defense against pathogens and other harmful substances. In addition to presenting an excellent mechanical barrier against invasion, the skin is populated by large numbers of harmless microorganisms that inhibit the multiplication of many foreign organisms that happen to land on it. Sweat and sebum, found on the sur-

face of the skin, also contain chemicals that destroy certain types of bacteria.

Pathogens that enter the body with inhaled air may be filtered out by hairs in the nose or trapped in the sticky mucous lining of the respiratory passageway. Such invaders may then be destroyed by phagocytes. Organisms that enter with food are usually destroyed by the acid secretions and enzymes of the stomach.

When pathogens succeed in invading the tissues other nonspecific defense mechanisms are activated. Certain phagocytic cells (including macrophages and some types of white blood cells) make up the **reticuloendothelial** (re-tik″-u-low-en-dow-**thee′**-lee-al) **system (RES)**. Some macrophages wander through the tissues phagocytizing foreign matter and releasing antiviral agents; others settle down in one place and destroy bacteria that pass by. Macrophages in different parts of the body

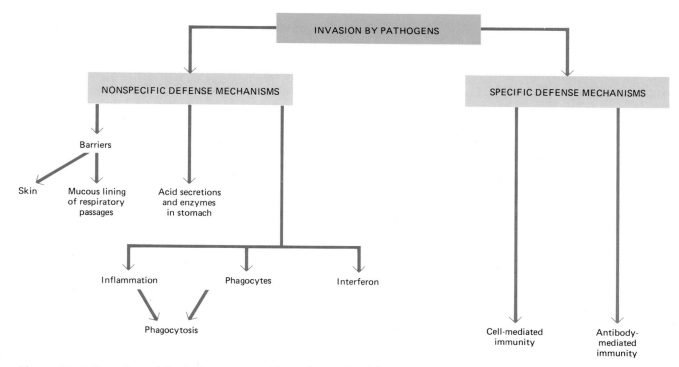

*Figure 14–1. Overview of the body's nonspecific and specific defense mechanisms.*

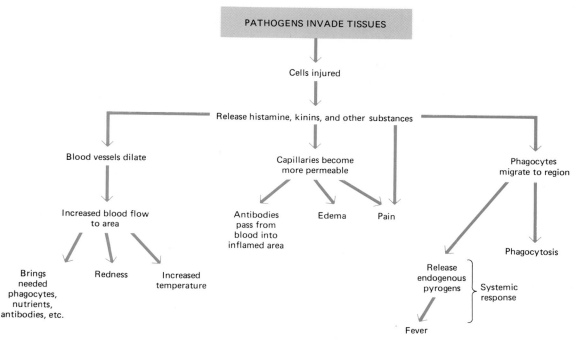

**Figure 14–2.** *The physiology of inflammation.*

function in specialized ways. For example, macrophages in the liver called **Kupffer cells** remove bacteria that have managed to get through the stomach's defenses and into the blood.

## Inflammation

When pathogens invade tissues, they trigger an **inflammatory response** (Fig. 14–2). Blood vessels in the affected area dilate, increasing blood flow to the area. This makes the skin look red and feel warm. Capillaries in the inflamed area become more permeable, permitting more plasma to leave the circulation and enter the tissues. As the volume of tissue fluid increases, **edema** (swelling) occurs. Thus the clinical characteristics of inflammation are redness, edema, heat, and pain.

The increased blood flow that occurs during inflammation brings great numbers of phagocytes (phagocytic cells) to the infected area. Increased permability of the blood vessels permits gamma globulins (plasma proteins that serve as antibodies) to leave the circulation and enter the tissues. As plasma leaves the circulation it also brings with it oxygen and nutrients.

Although inflammation is often a localized response, sometimes the entire body reacts. **Fever** is a common clinical symptom of widespread inflammatory response. Although the benefits of fever are not understood, elevated temperature is thought to inhibit bacterial iron uptake, which in turn slows bacterial multiplication. High fevers are harmful, however, often causing convulsions in young children. Other systemic effects of inflammation include loss of appetite, fatigue, and a general feeling of discomfort. The causes of these symptoms are not yet understood.

## Phagocytosis

One of the main functions of inflammation is to bring large numbers of phagocytes to the affected area. Once there, phagocytes ingest bacteria by flowing around them and engulfing them; this is **phagocytosis**. As a bacterium is ingested, it is neatly packaged within a vacuole formed by membrane pinched off from the cell membrane. One or more lysosomes adhere to the vacuole and release enzymes into it that kill the bacterium.

## Interferons

When infected by viruses or other intracellular parasites (some types of bacteria, fungi, and protozoa), certain types of cells respond by secreting proteins called **interferons** (in-tur-**feer**'-ons). These proteins trigger other cells to produce antiviral proteins. Viruses produced in cells exposed to interferon are not effective at infecting new cells.

As a result of recombinant DNA technology, interferon is now available commercially. In experimental trials interferon has been used successfully in some cases to boost patients' immunity against some viral infections. Some researchers are also optimistic that interferon may eventually prove effective in treating certain forms of cancer.

## SPECIFIC DEFENSE MECHANISMS

Nonspecific defense mechanisms rapidly destroy pathogens and prevent the spread of infection while specific defense mechanisms are being mobilized. Specific defense is the job of the lymphatic system, which can mobilize armies of highly specialized cellular soldiers and can wage sophisticated chemical warfare. The body's specific defense mechanisms are collectively referred to as **immune** (ih-**mewn'**) **responses**. The term immune is derived from a latin word meaning "safe." **Immunology** is the study of the body's defense mechanisms.

Specific immunity is possible because each individual is biochemically unique. All human beings have the same basic kinds of proteins, large carbohydrates, and nucleic acids, but just as no two individuals have identical fingerprints (unless they are identical twins and share the same genes), no two persons have identical macromolecules. Cells responsible for immunity "know" their own body compounds and "recognize" the macromolecules of invading pathogens as foreign. They distinguish between self and nonself. Entry of any foreign material stimulates these cells to launch immune responses in an effort to destroy the invader and preserve homeostasis.

Each type of pathogen has distinct macromolecules such as proteins or polysaccharides on its surface. Such macromolecules, called **antigens**, are capable of stimulating an immune response.

## T and B Lymphocytes

The principal warriors in specific immune responses are the trillion or so lymphocytes stationed strategically in the lymph tissue throughout the body. All lymphocytes can be traced back through their generations to stem cells in the bone marrow. However, before birth, descendants of the stem cells migrate to the lymph tissues, where they continue to proliferate throughout life. On their way to the lymph tissues one group of lym-phocytes stops temporarily in the thymus for processing. These become the **T lymphocytes**, or **T cells**. Their job is to attack foreign cells or viruses that enter the body. The rest of the lymphocytes, called **B lymphocytes**, or **B cells**, are responsible for the production of specific circulating antibodies.

## Cell-Mediated Immunity

In **cell-mediated immunity** lymphocytes attack invading pathogens directly. Cell-mediated immunity is the responsibility of T cells and macrophages. There are thousands of different varieties of lymphocytes, each capable of responding to a specific type of antigen. When an antigen gains entrance to the body, the types of lymphocytes able to react to that antigen become activated, or sensitized. It is thought that this activation process occurs when macrophages take up the antigens and present them to the lymphocytes.

Once stimulated, lymphocytes increase in size and then multiply by mitosis, each giving rise to a sizable clone of cells identical to itself (Fig. 14–3). T cells then differentiate to perform specific functions and the differentiated cells make their way to the site of invasion.

One type of differentiated T cell, the **killer T cell**, combines with antigens on the surface of an invading cell. Killer T cells release powerful substances that kill the foreign cell directly. **Helper T cells** stimulate macrophages, making them more adept at killing pathogens. Such stimulated macrophages are sometimes called angry macrophages.

T cells are especially adept at attacking viruses, parasites, fungi, and the type of bacteria that live within host cells. Once a host cell has been invaded by a pathogen, its macromolecules may be altered so that the immune system views it as foreign. Host cells inhabited by pathogens are thus destroyed by killer T cells. These lymphocytes also destroy cancer cells and, unfortunately, the cells of transplanted organs.

When T cells in the lymph nodes are sensitized and multiply, not all of them leave the lymph tissue and travel to the scene of battle. Some remain behind as **memory cells**. Should the invading pathogen ever attack again, the memory cells initiate a far swifter reaction than occurred during the first invasion, destroying pathogens so rapidly that they usually do not have time to establish themselves or even to cause symptoms of the disease. This explains why we do not usually become ill from the same type of infection more than once.

You may wonder, then, how someone can get a

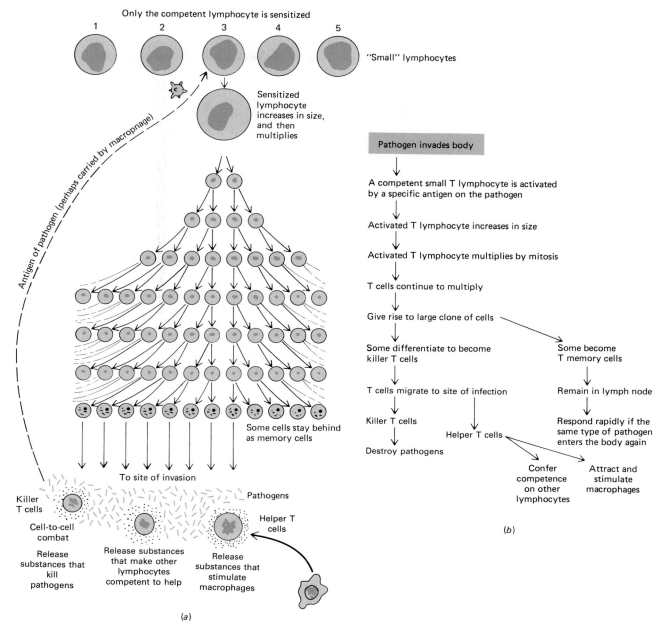

***Figure 14–3.*** *Cell-mediated immunity. When activated by an antigen, a T lymphocyte gives rise to a large clone of cells. Killer T cells and helper T cells migrate to the site of infection and act to destroy the invading pathogens.*

cold or influenza (the "flu") more than once. The answer is that there are many varieties of these infections, each caused by a slightly different virus. Furthermore, viruses frequently mutate, developing slightly different surface antigens in the process. (This appears to be a survival mechanism for them.) Even a slight change can nonetheless prevent recognition by memory cells, requiring the body to treat each different antigen as a new immunological challenge.

## Antibody-Mediated Immunity

The B lymphocytes are responsible for **antibody-mediated immunity** (Fig. 14–4). As with T lymphocytes, there are thousands of different kinds of B lymphocytes, each able to respond to a specific type of antigen. An important difference, though, is the way in which they respond. Instead of going out to meet the invader, as T lymphocytes do, B lymphocytes produce specific antibodies and send

## FOCUS ON
## How the Body Defends Itself Against Cancer

According to some investigators, cancer cells develop daily in each of us. Because they are abnormal cells, some of their surface proteins are different from those found on normal body cells. These different surface proteins act as antigens, stimulating an immune response that results in destruction of the abnormal cells. According to this **theory of immunosurveillance** (im″-mu-no-ser-**vay**′-lens), the mechanism sometimes fails, allowing uncontrolled growth of the abnormal cells.

Normally, killer T cells and macrophages attack cancer cells (see figure). Other cells, the **natural killer cells (NK cells)**, also attack cancer cells. Sometimes these phagocytes either fail to recognize cancer cells as foreign or are unable to destroy them. Studies indicate that patients with advanced cancer have far less NK cell activity than normal persons.

An exciting new approach in cancer research involves the production of **monoclonal** (mon″-oh-klown′-al) **antibodies**. In this procedure mice are injected with antigens from human cancer cells. After the mice have had time to make antibodies to the cancer cells, their spleens are removed, and cells containing the antibodies are extracted from the spleen tissue. Then these cells are fused with cancer cells from other mice. Cancer cells have an unlimited ability to divide, so these fused hybrid cells continue to divide indefinitely. Researchers can select the hybrid cells that are producing the antibodies they want and clone them in a separate tissue culture. Cells of this clone produce large amounts of the specific antibodies needed, thus the name monoclonal antibodies. These antibodies can be injected into the same cancer patients whose cancer cells were used to stimulate their production. Such antibodies are specific for destroying the cancer cells. The antibodies can also be tagged with toxic drugs that are delivered specifically to the cancer cells.

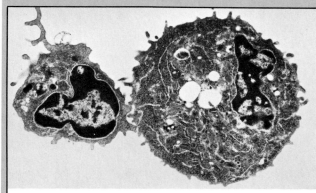
(a)

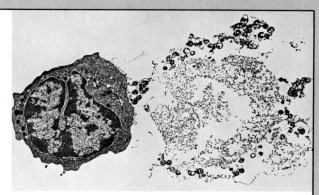
(b)

(a) An electron micrograph of a killer T cell (the smaller of the two cells) approaching a cancer cell. (b) After about 2 hours of contact, a killer T cell has destroyed a cancer cell. (Courtesy of Professeur Daniel Zagury.)

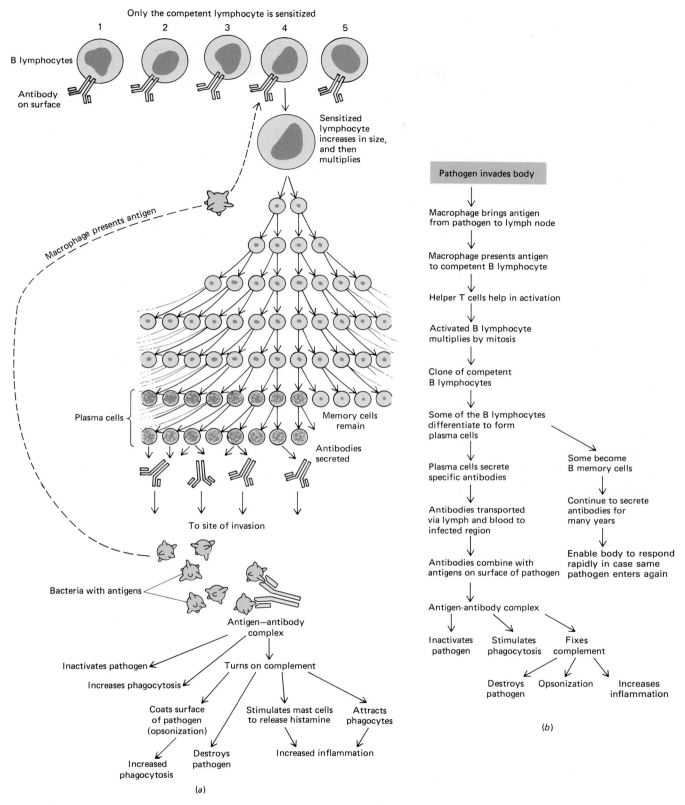

**Figure 14–4.** Antibody-mediated immunity. When activated by an antigen, a B lymphocyte gives rise to a large clone of cells. Many of these become plasma cells that secrete antibodies. The antibodies are transported to the site of infection by the blood or lymph. Antigen-antibody complexes form that directly inactivate some pathogens and also turn on the complement system. Some of the B lymphocytes become plasma cells that continue to secrete small amounts of antibody for years after the infection is over.

them out to do the job. As already defined, **antibodies** are highly specific proteins (also known as **immunoglobulins**), which are manufactured in response to specific antigens. They are among the body's most potent chemical weapons.

When a certain type of bacteria invades the body, bringing with it its own collection of antigens, some of the antigens find their way to the lymph tissue (either still attached to the pathogen or after being separated during phagocytosis.) Macrophages then present the antigens to the lymphocytes (Fig. 14–4). Helper T cells also play a role in the stimulation of B lymphocytes.

When the antigen comes into contact with the type of lymphocyte programmed to produce antibodies against it, the lymphocyte is activated. The activated lymphocyte begins to multiply, producing within a few days a large clone of immunologically identical lymphocytes (Fig. 14–4). Most of these cells increase in size and differentiate into **plasma cells**, the mature B cells that secrete large amounts of antibody. The secreted antibody is carried by the lymph to the blood and then transported to the infected region.

Some of the activated B lymphocytes do not fully differentiate but remain as memory cells, producing small amounts of antibody. Should the pathogen ever enter the body again, this circulating antibody (part of the gamma globulin fraction of the plasma) will immediately bind with it. At the same time, the memory cells will respond by quickly multiplying to produce new clones of the appropriate strain of plasma cells.

### Classes of Antibodies

Antibodies are grouped in five classes according to their structure. Using the abbreviation Ig for immunoglobulin, the classes are designated IgG, IgM, IgA, IgD, and IgE. Each class has different functions.

Normally about 75% of the antibodies in the body belong in the IgG group (part of the gamma globulin fraction of the blood). IgG is the only class of immunoglobulins that can cross the placenta (the organ of exchange between mother and developing child) to enter the fetal circulatory system. IgG is responsible for protecting the newborn baby from disease during the first 6 months or so of life.

### What Do Antibodies Do?

The principal job of an antibody is to identify a pathogen as foreign by combining with one or more antigens on its surface. Often antibodies

combine with several such antigens, creating a mass of clumped antigen-antibody complex (Fig. 14–4). The antigen-antibody combination activates several defense mechanisms.

1. The antigen-antibody complex may inactivate the pathogen or its toxin. For example, once an antibody has attached to the surface of a virus, the virus loses its ability to infect a new cell.
2. The combination of antibody with antigen on the surface of a pathogen stimulates phagocytes to destroy it.
3. Antibodies of the IgG and IgM groups exert most of their effect through the **complement system**. This is a sequence of about 11 proteins found in plasma and other body fluids. Normally the proteins are inactive but an antigen-antibody complex serves to stimulate the series of reactions that activate the system. The antibody is said to "fix" complement. Components of the complement system then function against invading pathogens by heightening the inflammatory response.

## Role of the Thymus

In some way the thymus confers **immunological competence** on T lymphocytes. This mens that they develop the ability to differentiate into cells that can carry out certain specific immune reactions to specific antigens. Apparently the thymus "instructs" the T lymphocytes just before birth and during the first few months of postnatal life.

The thymus secretes several hormones, including one called **thymosin** (**thy′**-mow-sin). Thymosin is thought to stimulate immature T cells to become immunologically active. Thymosin has been successfully administered to patients who have poorly developed thymus glands and, thus, low immunity. Investigators are currently injecting thymosin in certain cancer patients in the hope that it may stimulate cellular immunity, thereby helping to prevent the spread of the disease.

## Active and Passive Immunity

**Active immunity** develops from natural exposure to antigens (Table 14–1). If you had chickenpox as a young child, for example, you developed immunity that prevents you from contracting chickenpox again. Active immunity can also be developed by artificially exposing the body to the same antigens that occur on pathogens but that

THE BODY'S DEFENSE MECHANISMS 253

TABLE 14–1
**Active and Passive Immunity**

| Type of Immunity | When Developed | Memory Cells Developed? | How Long Does Immunity Last? |
|---|---|---|---|
| **Active** | | | |
| Naturally induced | Pathogens enter the body through natural encounter, e.g., person with measles sneezes on you | Yes | For many years |
| Artificially induced | After immunization, e.g., patient is vaccinated with measles vaccine | Yes | For many years |
| **Passive** | After injection with gamma globulin, or after transfer of antibodies from mother to developing baby | No | Only a few weeks or months |

have been rendered harmless in some way. This is the basis of clinical **immunization**.

By injecting an individual with antigens derived from a specific type of pathogen, the type of immune response can be planned. The body develops memory cells so that future encounters with the same kind of pathogen will be dealt with swiftly. The immune system cannot differentiate between antigens that enter the body accidentally and those that are purposely injected.

Effective vaccines can be produced in several different ways. A virus may be weakened (attenuated), so that it is not suffficiently potent to cause disease, and then ingested or injected. This is how the Sabin polio vaccine, smallpox vaccine, and measles vaccine are prepared. Diphtheria, whooping cough, and typhoid fever vaccines are prepared by killing the pathogens and using the dead organisms, which still bear the necessary antigens. In protecting against tetanus, botulism, and certain other diseases, vaccines are prepared from toxins secreted by the organisms. The toxin is altered so that it can no longer destroy tissues, but in such a way that its antigens are still intact. When injected with any of these kinds of vaccine, the body actively goes through the process of developing clones of specialized cells, producing antibodies, and developing memory cells.

In **passive immunity**, an individual is injected with antibodies actively produced by other humans or by animals. Passive immunity is borrowed immunity, so its effects are not lasting. It is used to boost one's defenses temporarily against a particular disease. For example, during the war in Vietnam viral hepatitis was rampant, so soldiers were injected with gamma globulin (containing the antibody to hepatitis virus) to help protect them from the disease. Unfortunately, such injected antibodies last only a few weeks because the body has not actively participated in an immune response and so has developed no memory cells and no lasting immunity.

Pregnant women confer passive immunity on their developing babies by producing antibodies for them. Babies who are breast-fed receive antibodies in their milk. These antibodies provide immunity to the pathogens responsible for gastrointestinal infection and perhaps to other pathogens as well.

## Rejection of Transplanted Organs

Hundreds of kidneys, hearts, and other organs have been transplanted from human donors to recipients during the past several years but with only limited success. Unfortunately, the immune system views transplanted tissues and organs as foreign and sets out to destroy them—usually effectively. The immune response aimed at transplanted tissues is referred to as **graft rejection**. T lymphocytes launch the attack and can destroy the grafted organ within a few days.

### Histocompatibility Antigens

Each of us has several groups of antigens referred to as **histocompatibility** (his″-toe-com-pat-ih-**bil**′-i-tee) **antigens** that affect transplants. Tissues with the same histocompatibility genes have the same histocompatibility antigens and thus are compatible. That is why tissue can be grafted from one part of a patient's body to another without fear of graft rejection. The less alike the histocompatibility antigens are, the less compatible are the tissues. Thus selection of a suitable donor is vitally important in transplantation procedures.

Only identical twins have identical histocompatibility genes and therefore identical antigens. Organs transplanted from one identical twin to another are therefore not perceived as foreign by the immune system of the recipient and are accepted. There is at least a one in four chance of making a good match between siblings. If two unrelated individuals are taken at random and typed, the chances are only about one in a thousand that their histocompatibility antigens will be well matched. Before transplants are undertaken, tissues from the patient and from potential donors are typed and attempts are made to match donor and recipient as closely as possible.

### Preventing Graft Rejection

Not many persons are fortunate enough to have an identical twin to supply spare parts. Most often transplanted organs are donated by unrelated persons. Furthermore, some parts, such as the heart, cannot be spared. Such organs come from recently deceased individuals.

To minimize the effects of graft rejection in less compatible matches, drugs and x-rays are used to kill T lymphocytes. These treatments kill all lymphocytes. As you might imagine, this suppresses not only graft rejection but also all immunological responses. Consequently many transplant patients succumb to pneumonia or other infections or to cancer.

An antibiotic called cyclosporin A is now being used in transplant patients. This drug appears to suppress T cells that have been activated by antigens on the graft but has little effect on B cells.

### Immunologically Privileged Sites

Certain locations in the body are known to be **immunologically privileged sites**. For example, because the cornea has almost no blood vessels associated with it and is evidently out of reach of the lymphocytes, corneal transplants are highly successful. Moreover, it is unlikely that antigens in the corneal graft would enter the blood and thus reach the lymph system. The uterus is another immunologically privileged site. There the human fetus is able to develop its own biochemical identity in safety.

## Hypersensitivity

Normally the immune system protects the body from pathogens with elegant efficiency but such a complex system sometimes malfunctions. **Hyper-**

**sensitivity** is an altered state of immune response that is harmful to the body.

### Allergic Reactions

About 15% of the population are plagued by allergic disorders such as allergic asthma or hayfever. There appears to be an inherited tendency to these disorders. Allergic persons have a tendency to produce antibodies against mild antigens, called **allergens**, that do not elicit a response in nonallergic individuals.

Let us examine a common immediate allergic reaction—a hayfever response to ragweed pollen (Fig. 14–5). When an allergic person inhales the microscopic pollen, allergens stimulate the release of an IgE antibody from sensitized plasma cells that may already be present in the nasal passages. The antibody attaches to receptors on the membranes of mast cells. Each mast cell has thousands of receptors on its surface to which the IgE molecules may attach. The other end of the antibody is left free to combine with the ragweed pollen allergen. When the allergen combines with the IgE antibody the mast cell releases histamine and other chemicals that cause inflammation. These substances cause vasodilation and increased capillary permeability, leading to edema and redness. The hayfever victims' nasal passages become swollen and irritated. Their noses run and eyes water, they sneeze, and they feel uncomfortable.

In **allergic asthma** the allergen-antibody reaction occurs in the bronchioles of the lungs. Mast cells release **slow-reacting substance of ananphylaxis (SRS-A)**, which causes smooth muscle to constrict. This can cause the airways in the lungs to constrict for several hours, making breathing difficult.

In some persons certain foods or drugs act as allergens and cause **hives**. The allergen-antibody reaction takes place in the skin and the excessive release of histamine is responsible for the swollen red welts of hives.

A dangerous kind of allergic reaction called **systemic anaphylaxis** may occur when an individual develops an allergy to specific drugs such as penicillin or to insect poison, for example, that in a bee sting. Within minutes after the drug is injected, a widespread reaction occurs involving the release of large amounts of histamine. So much histamine may be released into the circulation that extreme vasodilation and capillary permeability occur. Large amounts of plasma may be lost from the blood, causing circulatory shock, and death can occur within a few minutes.

*Figure 14–5.* A common type of allergic response.

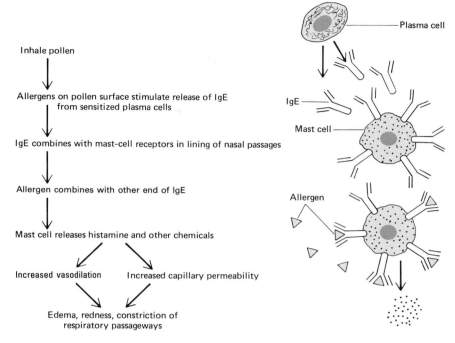

Inhale pollen

↓

Allergens on pollen surface stimulate release of IgE from sensitized plasma cells

↓

IgE combines with mast-cell receptors in lining of nasal passages

↓

Allergen combines with other end of IgE

↓

Mast cell releases histamine and other chemicals

↙        ↘

Increased vasodilation        Increased capillary permeability

↘        ↙

Edema, redness, constriction of respiratory passageways

Plasma cell

IgE

Mast cell

Allergen

The effects of histamines can be blocked by **antihistamines**. These drugs act by combining with the same receptor sites on cells targeted by histamines. When the antihistamine combines with the receptor, it prevents the histamine from combining and thus prevents its harmful effects. Antihistamines have proved helpful in alleviating the effects of many allergic responses such as hives and hayfever.

In serious allergic disorders patients are sometimes desensitized. They are injected with small amounts of the very antigen to which they are allergic. The purpose is to stimulate the production of IgG antibodies against the antigen. When the patient encounters the offending allergen again, IgG antibodies combine with the allergen, blocking its receptors so that IgE cannot combine with it. This less harmful immune response is substituted for the potentially harmful allergic reaction.

Multiple sclerosis is an example of an autoimmune disease that may be caused by the interaction of several factors. Genetic vulnerability to multiple sclerosis is thought to be inherited. If a person with genetic susceptibility is infected with a certain virus that infects the brain, the disease may develop. T lymphocytes and macrophages enter the brain and attempt to destroy the cells infected with the virus. In the process of destroying the infected cells, myelin is destroyed and the affected axons can no longer conduct impulses.

### Autoimmune Disease

We have seen that the body is normally able to distinguish between self and nonself. Occasionally, normal regulatory mechanisms malfunction and the body does launch an immune response against its own tissues, resulting in an **autoimmune disease**. Among the many diseases thought to result from such malfunctions are rheumatoid arthritis, multiple sclerosis (MS), myasthenia gravis, systemic lupus erythematosus (SLE), and perhaps infectious mononucleosis.

## SUMMARY

I. Nonspecific defense mechanisms that prevent entrance of pathogens include the skin, acid secretions in the stomach, and the mucous lining of the respiratory passageways.

II. Should pathogens succeed in traversing the "front line" defenses, other nonspecific defense mechanisms attempt to destroy the invading pathogens.

A. Macrophages of the reticuloendothelial system phagocytize pathogens that enter the lymph nodes, liver, spleen, or lungs.

B. Inflammation occurs as a response to infection. The inflammatory response brings needed phagocytic cells and antibodies to the infected area.

C. Neutrophils and macrophages migrate to

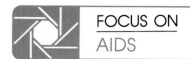

## FOCUS ON
### AIDS

First recognized in 1981, the **acquired immuno-deficiency syndrome (AIDS)** is a fatal disorder that kills its victims by destroying their immune systems. AIDS is caused by a virus identified as human T-lymphotropic virus type III (HTLV-III). The virus is ordinarily transmitted only through the blood or by sexual intercourse. AIDS is not spread by casual contact. The groups at highest risk for infection are homosexual and bisexual men (about 75% of cases) and those who abuse injected drugs (20% of cases). Effective blood-screening procedures have been developed to safeguard blood bank supplies, so that risk of infection from blood transfusion has been greatly reduced.

Many persons exposed to AIDS develop the AIDS-related complex (ARC); its symptoms include fever and weight loss. Patients with AIDS-related complex may eventually develop AIDS. Immunity is suppressed in AIDS patients owing to infection of one type of T cells ($T_4$ cells, which have helper and inducer functions) by the virus. The ability to resist infection is severely impaired and affected individuals die of a variety of rare infections and cancers.

Researchers are currently testing a variety of antiviral drugs in their search for an effective treatment for AIDS. Investigators are also trying to develop an effective vaccine against this disease.

the infected area and phagocytize pathogens.

   D. Certain cells release interferon when infected by viruses or other intracellular parasites.

III. Specific immunity depends on the body's ability to recognize its own unique macromolecules and to attack the foreign macromolecules (antigens) of pathogens.

IV. In cell-mediated immunity, specific T lymphocytes are activated by the presence of specific antigens. Activated T lymphocytes increase in size and then multiply, giving rise to a clone of identical cells.

   A. Some T cells differentiate to become killer T cells and migrate to the site of infection.

   B. Killer T cells kill pathogens and helper T cells stimulate macrophages.

   C. Some sensitized T cells remain in the lymph nodes as memory cells.

V. In antibody-mediated immunity, specific B lymphocytes are activated by the presence of specific antigens. Activated B lymphocytes multiply and give rise to cells that differentiate to become plasma cells. These plasma cells secrete specific antibodies.

   A. Antibodies diffuse into the lymph and are transported to the blood and then to the site of infection.

   B. Antibody combines with a specific antigen to form an antigen-antibody complex. This may activate several defense mechanisms, including the complement system.

VI. Active immunity, whether natural or artificial, involves exposure to an antigen and an active immune response, which includes the production of memory cells. This provides long-term protection. In passive immunity antibodies are borrowed from another person or animal that has produced them. Passive immunity is temporary.

VII. According to the theory of immunosurveillance, the immune system is continuously on guard for abnormal cells such as cancer cells and acts quickly to destroy them. When the immune system fails, diseases such as cancer can develop.

VIII. Because transplanted organs bring antigens with them, they stimulate graft rejection, an immune response launched mainly by T cells that destroy the transplant.

IX. In hypersensitivity the immune system becomes abnormally altered, causing harm to the body.

   A. In an allergic response, an allergen can stimulate production of IgE antibody, which combines with receptors on mast cells. When the allergen combines with the IgE antibody, the mast cells release histamine and other substances that cause inflammation and other symptoms of allergy.

   B. Autoimmune diseases may occur when the normal regulatory mechanisms fail and the body launches an immune response against its own tissues.

## POST TEST

1. Disease-causing organisms such as bacteria and viruses are correctly referred to as _____.
2. The clinical characteristics of inflammation are _____, _____, _____, and _____.
3. The increased blood flow characteristic of inflammation brings _____ to the infected area.
4. The process by which neutrophils and macrophages engulf bacteria is termed _____.
5. When certain types of cells are infected by viruses, they release a protein called _____.
6. Macromolecules that stimulate immune responses are called _____.
7. Plasma cells produce proteins called _____ that help destroy antigens.
8. B lymphocytes are responsible for _____ -mediated immunity.
9. T lymphocytes are responsible for _____ -mediated immunity.
10. Sensitized B or T cells that remain in the lymph nodes for many years after an infection are called _____ _____.
11. The main job of an antibody is to identify a pathogen as foreign by combining with _____ on its surface.
12. The _____ system is a group of about 11 proteins found in plasma and other body fluids.
13. The temporary immunity gained when one is injected with gamma globulin is called _____ immunity.
14. An example of artificially induced active immunity is _____.
15. The immune response aimed at transplanted tissues is called _____ _____.
16. In an allergic response mild antigens called _____ stimulate production of _____ _____, which attaches to receptors on the cell membranes of _____ cells.

## REVIEW QUESTIONS

1. Contrast nonspecific and specific types of defense mechanisms. Which type acts immediately?
2. How does the inflammatory response help to restore homeostasis?
3. What are the principal cells of the reticuloendothelial system?
4. How does interferon work?
5. Define (a) antigen (b) antibody.
6. Contrast the origins and actions of T and B lymphocytes.
7. Contrast cell-mediated immunity with antibody-mediated immunity, giving their principal differences.
8. Compare the immune response that occurs when someone with measles sneezes on you with the response stimulated when you are immunized against measles.
9. Why is passive immunity temporary?
10. Explain the theory of immunosurveillance. What happens when immunosurveillance fails?
11. What is graft rejection? How do physicians attempt to prevent it? Suppress it?

12. What are immunologically privileged sites?
13. What is meant by hypersensitivity?
14. List the events that take place in a common allergic response such as hayfever.
16. What is an autoimmune disease?

# V

# OBTAINING OXYGEN, NUTRIENTS, AND ENERGY

# 15

# The Respiratory System

LEARNING OBJECTIVES

**After you study this chapter you should be able to**
1. Trace a breath of air through the respiratory system from nose to alveoli.
2. Describe the structure of the lungs.
3. Summarize the mechanics of breathing.
4. Describe how respiration is regulated.
5. Describe how oxygen and carbon dioxide are exchanged in the lungs and in the tissues.
6. Outline the mechanisms by which oxygen and carbon dioxide are transported in the blood.
7. Describe the physiological effects of (a) hyperventilation and (b) surfacing too quickly from a deep-sea dive.
8. Describe the defense mechanisms of the respiratory system and the diseases that result from continued respiratory insult.

The respiratory system consists of the lungs and the series of tubes through which air reaches them. A breath of air enters the body through the nose, flows through the nasal cavities to the pharynx, through the larynx and into the trachea, commonly known as the windpipe (Fig. 15–1). Air then enters the bronchi (one bronchus enters each lung) and then passes into the many bronchioles of the lungs. These divide again and again until the air reaches the microscopic air sacs. From them oxygen diffuses into the blood within the capillaries that envelop each air sac.

## THE NASAL CAVITIES

Whether you breathe through your nose or mouth, air finds its way into the pharynx. Nose breathing is more desirable because of the "air conditioning" function of the nose. As air passes through the nose, it is filtered, moistened, and brought to body temperature. The nose also contains the receptors for the sense of smell.

Air passes into the nose through its two openings, the **nostrils**. The nostrils are fringed with coarse hair, which prevents large particles from

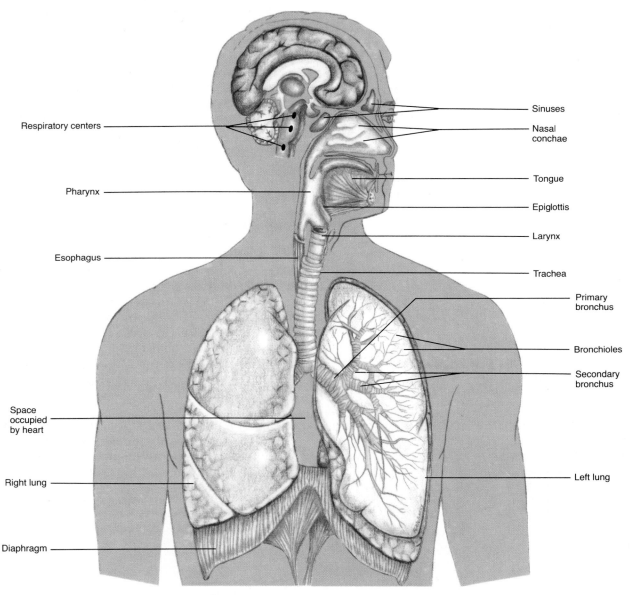

*Figure 15–1. The human respiratory system. The paired lungs are located in the thoracic cavity. The muscular diaphragm forms the floor of the thoracic cavity, separating it from the abdominal cavity below. An internal view of one lung illustrates its extensive system of air passageways. The microscopic alveoli are shown in later figures.*

entering the nose. The nostrils open into the two nasal cavities, which are separated by a partition, the **nasal septum**. The septum and walls of the nose consist of bone covered with a mucous membrane. Three bony structures, the **conchae**, project from the lateral walls of the nose. The conchae increase the surface area over which air must pass as it moves through the nose. The mucous membrane lining the nose has a rich blood supply that heats and moistens the lining and the air that comes into contact with it.

Mucous cells within the lining produce more than a pint of mucus a day, more in the event of allergy or infection. Inhaled dirt and other foreign particles are trapped in the layer of mucus that forms along the surface of the mucous membrane. Ciliated epithelial cells lining the membrane push a steady stream of mucus, along with its trapped particles, toward the throat. From these, the mucus is swallowed with the saliva. In this way foreign particles are delivered to the digestive system, which is far more capable of disposing of them than the delicate lungs.

Several sinuses (small cavities) in the bones of the skull communicate with the nasal cavities by small channels. They are lined with mucous membrane, which sometimes becomes inflamed and infected *(sinusitis)*.

## THE PHARYNX AND LARYNX

Posteriorly the nasal cavities are continuous with the throat, or **pharynx** (**far′**-inx). Air enters the **nasopharynx** (nay″-so-**far′**-inx), the superior part of the pharynx, and then moves down through the **oropharynx** behind the mouth. Finally, it passes through the **laryngopharynx** and enters the larynx.

The **larynx** (**lar′**-inx), or voice box, contains the vocal cords, muscular folds of tissue that project from its lateral walls. The vocal cords vibrate as air from the lungs rushes past them during expiration (breathing out). The narrow passageway through the larynx between the vocal cords is the glottis. During swallowing, a flap of tissue, the **epiglottis**, automatically closes off the larynx so that food cannot enter the lower airway. When this mechanism fails and foreign matter comes into contact with the sensitive larynx, a cough reflex is stimulated to expel the material from the respiratory system. Despite these mechanisms, choking sometimes occurs (see Focus on Choking).

The wall of the larynx is supported by cartilage that protrudes from the midline of the neck and is sometimes referred to as the Adam's apple. The

Adam's apple is more prominent in males than in females.

> Inflammation of the larynx, or *laryngitis*, is most often caused by a respiratory infection or by irritating substances such as cigarette smoke. Long-term smokers sometimes become permanently hoarse as a result of damage caused by chronic inflammation.

## THE TRACHEA AND BRONCHI

The **trachea** (**tray′**-kee-ah), or windpipe, is located anterior to the esophagus and extends from the larynx to the level of the fifth thoracic vertebra (about midchest). At that point it divides into right and left bronchi. Like the larynx, the trachea is kept from collapsing by rings of cartilage in its wall. The open parts of these C-shaped rings of cartilage face posteriorly toward the esophagus.

The larynx, trachea, and bronchi are lined by a mucous membrane that traps dirt and other foreign matter. Ciliated cells in this lining continuously beat a stream of mucus upward to the pharynx where it is swallowed. This cilia-propelled mucus elevator keeps foreign material out of the lungs.

One **bronchus** (**bronk′**-us) enters each lung. The structure of these main bronchi is similar to that of the trachea. Each bronchus branches again and again, giving rise to smaller and smaller bronchi and finally to tiny **bronchioles**. There are more than a million bronchioles in each lung. The network of branching and rebranching within the lungs is referred to as the *respiratory tree*.

## THE ALVEOLI

Each bronchiole leads into a cluster of tiny air sacs, the **alveoli**. The wall of an alveolus (al-**veé**-oh-lus) consists of a single layer of epithelial cells and sufficient elastic fibers to permit it to stretch and contract during breathing (Fig. 15–2). Each alveolus is enveloped by a network of capillaries so that gases diffuse easily between the alveolus and blood. Alveoli are coated by a thin film of **surfactant**, a substance that prevents them from collapsing.

## THE LUNGS

The lungs are large, paired, spongy organs that occupy the thoracic cavity. The right lung is di-

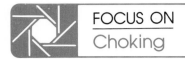

## FOCUS ON
### Choking

Choking kills an estimated 8000 to 10,000 people per year in the United States. Many of these have long suffered from some degree of paralysis or other malfunction of the muscles involved in swallowing, often without consciously realizing it. Swallowing is a complex process in which the mouth, pharynx, esophagus, and vocal cords must be coordinated with great precision. Functional muscular disorders of this mechanism can originate in a variety of ways—as birth defects, for example, or from brain tumors or vascular accidents involving the swallowing center of the brain stem.

Choking is more likely to occur in restaurants, where social interactions and unfamiliar surroundings are likely to distract one's attention from swallowing and where alcohol is more likely to be taken with the meal. A large number of choking victims have a substantial blood-alcohol content on autopsy, which suggests the possibility that in them a marginally effective swallowing reflex has been further and fatally compromised by the effects of alcohol on the brain.

Anyone who begins to choke and gasp during a meal should be asked if he or she can speak. If not, the person is probably suffering a laryngeal obstruction rather than a coronary heart attack. As a first step, deliver a strong blow to the victim's back with the open hand. If this fails, stand behind the victim, bring your arms around his or her waist, and clasp your hands just above the beltline. Your thumbs should be facing inward against the victim's body. Then squeeze abruptly and strongly in an upward direction. In most instances the residual air in the lungs will pop the obstruction out like a cork from a bottle. This is called the **Heimlich maneuver**. It can also be performed in a prone position. If the Heimlich maneuver must be performed in the prone position, place the victim face up. Kneel astride the victim's hips and, with one of your hands on top of the other, place the heel of bottom hand on the abdomen slightly above the navel but below the rib cage. Press into the victim's abdomen with a quick upward thrust. This may be repeated if necessary. If there is no response within 15 to 20 seconds, it may be necessary to start cardiopulmonary resuscitation (CPR).

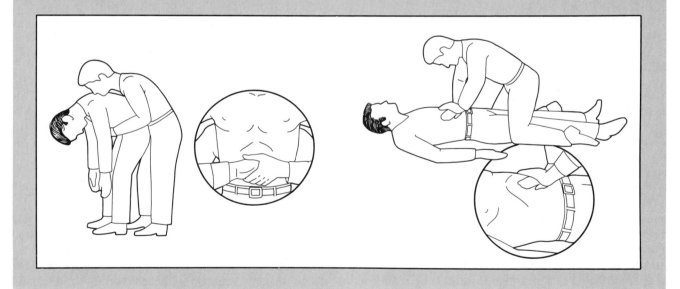

vided into three lobes, the left lung into two lobes. Each lung is covered with a **pleural membrane**, which forms a continuous sac enclosing the lung and continuing as the lining of the thoracic cavity. The part of the pleural membrane that encloses the lung is the **visceral pleura**, whereas the portion that lines the thoracic cavity is the **parietal pleura**.

Between the pleural membranes is a potential space, the **pleural cavity**. A film of fluid secreted by the pleural membranes fills the pleural cavity. This fluid permits the lungs to glide easily over the thoracic wall during breathing. Inflammation of the pleural membrane, called *pleurisy*, causes pain during breathing as the swollen membranes contact each other.

The thoracic cavity is completely enclosed. It is

**Figure 15–2.** *Structure of an alveolus. Note that the alveolar wall consists of extremely thin squamous epithelium, which permits gas exchange. The walls of the alveoli are shared and extensive capillary networks are sandwiched between them.*

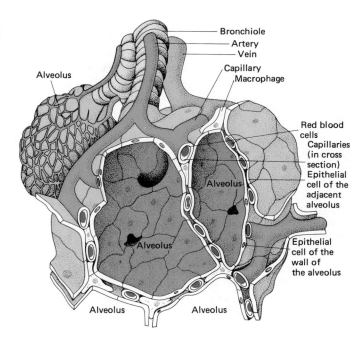

bounded on the top and sides by the chest wall, which contains the ribs, and its floor is the strong, dome-shaped **diaphragm**.

Inside, each lung consists mainly of bronchi, bronchioles, alveoli, blood vessels, and elastic tissue. Lymph tissue and nerves are also present. The bronchioles and alveoli are so numerous that the surface area available for gas exchange in the adult lungs approximates that of a tennis court.

## BREATHING

**Pulmonary ventilation**, or **breathing**, is the mechanical process of moving air into and out of the lungs. Breathing in is called **inspiration** (or inhalation); breathing out is **expiration** (exhalation).

During inspiration the diaphragm contracts and flattens and the intercostal muscles contract, increasing the size of the chest cavity (Fig. 15–3). Because the chest cavity is closed, when it expands, the film of fluid on the pleural membranes holds the lung surfaces against the chest wall. This causes the lungs to move outward along with the chest walls and increases the space within each lung. The air in the lungs at first tends to spread out to fill the increased space but then the pressure of the air in the lungs falls below the pressure of the air outside the body (that is, a partial vacuum occurs). As a result, air from the outside rushes in through the respiratory passageways and fills the lungs until the two pressures are again equal.

Expiration occurs when the diaphragm and intercostal muscles relax, permitting the elastic tissues of the lung to recoil. The size of the thoracic

**Figure 15–3.** *The mechanics of breathing. (a) Changes in the position of the diaphragm during inspiration and expiration result in changes in volume of the chest cavity. (b) Changes in position of the rib cage in expiration and inspiration. During inspiration the chest muscles pull the front ends of the ribs upward. The resulting increase in the volume of the chest cavity causes air to move into the lungs.*

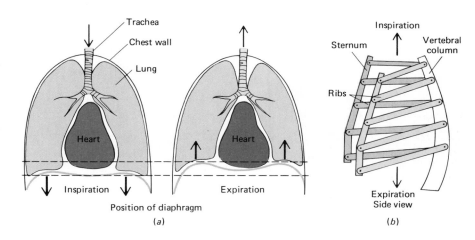

cavity decreases. Pressure increases inside the lung and its elastic fibers push against the air, forcing it to rush out of the lung. The millions of alveoli deflate and the lung is ready for another inspiration. During forced expiration several sets of muscles, including the abdominal muscles, contract.

## REGULATION OF RESPIRATION

The normal adult breathing rate is about 12 to 20 times per minute. When you are engaged in a strenuous game of racketball, you require more oxygen than when reading quietly. The rate, depth, and rhythm of breathing is regulated by respiratory centers in the medulla and pons. During exercise body tissues produce greater amounts of carbon dioxide. The carbon dioxide (after combining with water to form carbonic acid) causes the blood to be more acidic. Within the medulla there is an area that is sensitive to increased concentrations of carbon dioxide or to sharp decreases in oxygen concentration. There are similar receptors located in certain blood vessels (the carotid artery and aorta). When these receptors are stimulated, the medulla sends impulses that increase the rate and depth of breathing. Impulses from the medulla reach the diaphragm by way of the **phrenic nerves**.

Breathing is an involuntary process but the action of the respiratory centers can be consciously stimulated or inhibited. For example, you can inhibit breathing by holding your breath. You could not kill yourself by holding your breath, however, because when carbon dioxide builds up to a certain level, want to or not, you do breathe.

Underwater swimmers and divers not using scuba gear may voluntarily **hyperventilate** before going under water. Taking a series of deep breaths does not increase the oxygen in the blood but it does reduce the carbon dioxide content. This permits them to remain under water for a few extra moments before the urge to breathe becomes irresistible. Hyperventilation can result in dizziness and even unconsciousness. This is because a certain concentration of carbon dioxide in the blood is necessary to maintain normal blood pressure.

> When individuals have stopped breathing because of drowning, electrical shock, cardiac arrest, or other crisis, they can often be kept alive by mouth-to-mouth resuscitation until their own breathing reflexes can take over again. Cardiopulmonary resuscitation (CPR) is a method for helping those in respiratory and/or cardiac arrest. (For a summary of the procedure, see Focus on Cardiopulmonary Resuscitation.)

## GAS EXCHANGE

Breathing delivers oxygen to the alveoli of the lungs. However, if oxygen merely remained in the lungs, all the other body cells would quickly perish. The vital link between the alveoli and the body cells is the circulatory system. Each alveolus serves as a depot from which oxygen is loaded into the blood of the pulmonary capillaries.

Because the alveoli contain a greater concentration of oxygen than the blood entering the pulmonary capillaries, oxygen molecules diffuse from the alveoli into the blood (Fig. 15–4). Carbon dioxide moves from the blood, where it is more concentrated, to the alveoli, where it is less concentrated. Each gas diffuses through the thin lining of the capillary and the thin lining of the alveolus.

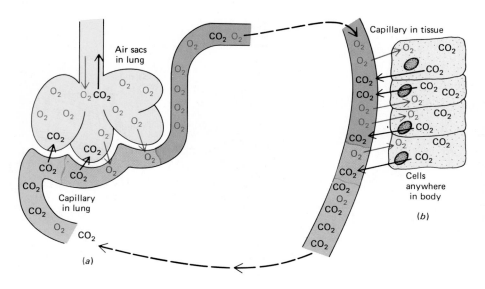

*Figure 15–4.* Gas exchange. (a) Exchange of gases between air sacs and capillary in the lung. The concentration of oxygen is greater in the air sacs than in the capillary, so oxygen moves from the air sacs into the blood. Carbon dioxide is more concentrated in the blood, so it moves out of the capillary and into the air sacs. (b) Exchange of gases between capillary and body cells. Here, oxygen is more concentrated in the blood, so it moves out of the capillary and into the cells. Carbon dioxide is more concentrated in the cells and so it diffuses out of the cells and into the blood.

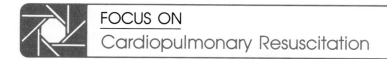

## FOCUS ON
## Cardiopulmonary Resuscitation

**Cardiopulmonary resuscitation**, or **CPR**, is a method for aiding victims of accidents or heart attacks who have suffered cardiac arrest and respiratory arrest. It should not be used if the victim has a pulse or is able to breathe. It must be started immediately, because irreversible brain damage may occur within about 3 minutes of respiratory arrest. Here are its ABCs:

**Airway**: clear airway by extending victim's neck; this is sometimes sufficient to permit breathing to begin again
**Breathing**: use mouth-to-mouth resuscitation
**Circulation**: attempt to restore circulation by using external cardiac compression

The procedure for CPR may be summarized as follows:

I. Establish unresponsiveness of victim.
II. Follow procedure for mouth-to-mouth resuscitation.
   1. Place victim on his or her back on firm surface.
   2. Clear throat and mouth and tilt head back so that chin points outward. Make sure that the tongue is not blocking airway. Pull tongue forward if necessary.
   3. Pinch nostrils shut and forcefully exhale into victim's mouth. Be careful, especially in children, not to overinflate the lungs.
   4. Remove your mouth and listen for air rushing out of the lungs.
   5. Repeat about 12 more times per minute. Do not interrupt for more than 5 seconds.
III. Follow procedure for external cardiac compression.
   1. Place heel of hand on lower third of breastbone. Keep your fingertips lifted off the chest. (In infants, two fingers should be used for cardiac compression: in children, use only the heel of the hand.)
   2. Place heel of the other hand at a right angle to and on top of the first hand.
   3. Apply firm pressure downward so that the breastbone moves about 4 to 5 cm (1.6 to 2 inches) toward the spine. Downward pressure must be about 5.4 to 9 kg (12 to 20 pounds) with adults (less with children). Excessive pressure can fracture the sternum or ribs, resulting in punctured lungs or a lacerated liver. This rhythmic pressure can often keep blood moving through the heart and great vessels of the thoracic cavity in sufficient quantities to sustain life.
   4. Relax hands between compressions to allow chest to expand.
   5. Repeat at the rate of at least 60 compressions per minute. (For infants or young children, 80 to 100 compressions per minute are appropriate.) If there is only one rescuer, 15 compressions should be applied, then two breaths, in a ratio of 15:2. If there are two rescuers, the ratio should be 5:1.

Table 15–1 shows the percentages of oxygen and carbon dioxide present in expired air compared with inspired air. There is over 100 times more carbon dioxide in expired air than in the air inspired from the environment. This is because carbon dioxide is produced by the cells of the body during cellular respiration (the chemical breakdown of fuel molecules).

## GAS TRANSPORT

When oxygen diffuses into the blood it enters the red blood cells and forms a weak chemical bond with hemoglobin, producing **oxyhemoglobin**.

Hemoglobin + oxygen → oxyhemoglobin

Because the chemical bond linking the oxygen with the hemoglobin is weak, this reaction is readily reversible. In tissues low in oxygen, oxyhemoglobin dissociates, releasing oxygen, which diffuses out of the capillaries and into the cells.

Oxyhemoglobin → oxygen + hemoglobin

Carbon dioxide is transported in the blood in

TABLE 15–1
**Composition of Inhaled Air Compared with That of Exhaled Air**

|  | % Oxygen ($O_2$) | % Carbon Dioxide ($CO_2$) | % Nitrogen ($N_2$) |
|---|---|---|---|
| Inhaled air (atmospheric air) | 20.9 | 0.04 | 79 |
| Exhaled air (alveolar air) | 14.0 | 5.60 | 79 |

Note: as indicated, the body uses about one-third of the inhaled oxygen. The amount of $CO_2$ increases more than 100-fold because it is produced during cellular respiration.

several ways. Most is transported as bicarbonate ions, which are produced when carbon dioxide chemically combines with water. Some of the carbon dioxide being transported is simply dissolved in plasma. Some is carried on the hemoglobin molecule.

## Diving and Flying

Adaptation to pressure change takes time. Divers who return to the surface too rapidly, or pilots who ascend to more than 35,000 feet too quickly, may develop **decompression sickness** ("the bends"). While deep below the surface, a diver breathes gases under high pressure. This pressure causes large amounts of nitrogen gas to dissolve in the blood and tissues. As the diver ascends to a region of lower pressure, the nitrogen dissolved in her or his tissues is liberated. If surfacing occurs too fast, nitrogen bubbles form in the tissues and blood and may block capillaries and cause other damage. The bubbles cause pain, paralysis, and even death—symptoms of decompression sickness.

## RESPIRATORY INSULTS: BREATHING DIRTY AIR

We breathe about 20,000 times each day, inhaling about 15 kg (35 pounds) of air—six times more than the food and drink we consume. Most of us breathe dirty urban air laden with particulates, carbon monoxide, and other harmful substances that are damaging to the respiratory system.

### Defense Mechanisms

A variety of defense mechanisms help protect the delicate lungs from the harmful substances we breathe. The hair around the nostrils, the ciliated mucous lining in the nose and pharynx, and the cilia-mucus elevator serve to trap foreign particles in inspired air. One of the body's most rapid defense responses to breathing dirty air is **bronchial constriction**. In this process the bronchial tubes narrow so that inhaled particles are more likely to land on their sticky mucous lining. Unfortunately,

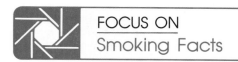

FOCUS ON
Smoking Facts

- Cigarette smoking is the largest single preventable cause of death and disability in the United States.
- The life of a 30-year-old who smokes 15 cigarettes a day is shortened by more than 5 years.
- If you smoke more than one pack per day, you are about 20 times more likely to develop lung cancer than a nonsmoker. According to the American Cancer Society, cigarette smoking causes more than 75% of all lung cancer deaths.
- If you smoke, you are more likely than a nonsmoker to develop atherosclerosis, and you double your chances of dying from cardiovascular disease.
- If you smoke, you are 20 times more likely to develop chronic bronchitis and emphysema.
- If you smoke, you are seven times more likely to develop peptic ulcers (especially malignant ulcers).
- If you smoke, you have about 5% less oxygen circulating in your blood.
- If you smoke when you are pregnant, your baby will weigh about 6 ounces less at birth, and there is double the risk of miscarriage, stillbirth, and infant death.
- Workers who smoke one or more packs of cigarettes per day are absent from their jobs because of illness 33% more often.
- Risks increase with the number of cigarettes

smoked, the number and depth of inhalations per cigarette, and smoking down to a short stub. Cigar and pipe smokers have lower risks than cigarette smokers because they do not inhale as much smoke. Cigarette smokers who switch to cigars and continue to inhale actually increase their risks.
- Nonsmokers confined in living rooms, offices, automobiles, or other places with smokers are adversely affected by the smoke. For example, when parents of infants smoke, the infant has double the risk of contracting pneumonia or bronchitis in its first year of life.
- When smokers quit smoking, their risk of dying from chronic pulmonary disease, cardiovascular disease, or cancer decreases. (Precise changes in risk figures depend on the number of years the person smoked, the number of cigarettes smoked per day, the age of starting to smoke, and the number of years since quitting.)
- Switching to low-tar, low-nicotine or filter brands does not help as much as one might think. Most smokers tend to compensate by increasing their consumption of cigarettes.
- If everyone in the United States stopped smoking, more than 300,000 lives would be saved each year.

when the bronchial passageways constrict, less air can pass through them to the lungs. This decreases the amount of oxygen available to the body cells. Chain smokers and those who breathe heavily polluted air may remain in a state of chronic bronchial constriction.

Neither the smallest bronchioles nor the alveoli are equipped with mucus or ciliated cells. Foreign particles that get through the respiratory defenses and find their way into the alveoli may remain there indefinitely or may be engulfed by macrophages. The macrophages may then accumulate in the lymph tissue of the lungs. Lung tissue of chronic smokers and those who work in dirty industries contains large blackened areas where carbon particles have been deposited.

## Respiratory Disease

Continued insult to the respiratory system results in disease. Chronic bronchitis and emphysema are **chronic obstructive pulmonary diseases (COPD)** that have been linked to smoking and breathing polluted air. More than 75% of patients with **chronic bronchitis** have a history of heavy cigarette smoking (see Focus on Smoking Facts). In chronic bronchitis, irritation from inhaled pollutants causes the bronchial tubes to secrete too much mucus. Ciliated cells, damaged by the pollutants, cannot effectively clear the mucus and trapped particles from the airways. The body resorts to coughing in an attempt to clear the airways. The bronchioles become constricted and inflamed and the patient is short of breath.

Victims of chronic bronchitis often develop **pulmonary emphysema**, a disease most common in cigarette smokers. In this disorder alveoli that have been inflamed owing to inhaled irritants attract neutrophils (white blood cells). Enzymes from neutrophil lysosomes damage the alveoli. Alveoli lose their elasticity and walls between adjacent alveoli are destroyed (Fig. 15–5). Surface area of the lung is so reduced that gas exchange is seriously impaired. Air is not expelled effectively and stale air accumulates in the lungs. The emphysema victim struggles for every breath and still the body does not get enough oxygen. To compensate, the right ventricle of the heart pumps harder and becomes enlarged. Emphysema patients frequently die of heart failure.

Cigarette smoking is also the main cause of **lung cancer**. More than 10 of the compounds in the tar of tobacco smoke have been shown to cause cancer. These carcinogenic substances irritate the cells lining the respiratory passages and alter their metabolic balance. Normal cells are transformed into cancer cells, which multiply rapidly and invade surrounding tissues.

## SUMMARY

I. In the nose air is filtered, humidified, and brought to body temperature.

II. From the nasal cavities air passes through the pharynx and into the larynx. The larynx protects the lungs by initiating a cough reflex when touched by foreign matter.

III. From the larynx inhaled air passes into the trachea and then into the right or left bronchus.

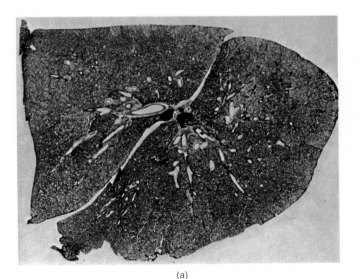
(a)

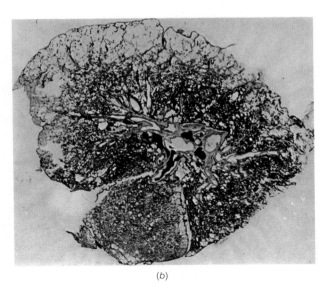
(b)

***Figure 15–5.*** *Freeze-dried lungs. (a) A normal lung. (b) A lung with advanced emphysema, in which alveoli have been destroyed and have run together. Alveolar walls have also been compressed hampering circulation. (From J. Turk and A. Turk: Environmental Science, 3rd ed. Philadelphia, Saunders College Publishing, 1984.)*

IV. Within the lungs the bronchi branch and re-branch giving rise to an extensive system of bronchioles.

V. Each bronchiole eventually terminates in a cluster of alveoli through which gas exchange takes place with the blood.

VI. The lungs are large, spongy organs covered with pleural membranes.

VII. Breathing is the mechanical process of moving air into and out of the lungs.

    A. When the diaphragm and intercostal muscles contract the thoracic cavity expands and pressure in the lung decreases. Air rushes into the lungs.

    B. When these muscles relax, pressure in the lung increases and air is expired.

VIII. Breathing is normally regulated by respiratory centers in the medulla and pons, which are sensitive to the concentration of carbon dioxide in the blood.

IX. Oxygen diffuses from the alveoli into the blood and is transported to the body cells in the form of oxyhemoglobin. As oxygen is needed by the cells, oxyhemoglobin dissociates and oxygen diffuses from the blood into the cells.

X. Carbon dioxide is transported mainly in the form of bicarbonate ions. In the lungs carbon dioxide diffuses from the blood in the pulmonary capillaries into the alveoli and then is expired.

XI. Divers who surface too rapidly or pilots who ascend too quickly may develop decompression sickness.

XII. Among the defense mechanisms of the respiratory system are the cilia-mucus elevator, bronchial constriction, and the action of macrophages. Continued insult to the respiratory system may result in chronic bronchitis, emphysema, or lung cancer.

## Post Test

1. Inhaled air passing through the pharynx would next enter the _____ and then pass through the _____.

2. Gas exchange takes place through the thin walls of the _____.

3. The floor of the thoracic cavity is formed by the _____.

4. The _____ seals off the larynx during swallowing.

5. When foreign matter contacts the larynx it may initiate a _____ _____.

6. The part of the pleural membrane that encloses the lung is the _____ _____.

7. A thin film of surfactant coats the _____.

8. Pulmonary ventilation is another term for _____.

9. Breathing in is called _____; breathing out is _____.

10. Oxygen is transported in the blood chemically bound to _____.

11. Impulses from the medulla reach the diaphragm by way of the _____ nerves.

12. A rapid response to inspiring dirty air is bronchial _____.

13. Label the diagram on the opposite page.

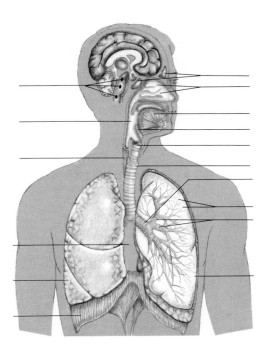

## REVIEW QUESTIONS

1. Trace a breath of inspired air from nose to alveoli, listing in sequence each structure through which the air must pass.
2. What are the advantages of having millions of alveoli rather than a pair of simple, balloonlike lungs?
3. Compare inspiration with expiration. How is breathing regulated?
4. The larynx is sometimes referred to as the watchdog of the lungs. Why do you think this is appropriate?
5. What are the advantages of breathing through the nose?
6. In what ways does the structure of the respiratory system permit gas exchange? (Hint: consider the thickness of alveolar and capillary walls as part of your answer.)
7. How does the respiratory system protect itself from harmful pollutants in the air we breathe? Describe several defense mechanisms.
8. What are some of the effects of continued respiratory insult?

# The Digestive System

## LEARNING OBJECTIVES

**After you study this chapter you should be able to**

1. List in sequence each structure through which a bite of food passes on its way through the digestive tract; label a diagram of the digestive system.
2. Describe in general terms the following steps in processing food: ingestion, digestion, absorption, and elimination.
3. Describe the wall of the digestive tract, distinguish between the visceral and parietal peritoneums, and describe their major folds.
4. Describe the structures of the mouth, including the teeth, and give their functions.
5. Describe the structure and function of the pharynx and esophagus.
6. Describe the structure of the stomach and its role in processing food.
7. Describe the anatomical features in the small intestine that increase its surface area and describe its functions.
8. Summarize the functions of the pancreas and liver.
9. Summarize carbohydrate, lipid, and protein digestion.
10. Describe the structure of an intestinal villus and explain its role in absorption of nutrients.
11. Describe the structure and functions of the large intestine and give its common disorders.

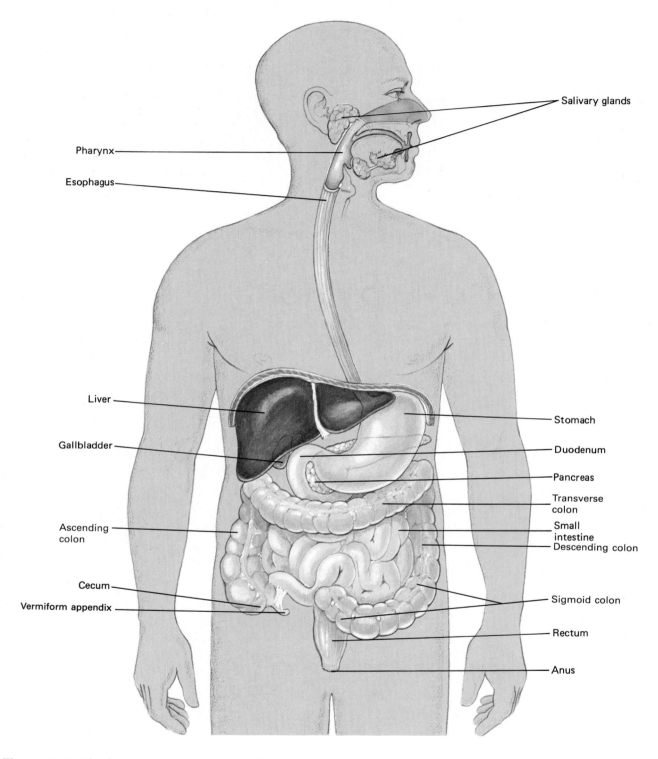

Salivary glands

Pharynx

Esophagus

Liver

Gallbladder

Stomach

Duodenum

Pancreas

Transverse colon

Ascending colon

Small intestine

Descending colon

Cecum

Vermiform appendix

Sigmoid colon

Rectum

Anus

*Figure 16–1.* The human digestive system. Note the complete digestive tract, a long, coiled tube extending from mouth to anus. Locate the three types of accessory glands.

After its entrance through the mouth, the food we eat takes a long and eventful journey through the digestive tract. The details of that journey are the subject of this chapter.

## THE DIGESTIVE TRACT

The **digestive tract**, also called the **alimentary** (al-eh-**men**′-tar-ee) **canal**, is a tube about 4.4 m (15 feet) long, extending from the mouth, where food is taken in, to the anus, the exit for elimination of unused food (Fig. 16–1). Below the diaphragm the digestive tract is often referred to as the **gastrointestinal** (gas″-trow-in-**tes**′-tah-nal) **(GI) tract**. The digestive tube is like a long coiled hose of varying diameter.

The parts of the digestive tract through which food passes in sequence are the mouth, pharynx (throat), esophagus, stomach, small intestine (subdivided into duodenum, jejunum, and ileum), and large intestine (subdivided into cecum, colon, and rectum). Three types of accessory digestive glands—salivary glands, liver, and pancreas—are not part of the digestive tract but secrete digestive juices into it.

## OVERVIEW OF FOOD PROCESSING

After appropriate foods are selected and obtained, they are **ingested**, that is, taken into the mouth, chewed, and swallowed. Because food is composed mainly of big pieces and large molecules (far too large to pass through the wall of the digestive tract) food must also be **digested**, that is, mechanically broken down and chemically split into small molecules. The chemical digestion of food breaks down long-chain organic molecules (such as polysaccharides or proteins). Each reaction is carried on with the help of a specific enzyme produced by cells of the digestive tract or its accessory glands. When small enough, the nutrient molecules pass through the wall of the intestine and into the blood or lymph, the process of **absorption**.

After nutrients are absorbed the blood **transports** them to the liver, where many are removed and stored. Those remaining in the blood are transported to the billions of cells of the body. Utilization of nutrients for metabolic activities takes place within each cell. Undigested and unabsorbed food is **eliminated** from the digestive tract by the process of **defecation** (def-eh-**kay**′-shun).

## WALL OF THE DIGESTIVE TRACT AND THE PERITONEUM

From esophagus to anus, the wall of the digestive tract has the same basic plan (Fig. 16–2). From the **lumen** (inner space) outward, four layers can be distinguished. The lining of the digestive tract is the **mucosa** (also called **mucous membrane**) (Fig. 16–2). It consists of epithelial tissue resting on a layer of loose connective tissue. In the esophagus and anal canal the epithelium is stratified squamous specialized for protection of underlying tissues. The columnar epithelium characteristic of other regions of the digestive tract is specialized for secretion of mucus or digestive juices or for absorption of nutrients. In the stomach and small intestine the mucosa is thrown into folds, which vastly increase its surface for digestion and absorption.

Beneath the mucosa lies a layer of connective tissue, the **submucosa**, rich in blood vessels and nerves. Under the submucosa is a layer of muscle. Rhythmic waves of contraction of these muscles push food along through the digestive tract, a process called **peristalsis** (per-ih-**stal**′-sis). Localized muscle contractions help to digest the food mechanically by breaking it apart and enhance chemical digestion by mixing food with the digestive juices.

The outer coat of the wall of the digestive tract is the **adventitia** (ad-ven-**tish**′-ee-ah). Below the level of the diaphragm this connective tissue coat is called the **visceral peritoneum**. By various folds it connects to the **parietal peritoneum**, the sheet of connective tissue that lines the walls of the abdominal and pelvic cavities. Between the visceral and parietal peritoneums is a potential space, the **peritoneal cavity**. Inflammation of the peritoneum, called **peritonitis**, can have serious consequences, because infection can easily spread to all the adjoining organs.

A large double fold of peritoneal tissue, the **mesentery** (**mes**′-un-terr″-ee), projects from the parietal peritoneum and attaches to the small intestine along much of its length, anchoring it to the posterior abdominal wall. The mesentery supports blood and lymph vessels, as well as nerves that supply the intestines.

Other important folds of peritoneum are the greater omentum, the lesser omentum, and the mesocolon (Fig. 16–3). The **greater omentum**, also known as the fatty apron, is a large double fold of peritoneum attached to the duodenum, stomach, and large intestine. It hangs down over the intestine like an apron. Large deposits of fat are found within the greater omentum, and strategically

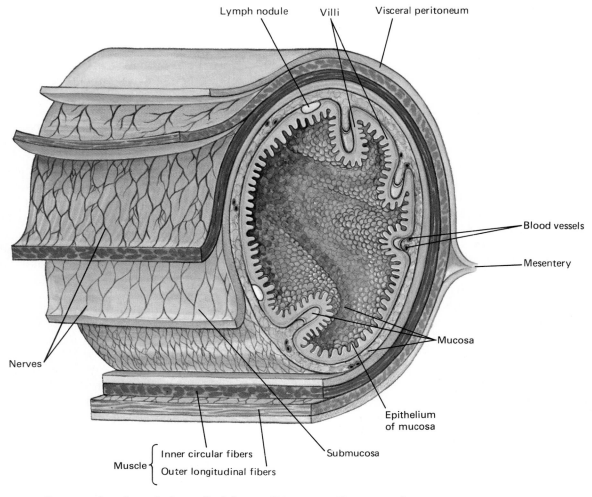

*Figure 16—2.* Cross section through the wall of the small intestine illustrating the mucosa, submucosa, muscle layers, and visceral peritoneum.

placed lymph nodes deal with infection and prevent its spread to the peritoneum. The **lesser omentum** suspends the stomach and duodenum from the liver. The **mesocolon** is a fold of peritoneum that attaches the colon to the posterior abdominal wall.

## THE MOUTH

The fleshy, sensitive lips guard the opening of the mouth, or **oral cavity**. The roof of the mouth is the **palate**. The flexible, muscular tongue on the floor of the mouth pushes the food about, which aids in chewing and swallowing. The movement of the tongue is limited posteriorly by the **lingual frenulum**, a fold of mucous membrane that attaches it to the floor of the mouth.

Food molecules on the tongue's surface find themselves among a myriad of hills and valleys formed by three types of projections called **papillae** on the tongue's surface. **Taste buds** in the papillae are sensitive to chemical differences among food molecules, enabling us to taste foods as sweet, sour, salty, or bitter (see also Chapter 9).

## The Teeth

The **teeth** are rooted in sockets (alveoli) of the alveolar processes, bony ridges that project from the mandible and maxilla. The **gingivae** (**jin'**-jeh-vee) (gums) cover the alveolar processes and extend slightly into each socket.

### The Structure of a Tooth

Each tooth consists of a **crown**, the part above the gum, and one or more **roots**, the portion beneath the gumline (Fig. 16—4). A section through a tooth, or an x-ray of it, shows that each tooth is

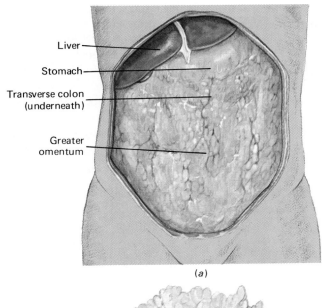

Liver

Stomach

Transverse colon
(underneath)

Greater
omentum

(a)

**Figure 16–3.** Folds of the peritoneum anchor the digestive organs to the abdominal wall and to one another. (a) Frontal view of abdomen. The greater omentum hangs down over the intestine like an apron. (b) Frontal view of abdomen. The transverse colon and greater omentum have been lifted to show the mesentery and mesocolon.

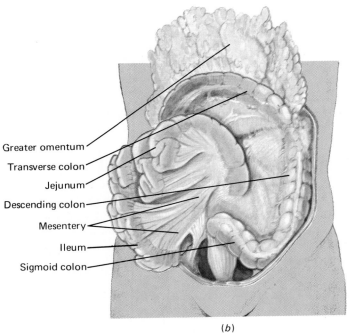

Greater omentum

Transverse colon

Jejunum

Descending colon

Mesentery

Ileum

Sigmoid colon

(b)

composed mainly of **dentin**, a calcified connective tissue that imparts shape and rigidity to the tooth. In the crown region the dentin is protected by a tough **enamel** covering. The bonelike enamel is the hardest substance in the body, comparable in hardness to quartz. Enamel helps protect the tooth against the wear and tear of chewing and against chemical substances that might dissolve the dentin. In the root region the dentin is covered by **cementum**, another bonelike substance.

The dentin encloses a **pulp cavity** filled with **pulp**, an extremely sensitive connective tissue containing blood vessels and nerves. Narrow extensions of the pulp cavity, called **root canals**, pass through the roots of the tooth. Each root canal has an opening at its base through which nerves and blood and lymph vessels enter the tooth.

### Deciduous and Permanent Teeth

By about 6 months of age the first of the temporary **deciduous teeth** (also called milk or baby teeth) show their crowns above the gums. New teeth erupt every few weeks thereafter so that a full set of 20 deciduous teeth is present by the time a child is about 2 years old (Fig. 16–5). These are fairly small teeth, and between the ages of 6 and 13 years they are slowly shed and replaced by larger **permanent teeth**.

The adult set of teeth consists of a maximum of 32 teeth. Because teeth are arranged bilaterally and are identical in the upper and lower jaw, it is traditional to describe the number of each type in one quadrant of the mouth. Closest to the midline are two **incisors** (a total of eight, four on top and four on bottom). The incisors are specialized for biting and cutting. Lateral to them are the **canines**, one in each quadrant. In humans the canines assist the incisors in biting but in many mammals they are enlarged and adapted for stabbing and tearing prey. The more posterior teeth are modified for grinding and crushing. In each quadrant there are two **premolars** and three **molars**. The third molars, called the *wisdom teeth*, often erupt after age

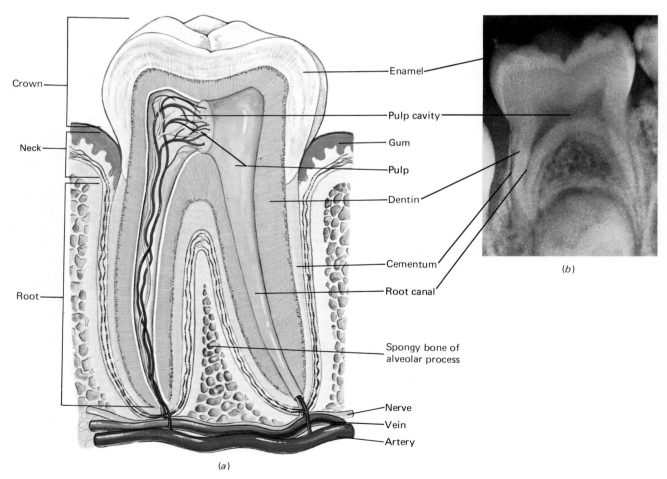

(a)

(b)

*Figure 16–4.* Structure of a tooth. (a) Sagittal section of a lower human molar. (b) X-ray of a healthy tooth.

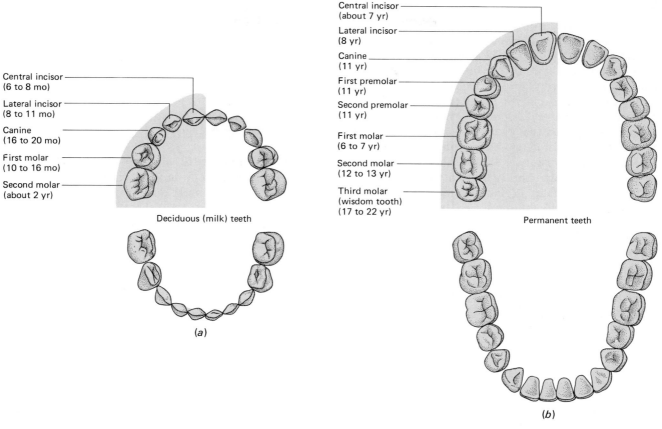

**Figure 16–5.** (a) Deciduous teeth. (b) Permanent teeth. Approximate time of eruption is shown in parentheses.

18. The human jaw is small in many persons, often not large enough to accommodate the wisdom teeth. In some cases they remain embedded in the bone and are described as impacted. Often they cause pain and must be surgically removed.

### Tooth Decay and Periodontal Disease

When allowed to accumulate, bacteria that normally inhabit the mouth form dental plaque on the surfaces of teeth. **Dental plaque** is a light-colored film formed from saliva and from food particles that have been acted on by bacteria. Plaque forms especially on the third of each tooth nearest to the gumline and also just beneath the gumline. Even after teeth are thoroughly cleaned, plaque begins to develop within 6 hours and at night it forms even more rapidly. If not removed periodically, plaque becomes calcified to form calculus. Dental plaque is an important factor in the cause of the two most common chronic diseases of the mouth: dental caries and periodontal disease.

**Dental caries** (kay′-rees) is the localized, progressive decay of teeth that produces cavities. Carbohydrates (especially sucrose) deposited on the teeth are decomposed by bacteria in the plaque. Some bacteria produce acids that can demineralize the outer surfaces of the teeth. Enamel cannot be repaired or replaced by the body's own action, and loss of enamel by decay or other trauma is permanent. Fortunately, enamel can be replaced to a large extent by artificial materials when tooth cavities are filled. Because dentin is sensitive tissue, cavities that extend into the dentin may be quite painful. If decay is untreated, bacteria can enter the pulp and cause infection.

Dental decay is the principal cause of tooth loss up to the age of 35. After that time tooth loss is most frequently attributed to **periodontal disease**. This condition affects the gums, producing **gingivitis** (jin-je-**vi**′-tis). Periodontal disease results from irritation and infection caused by dental plaque and calculus. As the disease progresses, the gums recede and bleed, and the teeth become loose as the bone tissue itself is slowly reabsorbed.

## Salivary Glands

The three main pairs of **salivary glands** are the parotid, submandibular, and sublingual glands. The **parotid glands**, largest of the salivary glands, are located in the tissue inferior and anterior to the ears. When one has mumps, the parotid glands become infected and swell. The **submandibular** (sub-man-**dib'**-u-lar) **glands** and **sublingual** (sub-**ling'**-gwal) **glands** lie below the jaw and under the tongue, respectively.

Saliva consists of two main components: (1) a serous (thin, watery) secretion containing the digestive enzyme **salivary amylase** and (2) a mucous secretion that lubricates the mouth. Salts, antibodies, and other substances that kill bacteria are also found in the saliva. Saliva lubricates the tissues of the mouth and pharynx, facilitating talking as well as chewing. By moistening food, saliva helps the tongue to convert the mouthful of food to a semi-solid mass called a **bolus** (**bow'**-lus), which can be swallowed easily.

**Swallowing: Through the Pharynx and Esophagus**

The bite of food that has been chewed, moistened, tasted, and fashioned into a bolus must now be swallowed, that is, moved from the mouth through the pharynx and down the esophagus.

## THE PHARYNX

The **pharynx**, or throat, is a muscular tube about 12 cm (4.8 inches) long that serves as the foyer of the respiratory, as well as the digestive, system. As we noted in Chapter 15, the three regions of the pharynx are the **oropharynx**, posterior to the mouth; the **nasopharynx**, posterior to the nose; and the **laryngopharynx**, which opens into the lar-

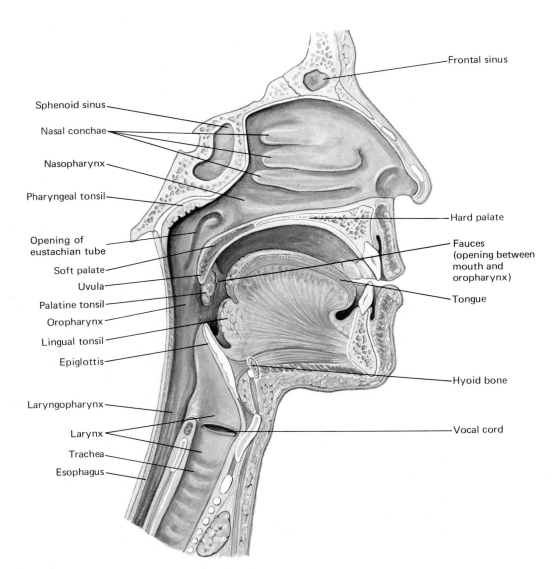

*Figure 16–6. Sagittal section of mouth, pharynx, and esophagus.*

ynx and esophagus. The opening leading from the mouth into the oropharynx is called the **fauces** (Fig. 16–6). The oropharynx and nasopharynx are partitioned by the **soft palate**, which hangs down like a curtain between them. The muscular soft palate is a posterior extension of the bony hard palate, which serves as the roof of the mouth. A small conical process, the **uvula**, hangs from the middle of the lower border of the soft palate.

In swallowing, the bolus is forced into the oropharynx by the tongue. Reflex movements of muscles in the wall of the pharynx propel the food into the esophagus. During swallowing, the opening to the larynx is closed by a small flap of tissue, the **epiglottis**. At the same time the soft palate is pulled upward to close off the nasopharynx. These actions prevent food from straying into the respiratory passageways.

## THE ESOPHAGUS

The **esophagus** (e-**sof'**-ah-gus) extends from the pharynx through the thoracic cavity, then passes through the diaphragm and empties into the stomach. The bolus is swept through the pharynx and into the esophagus by a wave of peristaltic contraction. As the bolus enters the esophagus, the peristaltic wave continues pushing the food down toward the stomach. Circular muscle fibers in the wall of the esophagus contract around the top of the bolus and relax below it, pushing it downward. Almost at the same time, longitudinal muscles around the bottom of the bolus and below it contract, shortening the tube (Fig. 16–7).

At the lower end of the esophagus is a circular muscle that acts as a sphincter, constricting the tube so that the entrance to the stomach is generally closed. This prevents the highly acidic gastric juice from splashing up into the esophagus. Occasionally gastric juice does spurt up into the esophagus and the wall of the esophagus becomes irritated. The resulting spasms may be perceived as heartburn, probably so named because the pain sensation seems to occur in the general region of the heart.

## THE STOMACH

When a peristaltic wave passes down the esophagus, the circular muscle at the bottom relaxes, permitting the bolus to enter the stomach. The **stomach** is a large, muscular organ that, when empty, is almost hotdog-shaped. Folds of the mucosa and submucosa called **rugae** give the inner

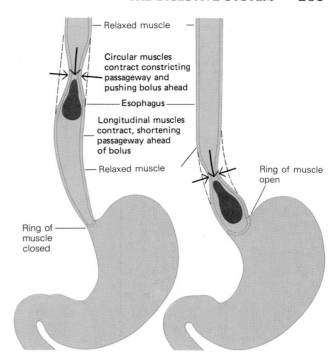

*Figure 16–7. Peristalsis. Food is moved through the digestive tract by waves of muscular contraction known as peristalsis.*

lining a wrinkled appearance (Fig. 16–8). As more and more food is chewed, swallowed, and delivered to the stomach, the rugae gradually smooth out, stretching the stomach and increasing its capacity to more than a liter (quart). As it fills, the stomach begins to look like a football. Contractions of the stomach mix the food thoroughly. Three layers of smooth muscle in its wall enable the stomach to mash and churn food and also move it along by peristalsis. The stomach is lined with simple columnar epithelium that secretes large amounts of mucus. Tiny pits mark the entrances to the millions of **gastric glands** that extend down deep into the mucosa. These glands secrete gastric juice containing hydrochloric acid and enzymes. The hydrochloric acid kills bacteria and breaks down the connective tissues in meat. Even after mixing with mucus and food, the pH of the hydrochloric acid is about 2. This is the pH at which the stomach's principal enzyme, pepsin, is most effective.

As food is digested over a 3- to 4-hour period, it is converted into a semisolid, soupy mixture called **chyme**. Peristaltic contractions slowly move the chyme toward the pylorus, the exit of the stomach. Although small amounts of water, salts, and lipid-soluble substances such as alcohol are absorbed through the stomach mucosa, comparatively little absorption takes place from the stomach.

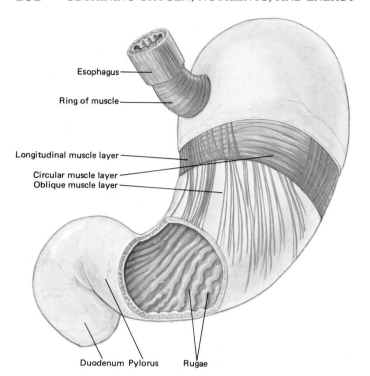

Esophagus

Ring of muscle

Longitudinal muscle layer

Circular muscle layer

Oblique muscle layer

Duodenum  Pylorus  Rugae

***Figure 16—8.*** *Structure of the stomach. From the esophagus, food enters the stomach, where it is mechanically and enzymatically digested.*

As digestion is completed, peristaltic waves propel a few milliliters of chyme at a time into the small intestine. The exit of the stomach is guarded by the **pyloric sphincter**, a strong ring of muscle that relaxes at appropriate times.

## THE SMALL INTESTINE

The **small intestine** is a long, coiled tube about 5 m (16 feet) long by 4 cm (1.5 inches) in diameter. The first 22 cm or so of the small intestine is the **duodenum** (du″-o-dee′-num), which is curved like the letter C. As the tube turns downward it is called the **jejunum** (je-joo′-num), which extends for about 2 m (6 feet) before becoming the **ileum**. The inner wall of the small intestine is marked throughout by circular folds of the mucous membrane.

The velvety appearance of the intestinal lining is due to millions of tiny fingerlike projections of the mucous membrane, the intestinal **villi** (**vill′**-i) (Fig. 16–9). Like the circular folds, the villi increase the surface area of the small intestine for digestion and absorption of nutrients. The intestinal surface is further expanded by thousands of **microvilli**, which are folds of cytoplasm on the exposed borders of the epithelial cells.

If the intestinal lining were smooth, like the inside of a garden hose, food would move so rapidly through the intestine that many valuable nutrients would be wasted. The combined effects of the circular folds, the villi, and the microvilli, however, increase the surface area of the small intestine by about 600 times. In fact, if the lining of the intestine could be completely unfolded and spread out, its surface would approximate the size of a tennis court!

Between the villi are the **intestinal glands**, which dip deeply into the mucosa. These glands secrete large amounts of fluid that serve as a medium for digestion and absorption of nutrients. Contrary to popular belief, most chemical digestion takes place in the duodenum rather than in the stomach. By the time the chyme enters the duodenum most food molecules are partially digested but are still too large to pass through the intestinal wall.

Bile from the liver and enzymes from the pancreas are released into the duodenum and act on the chyme. Then enzymes produced by the epithelial cells lining the duodenum complete the job of breaking down food molecules so that they can be absorbed.

## THE PANCREAS

The **pancreas** is a large, elongated gland that lies in the abdomen inferior to the stomach; its head is embraced by the C-shaped curve of the duodenum (Fig. 16–10). The pancreas is both an exocrine and

Tom described his recent recurrent abdominal pain to his physician. He complained of a burning, gnawing sensation that recurred during the day whenever his stomach was empty. Sometimes the pain awakened him during the night. Eating or ingestion of antacids relieved the pain.

Dr. Pepto arranged for Tom to have an upper GI series. As Tom drank the cup of strawberry-flavored barium, x-ray films of his upper GI tract were taken. These films demonstrated the barium progressively filling his upper GI tract. The barium outlined the small duodenal crater, enabling the diagnosis of **peptic ulcer** disease (see figure).

Dr. Pepto explained that gastric juice had digested a small bit of the lining of the duodenum, leaving an open sore, the peptic ulcer. Sometimes peptic ulcers occur in the stomach or lower portion of the esophagus. Normally, protective mechanisms prevent the gastric juice from damaging the wall of the digestive tract. Cells of the gastric mucosa secrete an alkaline mucus that coats the wall and neutralizes the acidity of the gastric juice along the lining. In addition, the epithelial cells lining the digestive tract fit tightly together, preventing gastric juice from leaking between them and onto the tissue beneath. Should some of the epithelial cells become damaged, they are quickly replaced. The life span of an epithelial cell in the gastric mucosa is only about 3 days.

Tom learned that about 1 in 10 persons suffers from a peptic ulcer sometime during life. Treatment is important because peptic ulcers are not only often painful but also may bleed, leading to anemia. If the ulcer extends deeply into the wall of the digestive tract, large blood vessels may be damaged, resulting in hemorrhage. Occasionally, a peptic ulcer extends all the way through the wall. This is a **perforated ulcer**. Bacteria and food may pass through the opening to the peritoneum, leading to peritonitis. Perforation is the main cause of death from ulcers.

Dr. Pepto instructed Tom to avoid the use of alcohol and aspirin because these substances reduce the resistance of the mucosa to digestion of gastric juice. He also suggested that Tom avoid eating pepper or drinking coffee, tea, colas, and other beverages with caffeine because caffeine stimulates gastric secretion. Tom was also told to stop smoking cigarettes because smoking decreases healing rates for peptic ulcers. Tom was put on a regimen of liquid antacids and told that if he followed instructions there was an 80% chance that his ulcer would heal in about 6 weeks.

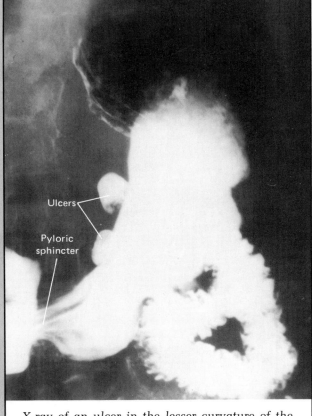

*X-ray of an ulcer in the lesser curvature of the stomach. (Courtesy of Dr. Jon Ehringer.)*

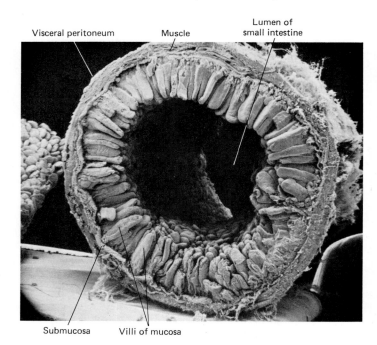

Visceral peritoneum   Muscle   Lumen of small intestine

Submucosa   Villi of mucosa

***Figure 16–9.*** *Scanning electron micrograph of a cross section of the small intestine (approximately ×30). (From Kessel, R.G., and Kardon, R.H.: Tissues and Organs: A Text–Atlas of Scanning Electron Microscopy. San Francisco, W.H. Freeman and Co., 1979. © 1979.)*

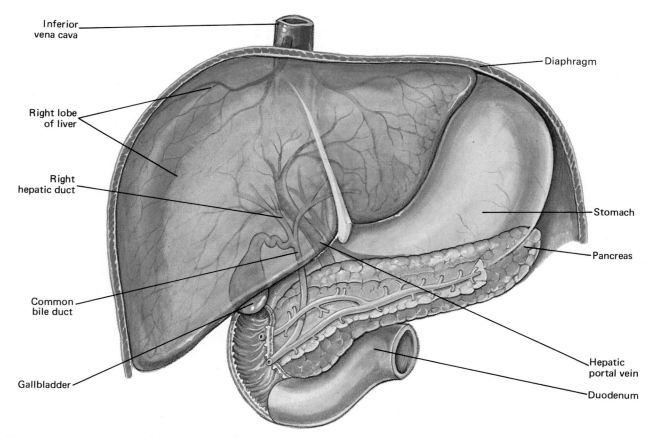

Inferior vena cava

Right lobe of liver

Right hepatic duct

Common bile duct

Gallbladder

Diaphragm

Stomach

Pancreas

Hepatic portal vein

Duodenum

***Figure 16–10.*** Structure of the liver and pancreas. Note the gallbladder and ducts.

an endocrine gland. Its exocrine portion secretes **pancreatic juice**, an alkaline fluid containing a number of digestive enzymes. The pancreatic duct joins the bile duct coming from the liver, forming a single duct that passes into the duodenum. Frequently an accessory pancreatic duct is present.

> If the pancreas becomes damaged and malfunctions (usually as a result of increased secretion and blockage of ducts), the pancreatic tissue may be digested by its own enzymes. This condition, called **acute pancreatitis**, is frequently associated with alcoholism.

## THE LIVER

Just inferior to the diaphragm lies the liver, the largest and one of the most complex organs in the body (Fig. 16–10). A single liver cell can carry on more than 500 separate metabolic activities. The right lobe of the liver is larger than its left lobe and has three main parts. Each liver lobe is divided into thousands of microscopic **lobules**, the functional units of the liver. A lobule consists of several plates of liver cells.

Oxygenated blood is brought to the liver by the *hepatic arteries*. However, the liver also receives blood from the *hepatic portal vein*, which delivers nutrients just absorbed from the intestine. Small branches of the hepatic arteries and the hepatic portal vein deliver blood to the tiny *hepatic sinusoids*, allowing blood from the hepatic arteries and hepatic portal vein to mix. The liver sinusoids are partially lined with phagocytic **Kupffer cells**, which remove bacteria and other foreign matter and worn-out blood cells. Blood from the liver sinusoids is eventually delivered to the hepatic veins that conduct blood toward the heart.

### Functions of the Liver

The numerous functions of the liver include the following:

1. Secretes bile, which is important in the digestion of fats. **Bilirubin** (bil-eh-**roo'**-bin), a pigment released when red blood cells are broken down, is excreted in the bile.
2. Removes nutrients from the blood.
3. Converts glucose to glycogen and stores it; then when glucose is needed, it breaks down the glycogen and releases glucose into the blood.
4. Stores iron and certain vitamins.
5. Converts excess amino acids to fatty acids and urea.
6. Performs many important functions in the metabolism of proteins, fats, and carbohydrates.
7. Manufactures many of the plasma proteins found in the blood.
8. Detoxifies many drugs and poisons that enter the body.
9. Phagocytizes bacteria and worn-out red blood cells.

## The Gallbladder

Bile is stored in the pear-shaped **gallbladder** (Fig. 16–10). The hormone cholecystokinin (CCK) is secreted by the intestinal mucosa, mainly when fat is present in the duodenum. This hormone stimulates the gallbladder to contract, releasing bile into the cystic duct. The cystic duct from the gallbladder joins the duct from the liver to form the **common bile duct**, which (together with the duct from the pancreas) opens into the duodenum.

## CHEMICAL DIGESTION

As chyme is moved through the intestine by peristaltic contractions, digestion of nutrients is completed and the nutrients are absorbed. Secretion of digestive juices is stimulated by hormones and chyme. For example, the hormone gastrin, which is released by the stomach mucosa, stimulates the gastric glands to secrete. The intestinal glands are stimulated to release their fluid mainly by local reflexes initiated when the small intestine is distended by chyme.

### Digestion of Carbohydrates

Large carbohydrates such as starch and glycogen consist of long chains of glucose molecules. Starch digestion begins in the mouth as salivary amylase degrades some of the long starch molecules to smaller compounds of dextrin and then to the sugar maltose.

In the duodenum, pancreatic amylase (in the pancreatic juice) splits the remaining starch molecules to maltose units. Then maltase released by the epithelial cells lining the duodenum breaks down each maltose molecule to two molecules of glucose (Table 16–1). The sugars sucrose and lactose (both disaccharides) are also degraded by enzymes released by the epithelial cells lining the duodenum.

TABLE 16–1
**Summary of Digestion**

| Location | Source of Enzyme | Digestive Process |
|---|---|---|
| *Carbohydrate Digestion* | | |
| Mouth | Salivary glands | Polysaccharides (e.g., starch) $\xrightarrow{\text{salivary amylase}}$ maltose + small polysaccharides |
| Stomach | | Action continues until salivary amylase is inactivated by acidic pH |
| Small intestine | Pancreas | Undigested polysaccharides and small polysaccharides $\xrightarrow{\text{pancreatic amylase}}$ maltose |
| | Intestine | Disaccharides degraded to simple sugars as follows: |
| | | Maltose (malt sugar) $\xrightarrow{\text{maltase}}$ glucose + glucose |
| | | Sucrose (table sugar) $\xrightarrow{\text{sucrase}}$ glucose + fructose |
| | | Lactose (milk sugar) $\xrightarrow{\text{lactase}}$ glucose + galactose |
| *Protein Digestion* | | |
| Stomach | Stomach (gastric glands) | Protein $\xrightarrow{\text{pepsin}}$ polypeptides |
| Small intestine | Pancreas | Polypeptides $\xrightarrow{\text{trypsin, chymotrypsin}}$ tripeptides + dipeptides<br>A—A—A—A—A   A—A—A   A—A<br>A—A—A—A—A |
| | | Dipeptides $\xrightarrow{\text{peptidase}}$ free amino acids<br>A—A   A   A   A |
| | Small intestine | Tripeptides + dipeptides $\xrightarrow{\text{peptidases}}$ free amino acids<br>A—A—A  A—A   A   A   A   A   A   A   A |
| *Lipid Digestion* | | |
| Small intestine | Liver | Glob of fat $\xrightarrow{\text{bile}}$ emulsified fat |
| | Pancreas | Fat (triacylglycerol) $\xrightarrow{\text{lipase}}$ fatty acids + glycerol   E |

○ , Monosaccharide; ⊏ , triacylglycerol; E , glycerol; ∿ , fatty acid; A, amino acid units or, when standing alone, a free amino acid.

Many plant foods are rich in starch. However, this starch is not readily available to us because it is encased within the cellulose cell walls of plant cells. Because humans do not have enzymes that digest cellulose, much of this starch passes through the digestive tract without being digested. Cooking destroys the cellulose walls so that the starch can be more easily reached by amylase and other enzymes.

Glucose is the major product of carbohydrate digestion, accounting for about 80% of the monosaccharides (simple sugars) obtained from food. Carbohydrate digestion is summarized in Table 16–1.

## Digestion of Proteins

You may recall from Chapter 2 that proteins consist of molecular subunits called amino acids that are linked together by peptide bonds. The goal of protein digestion is to break the peptide bonds and release free amino acids. Protein digestion begins in the stomach with the enzyme pepsin. Pepsin reduces most proteins to intermediate-sized polypeptides. In the duodenum, the enzymes trypsin and chymotrypsin in the pancreatic juice reduce these peptides to smaller peptides (tripeptides and dipeptides). Then peptidases from the intestinal epithelial cells split some of these peptides into free amino acids. Free amino acids are absorbed into the intestinal epithelial cells. Protein digestion is summarized in Table 16–1.

## Digestion of Lipids

Lipid digestion begins in the duodenum with the action of bile. Bile emulsifies (mechanically breaks down) fat by a detergent action that breaks it apart into smaller particles. These particles are acted on by an enzyme in the pancreatic juice called pancreatic lipase. Pancreatic lipase breaks down the fat molecules to free fatty acids and glycerol. Fat digestion is summarized in Table 16–1.

## ABSORPTION

After food has been digested, the nutrients are absorbed by the intestinal villi. The structure of a villus is illustrated in Figure 16–11. Within each villus is a network of capillaries that branches from an arteriole and empties into a venule. A central lymph vessel called a **lacteal** (**lak′**-tee-al) is also present. To reach the blood or lymph, a nutrient molecule must pass through the single layer of epithelial cells lining the villus and through the single layer of cells forming the wall of the capillary or the lacteal.

Amino acids and simple sugars are absorbed through the epithelial cells lining the intestine and into the blood. They are transported directly to the liver by the hepatic portal vein. Fatty acids, on the other hand, are absorbed into the lacteals and circulate through the lymph system before entering the blood.

## THE LARGE INTESTINE

The **ileocecal** (il″-e-o-**see′**-kal) **valve**, a sphincter between the small and large intestines, is normally closed so that chyme in the large intestine cannot move backward into the ileum. In response to a peristaltic contraction bringing chyme toward it, the ileocecal valve opens, allowing the chyme (containing undigested and unabsorbed substances) to enter the large intestine.

One to 3 days or even longer may be required for the slow journey through the **large intestine**. Bacteria inhabiting the large intestine devour the last remnants of the meal and return the favor by producing certain vitamins that can be absorbed and utilized. Some bacteria may digest some of the cellulose, releasing more nutrients for absorption. As the chyme slowly passes through the large intestine, water and sodium will be absorbed and it will assume the consistency of normal feces.

Although only about a little more than 1.5 m (about 5 feet) long, the large intestine is called large because its diameter is considerably greater than that of the small intestine. The small intestine joins the large intestine about 7 cm above the end of the large intestine, thereby creating a pouch called the **cecum** (**see′**-kum). The **vermiform appendix**, a worm-shaped blind tube rich in lymph tissue, projects from the end of the cecum. The function of the appendix is unknown. It is usually considered a vestigial structure, perhaps important as an incubator for bacteria that digested cellulose in the vegetarian past of the human species. Inflammation of the appendix, known as **appendicitis**, can lead to peritonitis and other complications if not diagnosed and treated promptly.

From the cecum to the rectum the large intestine is known as the **colon**. The **ascending colon** extends from the cecum straight up to the lower border of the liver. As it turns horizontally it becomes the **transverse colon**, which extends across the abdomen below the liver and stomach, anterior to the small intestine. On the left side of the abdomen the **descending colon** turns downward, giving

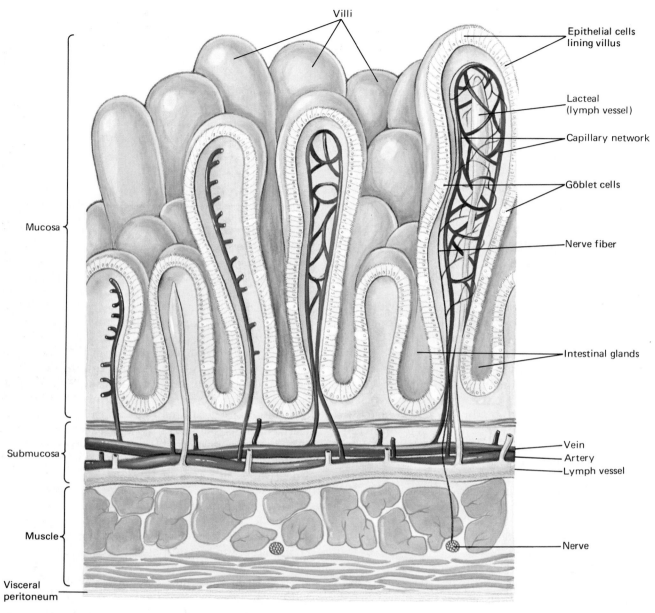

**Figure 16–11.** *The surface of the small intestine is studded with villi and tiny openings into the intestinal glands. Here, some of the villi have been opened to show the blood and lymph vessels within.*

rise finally to the S-shaped **sigmoid colon**, which empties into the short **rectum**. The rectum is the last 12 cm or so of the digestive tract. It terminates in the **anus**, the opening for elimination of feces. The final 4 cm of the rectum are called the **anal canal**.

The mucosa of the large intestine lacks villi and produces no digestive enzymes. The surface epithelium consists of cells specialized for absorption and goblet cells that secrete mucus.

The functions of the large intestine may be summarized as follows:

1. Absorption of sodium and water. Sodium is absorbed by active transport and water follows by osmosis.
2. Incubation of bacteria. Because the movements of the large intestine are quite sluggish, bacteria have time to grow and reproduce there. Some types of bacteria maintain a mutualistic relationship with their human host, in that they produce certain vitamins (for example, vitamin K and some of the B vitamins) in exchange for food and shelter. When there is a normal balance of intestinal bacte-

ria, growth of harmless bacteria tends to prevent growth of pathogenic varieties. When the normal ecology of the large intestine is upset, however, as sometimes happens when one takes certain antibiotics, harmful bacteria may multiply and cause disease.

3. Elimination of wastes. Undigested and unabsorbed food as well as sloughed-off cells from the intestinal epithelium and bile pigments are eliminated from the body by the large intestine in the form of feces.

After meals the motility of the large intestine increases. Distension of the stomach with food also initiates contractions of the rectum, stimulating the desire to **defecate** (expel feces).

Two sphincters, an internal anal sphincter (composed of smooth muscle) and an external anal sphincter (voluntary muscle), in the wall of the anal canal guard the anal opening. When the rectum is distended with feces, the internal sphincter relaxes but the external sphincter remains tonically contracted until relaxed voluntarily. Thus defecation is a reflex action that can be voluntarily inhibited by keeping the external sphincter contracted.

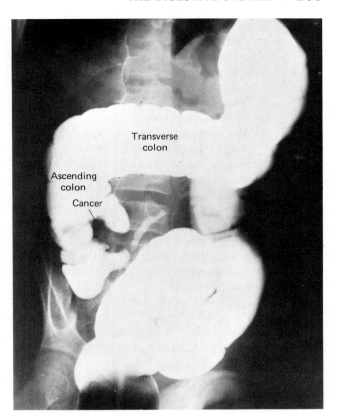

***Figure 16-12.*** *X-ray of the large intestine of a patient with cancer of the colon. The lumen of the large intestine has been filled with a suspension of barium sulfate, which makes irregularities in the wall visible. The cancer is evident as a mass that projects into the lumen.*

When chyme passes through the intestine too rapidly, defecation becomes more frequent and the feces are watery. This condition, called **diarrhea**, may be caused by pathogens that irritate the lining of the large intestine, increasing motility and decreasing absorption. Emotional tension and certain foods such as prunes also stimulate intestinal motility and can lead to diarrhea. Prolonged diarrhea results in loss of water and needed electrolytes such as sodium and potassium. Dehydration, especially in infants, may be serious, even leading to death.

**Constipation** refers to abnormally slow movement of feces through the large intestine. In this case, more water than usual is removed from the chyme, so that the feces are hard and dry. Constipation is often caused by a diet containing insufficient bulk but emotional factors may also produce this condition.

**Cancer of the colon** is one of the most common causes of cancer deaths in the United States (Fig. 16–12). Research indicates that this type of cancer may be related to diet, because the disease is more common in those whose diets are low in fiber. It has been suggested that less fiber results in less frequent defecation, allowing prolonged contact between the mucosa of the colon and carcinogens such as nitrites (used as preservatives) in foods. Cancer in the large intestine produces symptoms at an early stage and is potentially curable by surgery when treatment is undertaken quickly.

## SUMMARY

I. In sequence, a bite of food passes through the mouth, pharynx, esophagus, stomach, small intestine (duodenum, jejunum, ileum), and large intestine (cecum, colon, rectum) and unabsorbed food passes out through the anus.

II. The digestive system functions in the ingestion, digestion, and absorption of nutrients. Food that is not absorbed is eliminated by the process of defecation.

III. The lining of the digestive tract is its mucosa; beneath that is a layer of connective tissue (submucosa); then, a layer of muscle occurs; the outer coat of the wall is the adventitia. Below the diaphragm the adventitia is called the visceral peritoneum.

A. The parietal peritoneum lines the walls of the abdominal and pelvic cavities.

B. The two peritonea are connected by various folds, including the greater omentum, the lesser omentum, and the mesocolon.

IV. Mechanical digestion and chemical digestion of carbohydrates begin in the mouth.
   A. The teeth grind and crush the food.
      1. The crown of a tooth is covered by tough enamel.
      2. Beneath the enamel is the dentin that makes up most of the tooth.
   B. Saliva contains salivary amylase, which chemically digests large carbohydrates (polysaccharides) to dextrins.

V. In swallowing, reflex movements propel the bolus through the pharynx and into the esophagus. Peristaltic contractions push the food through the esophagus to the stomach.

VI. Food is further processed in the large muscular stomach.
   A. Three layers of smooth muscle within the stomach wall enable the stomach to contract in many directions, mashing and churning the food and reducing it to chyme.
   B. Gastric glands in the stomach wall secrete gastric juice.
      1. Pepsin in the gastric juice chemically digests proteins.
      2. Hydrochloric acid kills bacteria and helps break down connective tissues in the meat we eat.

VII. Most chemical digestion takes place within the duodenum.
   A. Bile from the liver and pancreatic juice from the pancreas are released into the duodenum and mixed with the chyme.
   B. Cells of the small intestine produce enzymes needed for the final digestion of proteins, fats, and carbohydrates.

VIII. The pancreas releases enzymes that chemically digest proteins, lipids, and carbohydrates.

IX. The liver is made up of thousands of lobules consisting of plates of liver cells. The liver performs many functions.
   A. The liver receives blood from both the hepatic arteries and the hepatic portal vein.
   B. As blood courses through the hepatic sinusoids, nutrients are removed from it for storage in the liver and Kupffer cells remove bacteria.
   C. Bile produced in the liver is stored in the gallbladder.

X. Secretion of digestive juices is stimulated by the presence of chyme and by hormones. Food is slowly digested as it moves through the digestive tract.
   A. Carbohydrate digestion begins in the mouth, where salivary amylase breaks down starches to dextrins and maltose. In the duodenum pancreatic amylase continues the digestion of carbohydrates to maltose. Then specific disaccharides in the duodenum break down disaccharides to monosaccharides such as glucose.
   B. Chemical digestion of proteins begins in the stomach with the action of pepsin. In the duodenum enzymes from the pancreas continue to reduce proteins to polypeptides and then dipeptides. Finally, peptidases produced by the epithelial cells lining the duodenum break down the dipeptides to free amino acids.
   C. Lipid digestion begins in the duodenum with emulsification by bile; then lipase from the pancreas enzymatically degrades the fat to fatty acids and glycerol.

XI. Absorption takes place through the villi of the small intestine.
   A. Glucose and amino acids are absorbed through the epithelial cells lining the villi; then these nutrients enter the blood through capillaries in the villi and are transported to the liver.
   B. Fatty acids are absorbed into the epithelial cells of the villi and then pass into the lacteal within the villus.

XII. Indigestible materials such as cellulose and unabsorbed nutrients pass into the large intestine.
   A. Excess water and sodium are absorbed from the chyme as it passes through the large intestine.
   B. Undigestible material, unabsorbed food, and bile pigments that have been excreted by the liver are eliminated by the large intestine in the form of feces.

## POST TEST

1. The process of taking food into the mouth, chewing, and swallowing it is called _____.

2. _____ consists of mechanically and chemically breaking down food into molecules small enough to be absorbed.

3. The inner lining of the wall of the digestive tract is the _____.

4. Inferior to the diaphragm, the adventitia is called the _____
_____.

5. Rhythmic waves of contraction that push food along through the digestive tract are referred to as _____.

6. The double fold of peritoneum that hangs down over the intestine like an apron is called the _____ _____.

7. The normal maximum number of teeth in the adult mouth is _____.

8. The portion of a tooth above the gumline is the _____; the part below the gum is the _____.

9. Each tooth is composed mainly of _____, which in the crown region is covered by _____.

10. The largest salivary glands are the _____.

11. Salivary amylase breaks down _____ to _____ and _____ _____.

12. The folds in the mucosa and submucosa of the stomach are called _____.

13. Two substances produced by the gastric glands are _____ and _____ _____.

14. The three divisions of the small intestine are the _____, _____, and _____.

15. The circular folds, the _____ and the _____, all increase the surface area of the small intestine.

16. Bile is stored in the _____.

17. Gastrin is released by the _____ _____ and stimulates the _____ _____.

18. The end products of protein digestion are _____ _____.

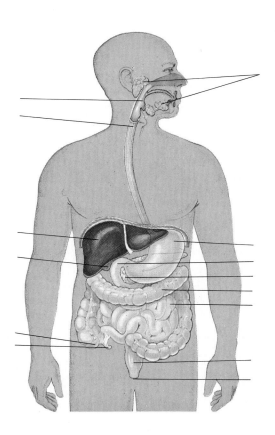

19. Nutrients are absorbed by the intestinal _____.
20. Chyme passing through the transverse colon would next enter
    the _____  _____.
21. Label the diagram on the previous page.

## REVIEW QUESTIONS

1. Trace the passage of a bite of food containing primarily cellulose through
   the digestive tract, listing each structure through which it must pass and describing what happens to the cellulose in each place.
2. Trace the passage of a protein food through the digestive tract, describing
   how it changes along the way. Do the same for a lipid and a carbohydrate.
3. Describe (or label on a diagram) the structure of a tooth.
4. What mechanisms protect the lining of the digestive tract from ulcer formation? (See Focus on Peptic Ulcers, A Case Study).
5. What structures increase the surface area of the small intestine? Why is it
   important to increase the surface area?
6. Draw a diagram of a villus and label its parts.
7. List the three types of accessory glands that release secretions into the digestive tract and give the composition and functions of each type of secretion.
8. Describe several functions of the liver.
9. Foods of plant origin are not very digestible, yet they are considered important for normal digestive tract function. Why?

# Nutrition and Metabolism

LEARNING OBJECTIVES

**After you study this chapter you should be able to**
1. Compare anabolism and catabolism; distinguish between basal metabolic rate and total metabolic rate.
2. Identify each of the basic nutrients, give its role in the body, and describe the effects of its dietary deficiency.
3. Identify minerals required by the body (as listed in Table 17–2) and give their functions in the body.
4. Describe the actions and effects of deficiency of the vitamins listed in Table 17–3.
5. Identify the principal types of carbohydrates ingested and their fate in the digestive tract (that is, what form they are in when they are absorbed). Describe the fate of glucose after its absorption.
6. Identify foods that are rich in saturated fats and cholesterol and those rich in polyunsaturated fats and trace the fate of lipids in the body.
7. Explain why essential amino acids must be included in the diet and describe the fate of amino acids in the body.
8. Give the basic energy equation for maintaining

body weight and tell what happens when it is altered in either direction.

9. Give the effects of obesity on health, its causes, and its cure based on energy considerations.

---

Nutrients are the chemical substances in food that are used by the body to make new cells and tissues, as fuel for needed energy, and in many types of metabolic activities. Nutrients essential to good health are provided by a balanced diet consisting of water, minerals, vitamins, carbohydrates, lipids, and proteins.

## METABOLISM

The cells of the body are in a constant state of activity. They continuously synthesize, use, and then degrade molecules. They proliferate, function, die, and are replaced by new cells. The term **metabolism** (meh-**tab**'-oh-lizm) refers to all of these chemical and energy transformations that take place in the body.

Chemical reactions either require energy or release energy. Thus metabolism can be divided into two broad phases: anabolism and catabolism. **Anabolism** (ah-**nab**'-oh-lizm) is the building, or synthetic, aspect of metabolism. Through anabolic reactions nutrients are converted into complex living matter. Just as assembling, maintaining, and operating an automobile requires energy, building and maintaining a body also necessitates continuous input of energy.

The energy for anabolic activities comes from using energy-containing nutrients as fuel. As these are "burned," or oxidized, energy stored within their chemical bonds is released. This breaking-down aspect of metabolism is known as **catabolism** (kah-**tab**'-oh-lizm).

**Metabolic rate** is measured as the amount of energy (heat) liberated by the body during metabolism. Nutritionists measure the energy value of food in Calories (Cal) per gram of food. Metabolic rate is expressed either in Calories of heat energy expended per hour per day or as a percentage above or below a standard normal level. Almost all the energy expended by the body is ultimately converted to heat.

The **basal metabolic rate (BMR)** is the body's basic cost of metabolic living, the rate of energy use in the body during resting (basal) conditions. An individual's **total metabolic rate** is the sum of his or her BMR and the energy used to carry on all daily activities. Obviously a laborer or someone

**TABLE 17–1**
**Approximate energy expenditure for various activities**

| Activity | Calories/Hour Above BMR Requirements |
|---|---|
| Sitting at rest | 100 |
| Walking | 130–200 |
| Jogging | 500–800 |
| Bicycling (moderate speed) | 400 |
| Swimming (moderate) | 500–700 |
| Typewriting rapidly | 140 |

who engages in a daily exercise program would have a greater total metabolic rate than one who sits behind a desk all day. Table 17–1 gives the amounts of energy expended per hour for several different types of activities.

## WATER AND WHY WE NEED IT

An average adult requires a daily intake of about 2.4 l (2.5 quarts) of water. About two-thirds of this amount is ingested in the form of water itself or other fluids. Solid foods, which actually consist of from 65 to 90% water by weight, provide the rest. That expensive roast beef is actually about 60% water by weight and a raw apple about 85% water.

Water is required as a principal component of the body, which is itself more than 60% water by weight. All chemical reactions in the body take place in a watery medium. Water is an almost universal solvent, meaning that almost all chemical compounds dissolve in it. The molecular motion of the dissolved molecules permits them to contact one another and interact. In many metabolic reactions water serves as an active ingredient.

Water is also used to transport materials within cells and from one place in the body to another. Blood plasma (which is more than 90% water) transports nutrients, hormones, wastes, and other substances. Urine and sweat (both more than 95% water) carry wastes from the body. Water has the capacity to absorb considerable amounts of heat without rapidly changing its own temperature. Because of this property, water helps to maintain the constant temperature of the body. In addition, as water evaporates from the skin as sweat and from the lungs as water vapor, it rids the body of excess heat.

## MINERALS

**Minerals** are inorganic nutrients ingested in the form of salts dissolved in food and water. Sodium, chlorine, potassium, magnesium, calcium, sulfur, phosphorus, iron, iodine, and fluorine are all minerals known to have important functions in the body. A number of others are known as **trace elements** (for example, selenium and cobalt) because they are required in very small amounts. (See also Table 2–1.)

A salt content of about 0.9% is needed to maintain an appropriate fluid balance in the body. As salts are lost from the body in sweat, urine, and feces, they must be replaced by dietary intake. Some minerals are needed to activate metabolic reactions. Others are essential components of important body chemicals. For example, iron is needed as a component of hemoglobin and iodine as an ingredient of thyroid hormones. Iron, calcium, and iodine are the minerals most likely to be deficient in the diet. Table 17–2 lists some important minerals and gives their functions in the body.

TABLE 17–2
**Some Important Minerals and Their Functions**

| Mineral | Functions | Sources |
|---|---|---|
| Calcium | Component of bones and teeth; essential for normal blood clotting; needed for normal muscle and nerve functions | Dairy products, green leafy vegetables |
| Phosphorus | As calcium phosphate, an important structural component of bone; essential in energy transfer and storage (component of ATP) and in many other metabolic processes; component of DNA and RNA; performs more functions than any other mineral; antacids can impair absorption | Beef, dairy products |
| Sulfur | Component of many proteins (e.g., insulin) | High-protein foods, such as meat, fish, legumes, nuts |
| Potassium | Influences muscle contraction and nerve excitability | Occurs in fruits and many other foods |
| Sodium | Important in fluid balance; essential for conduction of nerve impulses | Occurs in most foods; sodium chloride (table salt) added as seasoning; too much is ingested in average American diet; excessive amounts may lead to high blood pressure |
| Chlorine | Important in fluid balance and acid-base balance | Most foods; ingested as sodium chloride |
| Copper | Component of many enzymes; essential for hemoglobin synthesis | Liver, eggs, fish, whole wheat flour, beans |
| Iodine | Component of thyroid hormones (hormones that stimulate metabolic rate) | Seafoods, iodized salt, vegetables grown in iodine-rich soil; deficiency results in goiter (abnormal enlargement of thyroid gland) |
| Cobalt | As component of vitamin $B_{12}$, essential for red blood cell production | Meat, dairy products; strict vegetarians may become deficient in this mineral |
| Manganese | Necessary to activate an enzyme essential for urea formation; activates many other enzymes | Whole-grain cereals, egg yolks, green vegetables; poorly absorbed from intestine |
| Magnesium | Appropriate balance between magnesium and calcium ions needed for normal muscle and nerve function; component of many coenzymes | Occurs in many foods |
| Iron | Component of hemoglobin, important respiratory enzymes, and other enzymes essential to oxygen transport and cellular respiration | Meat (especially liver), nuts, egg yolk, legumes; mineral most likely to be deficient in diet; deficiency results in anemia |
| Fluorine | Component of bones and teeth; makes teeth resistant to decay | Where it does not occur naturally, fluorine may be added to municipal water supplies (fluoridation); excess causes tooth mottling |
| Zinc | Component of at least 70 enzymes; component of some peptidases, and thus important in protein digestion; may be important in wound healing | Occurs in many foods |

## VITAMINS

**Vitamins** are organic compounds required for certain biochemical processes. Many, especially the B vitamins, serve as **coenzymes**, compounds that function with specific enzymes in regulating chemical reactions.

Two groups of vitamins are (1) the **fat-soluble vitamins**, including vitamins A, D, E, and K, and (2) the **water-soluble vitamins**, which include vitamin C and those belonging to the B complex (a group of several types of B vitamins). Table 17–3 gives the recommended daily allowance, sources, actions, and effects of various vitamin deficiencies (Fig. 17–1).

Controversy rages over the issue of vitamin supplements. Many nutritionists think that a balanced diet provides all the vitamins needed. Others argue that most of us do not eat a balanced diet and are likely to suffer from vitamin deficiencies. Debate also continues over intake of large amounts of specific vitamins. You may be familiar with assertions that vitamin C helps prevent the common cold and that vitamin E protects against vascular disease. More recently claims have been made that vitamins C, E, and A may help protect against certain types of cancer. The truth is that there is still a great deal to learn about the actions of vitamins. Much more research is needed before their complex biochemical roles will be understood. Meanwhile moderation is recommended.

**Hypervitaminosis**, a condition resulting from ingestion of excessive amounts of vitamin A or D, is being seen with increasing frequency. Because vitamins A and D are fat-soluble, they are not easily excreted in the urine. Instead, they tend to accumulate in fatty tissues of the body (mainly in the liver), where they can build up to harmful levels. Hypervitaminosis A results in loss of hair and skin disorders. Hypervitaminosis D results in weakness, fatigue, loss of weight, and other symptoms. Even vitamin C in excessive amounts can be harmful, especially in children.

## CARBOHYDRATES

**Carbohydrates** are the body's principal fuel. Our cells "burn" them to obtain energy needed for metabolic activities, growth, repair, and physical activity. In the average American diet carbohydrates provide about 50% of the Calories ingested daily.

Foods rich in carbohydrates include rice, potatoes, corn, and other cereal grains. These are the least expensive foods; thus the proportion of carbohydrates in a family's diet may reflect economic status. Poor people often subsist on diets that are almost exclusively carbohydrate, whereas more af-

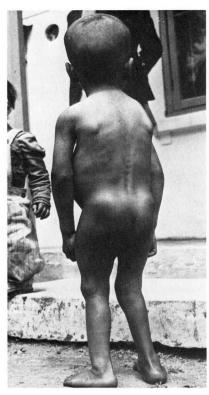

*Figure 17–1. Child with rickets, a condition that results from deficiency of vitamin D during childhood. This deficiency decreases the body's ability to absorb and use calcium and phosphorus and produces soft, malformed bones. Note the bowed legs. (United Nations, Food and Agricultural Organization photo.)*

fluent persons enjoy more expensive protein-rich foods such as meat and dairy products.

Most carbohydrates are ingested in the form of starch and cellulose, both polysaccharides. Starch is the form in which plant cells store glucose, and in the digestive tract it is eventually degraded to glucose. Cellulose is the material that makes up the cell walls surrounding plant cells. Humans do not have the enzymes needed to digest cellulose. However, it is an important part of dietary fiber, providing bulk needed for proper function of the large intestine.

In affluent societies about 25% of the carbohydrate intake (more in children) is in the form of the disaccharide sucrose (cane or beet sugar). Sucrose is the so-called refined sugar that we put in our coffee and desserts.

Most carbohydrates are absorbed in the form of glucose; those that are not are rapidly converted into glucose in the liver. Once absorbed, glucose is transported to the liver. As the glucose-rich blood flows through the liver, the liver cells remove excess glucose (Fig. 17–2).

One of the most important jobs of the liver is to help regulate the blood-sugar level. The cells of

TABLE 17–3
**The Vitamins**

| Vitamins (U.S. RDA[1]) | Actions | Effect of Deficiency | Sources |
|---|---|---|---|
| **Fat-Soluble** | | | |
| A (5000 IU[2]) | Component of retinal pigments, essential for normal vision; essential for normal growth and health of epithelial tissue; promotes normal growth of bones and teeth; excessive amounts harmful | Failure of growth; night blindness; atrophy of epithelium; epithelium subject to infection; scaly skin | Liver, fish-liver oils, egg, yellow and green vegetables |
| D (400 IU) | Promotes calcium absorption from digestive tract; essential to normal growth and maintenance of bone; excessive amounts harmful | Bone deformities; rickets in children; osteomalacia in adults | Liver, fish-liver oils, egg yolk, fortified milk, butter, margarine |
| E (30 IU) | Inhibits oxidation of unsaturated fatty acids that help form cell membranes; precise biochemical role not known | Increased catabolism of unsaturated fatty acids, so not enough are available for maintenance of cell membranes and other membranous organelles; prevents normal growth | Oils made from cereals, seeds, liver, eggs, fish |
| K (probably about 1 mg) | Essential for blood clotting | Prolonged blood-clotting time | Normally supplied by intestinal bacteria; green leafy vegetables |
| **Water-Soluble** | | | |
| C (ascorbic acid) (60 mg) | Needed for synthesis of collagen and other intercellular substances; aids formation of bone matrix and tooth dentin; may help body withstand injury from burns and bacterial toxins; possible role in preventing common cold or in the development of acquired immunity(?); harmful in excessive dose | Scurvy (wounds heal slowly and scars become weak and split open; capillaries become fragile; bone does not grow or heal properly) | Citrus fruits, strawberries, tomatoes |
| B complex vitamins | | | |
| Thiamine (B₁) (1.5 mg) | Required as coenzyme in many enzyme systems; important in carbohydrate and amino acid metabolism | Beriberi (weakened heart muscle, enlarged right side of heart, nervous system and digestive tract disorders) | Liver, yeast, cereals, meat, green leafy vegetables |
| Riboflavin (B₂) (1.7 mg) | Used to make coenzymes essential in cellular respiration | Dermatitis, inflammation of mouth and cracking at corners; mental depression | Liver, cheese, milk, eggs, green leafy vegetables |
| Niacin (nicotinic acid) (20 mg) | Component of important coenzymes essential to cellular respiration | Pellagra (dermatitis, diarrhea, mental symptoms, muscular weakness, fatigue) | Liver, meat, fish, cereals, legumes, whole-grain and enriched breads |
| Pyridoxine (B₆) (2 mg) | Needed for amino acid synthesis and protein metabolism | Dermatitis, digestive tract disturbances, convulsions | Liver, meat, cereals, legumes |
| Pantothenic acid (10 mg) | Important in cellular metabolism | Deficiency extremely rare | Widespread in foods |
| Folic acid (0.4 mg) | Required for reactions involved in nucleic acid synthesis and for maturation of red blood cells | A type of anemia | Produced by intestinal bacteria; liver, cereals, dark-green leafy vegetables |
| Biotin (0.3 mg) | Needed for fat metabolism | Deficiency unknown | Produced by intestinal bacteria; liver, chocolate, egg yolk |
| B₁₂ (6 mg) | Important in nucleic acid metabolism | Pernicious anemia | Liver, meat, fish |

[1]RDA, The recommended dietary allowance, established by the Food and Nutrition Board of the National Research Council, to maintain good nutrition for healthy persons.
[2]International Unit, The amount that produces a specific biological effect and is internationally accepted as a measure of the activity of the substance.

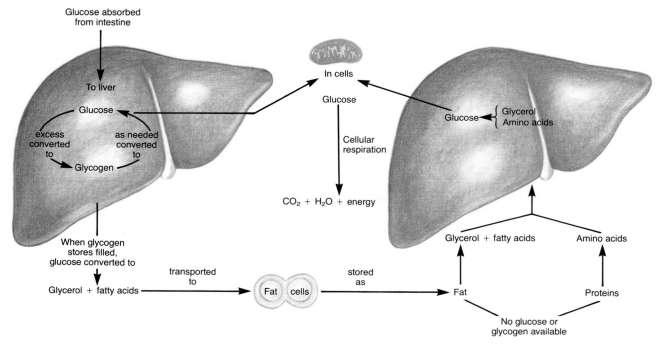

**Figure 17–2.** *The fate of glucose in the body.*

the body are extremely dependent on a constant supply of glucose delivered by the blood. Brain cells are especially dependent because they are unable to store glucose themselves. If deprived of this vital source of energy for even a few minutes, they cease to function. When after a meal the glucose concentration in the blood is above the homeostatic level, the liver cells remove and store the excess as glycogen. Then, between meals, when the glucose level begins to fall, the liver cells release glucose back into the blood. (You should recall that these metabolic activities are regulated by insulin and glucagon.) The amount of glycogen stored in the liver is sufficient to maintain the blood-glucose level for several hours. After the glycogen runs out, liver cells begin to convert amino acids and fat into glucose.

The normal fasting level of blood glucose is about 90 mg/100 ml (or 90 mg%). This means that there are 90 mg of glucose per 100 ml of blood. After a carbohydrate-rich meal the level may increase briefly to about 140 mg/100 ml. If the liver did not remove the excess, the level would rise to more than three times normal after a carbohydrate-rich meal and then fall drastically between meals or during the night.

When too much carbohydrate-rich food is eaten, the liver cells may become fully packed with glycogen and still have more glucose to manage. In this situation liver cells (and also fat cells) convert excess glucose to fat.

Glucose is the principal fuel used in **cellular respiration**, the complex series of chemical reactions by which the cell breaks down organic compounds to obtain the energy trapped within their chemical bonds. During cellular respiration glucose is degraded to carbon dioxide and water. A summary equation for cellular respiration follows:

$$C_6H_{12}O_6 + 6\ O_2 \rightarrow 6\ CO_2 + 6\ H_2O + energy$$
Glucose Oxygen Carbon Water
       dioxide

The energy is packaged within the remarkable chemical compound called **adenosine triphosphate (ATP)**.

## LIPIDS

Cells use **lipids** as fuel, as components of cell membranes, and as parts of steroid hormones and certain other substances. Lipids account for about 40% of the Calories in the average American or Canadian diet. In poor countries this percentage falls to less than 10% because most lipid-rich foods—meats, eggs, and dairy products—are relatively expensive.

Most lipids are ingested as fats. Fats may be saturated (that is, fully loaded with hydrogens) or unsaturated (containing two or more double bonds so that hydrogen atoms can be added). As a rule, meat and other animal foods are rich in both saturated fats and cholesterol, whereas plant foods contain unsaturated fats and no cholesterol. Commonly used polyunsaturated vegetable oils are corn, soya, cottonseed, and safflower oils. Butter contains mainly saturated fats.

The average American diet provides about 700 mg of cholesterol each day, whereas only about 300 is recommended. Egg yolks, butter, and meat are rich in cholesterol.

> Diets high in saturated fats and cholesterol are thought to increase the chances of developing atherosclerosis, a progressive disease in which the arteries become occluded with fatty material. As was discussed in Chapter 13 atherosclerosis leads to heart disease. On the other hand, ingestion of polyunsaturated fats tends to decrease blood-cholesterol levels, thus affording some protection against the development of atherosclerosis. For these reasons many people now use vegetable oils and polyunsaturated margarines instead of butter and lard, skim milk instead of whole milk, and ice milk instead of ice cream.

## Fate of Lipids

Lipids are absorbed into the lymph but soon enter the blood. As blood flows through adipose tissues, most of it is taken up by fat cells and stored as fat. The stored fat is then mobilized from adipose tissue as needed. Fat is continuously mobilized and then replaced. The fat molecules you have stored in your fat cells today are not the same ones that were there last week, although the total amount is probably much the same!

Lipids are transported in the blood in combination with protein. The lipoprotein particles are assembled by the liver. One type of lipoprotein, called low-density lipoprotein, contains mainly cholesterol. A high plasma concentration of this lipoprotein is associated with the development of atherosclerosis.

## Using Fat As Fuel

Each gram of fat contains about twice as many Calories as a gram of glucose or amino acids. Although the amount of glycogen that the body can store is limited, a look around should convince you that there is almost no limit to the amount of fat a person can store. Most of it is stored in the adipose tissues found in the subcutaneous areas of the body. This body fat represents an important fuel reserve and most cells can utilize fatty acids as fuel almost interchangeably with glucose. In

fact, between meals most cells shift their energy metabolism so that fat is used as fuel instead of glucose. In this way glucose is reserved for nerve cells, which are not able to utilize lipids as fuel under ordinary circumstances.

## PROTEINS

Protein consumption is often an index of a country's (or an individual's) economic status, because high-quality protein is the most expensive and least widely available of all nutrients. Protein poverty is one of the world's most serious health problems. Millions of human beings suffer poor health, disease, and even death as a result of protein malnutrition (Fig. 17–3).

Why are **proteins** so critical as nutrients? Ingested proteins are degraded in the digestive tract to their molecular subunits, amino acids, which are then absorbed and utilized by the cells to make the types of proteins needed. They are essential as building blocks of cells; indeed, 75% of body solids consist of protein. Proteins also serve as enzymes and as other vital compounds, such as hemoglobin.

Of the 20 or so amino acids important in nutri-

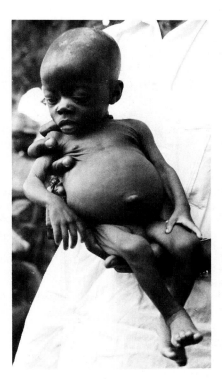

*Figure 17–3.* Child suffering from kwashiorkor, a disease caused by severe protein deficiency. Note the characteristic swollen belly, which results from fluid imbalance. (United Nations, Food and Agricultural Organization photo by P. Pittet.)

tion, the body is able to make several from organic components. About eight of the amino acids (10 in children) cannot be synthesized by the body cells at all, or at least not in sufficient quantity to meet the body's needs. These, which must be provided in the diet, are called the **essential amino acids**.

Not all proteins contain the same kinds or quantities of amino acids, and many proteins lack some of the essential amino acids. The highest-quality proteins (those that contain the most appropriate distribution of amino acids for human nutrition) are found in eggs, milk, meat, and fish. Some foods, such as gelatin or soybeans, contain all the essential amino acids but do not contain them in nutritionally adequate proportions. Most plant proteins are deficient in one or more of the essential amino acids.

About 56 g of protein per day (half of a Quarter Pounder) is the recommended daily amount for adults. In the United States and other developed countries most persons eat far more protein than necessary. It has been estimated that the average American eats about 300 pounds of meat and dairy products per year. In underdeveloped countries an average of only 2 pounds per person per year is consumed.

Most humans depend on cereal grains as their staple food, usually rice, wheat, or corn. None of these foods provides an adequate proportion of total amino acids or distribution of essential amino acids, especially not for growing children. In some underdeveloped countries starchy crops such as sweet potatoes are the main food. The total protein content of these foods is less than 2%—far below minimum needs. (See Focus on the Vegetarian Diet.)

## Fate of Amino Acids

Whereas glucose and fats are mainly used in catabolism, amino acids are utilized mainly in the anabolic (building) processes of the body (Fig. 17–4). They are the building blocks used to make proteins needed for cell parts, to make new cells, and to synthesize enzymes. In the muscle cells they are assembled into myosin and actin, the proteins needed for muscle contraction. In the liver they are used to produce plasma proteins and they are used by red blood cells to make hemoglobin.

Although small numbers of amino acids accumulate in the cytoplasm of all cells, there is no

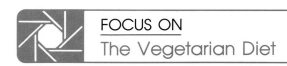

## FOCUS ON
## The Vegetarian Diet

Most of the world's population depends almost exclusively on plant foods for proteins and other nutrients. However, besides being deficient in some of the essential amino acids, plant foods have a lower percentage of protein than animal foods. Meat contains about 25% protein; the new high-yield grains contain 5% to 13%. Another problem is that plant protein is less digestible than animal protein. Because we cannot digest the cellulose cell walls, much of the protein encased within the cells passes on through the digestive tract as part of the bulk.

Yet another problem with the vegetarian diet is that the body has no mechanism for storing amino acids. Cells cannot make a protein storage compound comparable to glycogen, and they have no protein depot, in the sense that fat is stored in adipose tissue. One might almost say that all the essential amino acids must be ingested in the same meal. For example, if corn is eaten for lunch and beans for dinner, the body will not have all the essential amino acids at the same time and will not be able to manufacture needed proteins.

Does this mean, then, that vegetarian diets are always unhealthful? Not at all. Given a variety of plant foods and some knowledge of nutrition, a vegetarian can plan a diet that provides all the needed

amino acids. The main task is to select foods that complement one another. For example, if beans and corn or beans and rice are eaten together in the proper proportions, they will provide the required essential amino acids. When dairy products are available, they should be eaten with the plant foods. For example, when cereal is eaten with milk, the meal has a much greater nutritional value. Macaroni and cheese is another example.

Soybeans, peanuts, and other legumes have more than twice the protein content of the cereal grains. Unfortunately, yields per acre of these crops are much lower than yields per acre of cereal grains. Also, most of the legumes produced are used as livestock feed, rather than for human consumption. In fact, in the United States 91% of the cereal, legume, and other vegetable protein suitable for human use is fed to livestock. This represents a tremendous and serious loss of protein to human beings, because for every 5 kg (11 pounds) of vegetable and fish protein fed to livestock in addition to their forage intake, only 1 kg (2.2 pounds) of animal protein is produced. Meat is expensive economically because it is ecologically expensive. As the human population continues to expand, more and more of us will have to turn to vegetarian diets.

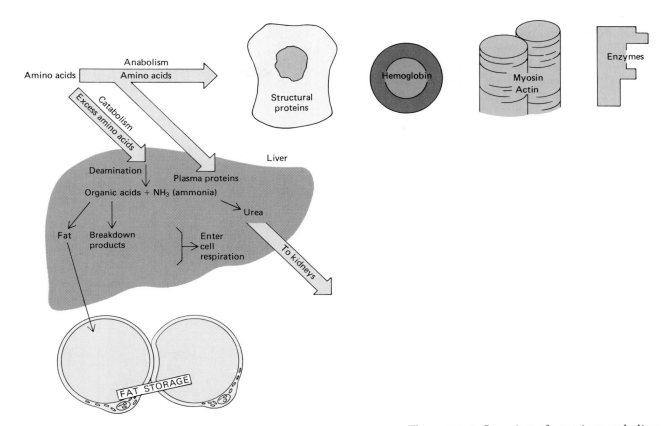

**Figure 17–4.** *Overview of protein metabolism.*

mechanism for storing large quantities. Excess amino acids are removed from the blood by the liver cells and **deaminated**, that is, the amino group is removed from each amino acid. As they are cleaved from the amino acid, the amino groups are converted into ammonia. However, ammonia is toxic and is quickly converted to urea. The urea then passes into the blood and is excreted by the kidneys. After deamination the remaining portion of the amino acid may be converted into carbohydrate or lipid and either used as fuel or stored as fat.

## Nitrogen Balance

The amount of nitrogen in the urine reflects the amount of amino acid (and protein) breakdown. When the amount of nitrogen in the diet and the amount excreted in the urine of an adult are the same, the person is said to be in **nitrogen balance**. During starvation and certain disorders large amounts of protein are degraded, and the body excretes more nitrogen than it takes in, a state of negative nitrogen balance. When a child is growing or

when an individual is recovering from an illness, intake of protein is greater than nitrogen excretion and the body is said to be in positive nitrogen balance.

## ENERGY BALANCE AND BODY WEIGHT

Nutritional balance requires both adequate amounts of all the essential nutrients and sufficient Calories to support the energy needs of the body. An average-sized man who does not engage in any exercise program and who sits at a desk all day expends about 2000 Cal daily. If he ingests 2000 Cal in the food he eats each day, he will be in a state of energy balance, that is, his energy input will equal his energy output. This is an important concept, for when energy (Calorie) input equals energy output, body weight remains constant. When energy output is greater than energy input, stored fat is burned and body weight decreases. On the other hand, when energy input is greater than energy output, the excess fuel is stored as fat and the individual gains weight.

## Obesity

Some 40 million Americans eat too much. **Obesity**, the excess accumulation of body fat, is a serious form of malnutrition in affluent societies. An overweight person places an extra burden on her or his heart, because it has to work harder to pump blood through the excess adipose tissue. Obese persons are also more likely to develop atherosclerosis, hypertension, hernia, and gallbladder disease. They also present greater surgical risks. According to insurance statistics, men who are 20% or more overweight have a 43% greater risk of dying from heart disease, a 53% greater risk of dying from cerebral hemorrhage, and more than a 150% greater chance of dying from diabetes.

### Causes of Obesity

Overeating is the only way to become obese. People gain weight when they take in more Calories in food than they expend in daily activity. (Although water retention does increase body weight, it does not affect fat storage; you can get rid of excess water faster and more easily than excess fat.) It has been estimated that for every 9.3 Cal of excess food taken into the body, 1 g of fat is stored. (An excess of about 140 Cal per day for a month will result in gaining 1 pound.) A person who has gained weight will maintain that weight even if food intake is reduced so that energy intake and output are balanced. The only way to lose weight is to shift the energy balance so that output is greater than input.

A 16-year-old athlete requires a much larger food intake to support his or her growth and physical activity than he or she does 10 years later as an accountant who spends most of the day sitting at a desk. Those who continue eating at the same level even after their activities have become less strenuous (requiring less energy) are destined to become overweight.

Most overweight people overeat because of a combination of poor eating habits and psychological factors. Childhood obesity is thought to be a contributing factor to adult obesity. The number of fat cells in the body is thought to be determined early in life. Babies and children who are overfed develop up to five times the normal number of fat cells.

Fat cells are like tiny balloons that can be inflated with fat (Fig. 17–5). They can blow up to about 50% their normal size as fat accumulates within. Then, as fat is mobilized, they shrink (or deflate). If you were an overweight child, you have thousands of extra fat cells just waiting to fill with fat. Some investigators think that persons with ex-

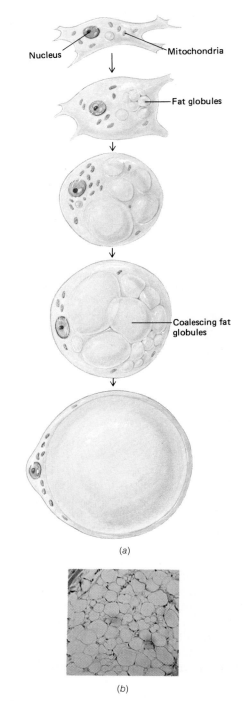

*Figure 17–5.* Storage of fat in a fat cell. (a) As more and more fat droplets accumulate in the cytoplasm, they form a large globule of fat. Such a fat globule may occupy most of the cell, pushing the cytoplasm and organelles to the periphery. (b) Photomicrograph of adipose tissue (approximately ×100). The fat droplets were dissolved by chemicals used to prepare the tissue, leaving large spaces. Because of these spaces, the cells tend to collapse and no longer appear round.

cessive numbers of fat cells have a higher setting of the appetite-regulating centers in the hypothalamus.

As more is learned about metabolism, it is likely

that factors that encourage obesity will be discovered. For example, it has been suggested that some people may have more efficient digestive tracts than others—that is, food may be more efficiently processed in them, resulting in absorption of a larger percentage of nutrients. Those who process food less efficiently waste more nutrients. They can afford to eat more because a lower percentage of Calories is actually absorbed. Despite these possible individual differences, however, one can control weight by adjusting food intake to meet energy needs.

### Cures

The only cure for obesity is to shift energy relationships so that energy intake is less than energy output. The body then must draw on its fat stores for the needed Calories. As the fat is mobilized and "burned," body weight decreases. This is best accomplished by a combination of increased exercise (that is, energy expenditure) and decreased total caloric intake.

Most nutritionists agree that the best reducing diet by far is a well-balanced diet, having a normal proportion of fats, carbohydrates, and proteins. In other words, eat everything but in smaller quantities.

Many people have become rich by promoting imaginative reducing diets, books, slenderizing devices, and formulas that appeal to millions of overweight individuals looking for an easy way to shed excess poundage. These gimmicks are of only psychological value; they may encourage the overweight to reduce food consumption. However, they often have drawbacks that can damage one's health and in a few cases may even cause death.

For example, high-protein diets tax the kidneys, which must excrete excessive amounts of urea, and may cause permanent kidney damage. There is no truth to the claims that you can eat all you want of one particular type of nutrient (for example, protein), for as you know, an excess of protein or carbohydrate is converted to fat and stored. Yet another disadvantage of many popular reducing diets is that they cannot be maintained for long periods of time. After a few weeks the dieter slips back into old eating habits and may rapidly regain the weight lost.

## SUMMARY

I. A balanced diet includes water, minerals, vitamins, carbohydrates, lipids, and proteins.
II. Metabolism is the sum of all the chemical and energy transformations that take place in the body.
   A. Anabolism is the synthetic aspect of metabolism, such as making proteins.
   B. Catabolism is the breaking-down aspect of metabolism, such as burning nutrients as fuel.
   C. Basal metabolic rate (BMR) is the amount of energy utilized by the body under resting conditions. Total metabolic rate is the sum of BMR and the energy needed to carry on one's daily activities.
III. Water is a vital component of the body; it is used as a medium in which chemical reactions take place and to transport materials.
IV. Some of the minerals required by the body are iron (a component of hemoglobin and other enzymes); iodine (a component of thyroid hormones); calcium and phosphorus (components of bone and teeth, essential for many body activities); and sodium and chlorine (needed for maintaining appropriate fluid balance). See Table 17–2.
V. The actions, sources, and effects of various vitamin deficiencies are listed in Table 17–3.
   A. The water-soluble vitamins are vitamin C and the B complex vitamins.
   B. The fat-soluble vitamins are vitamins A, D, E, and K.
VI. Most carbohydrates are ingested as starch or cellulose. During digestion they are broken down into the sugar glucose. The liver is important in maintaining blood-glucose levels.
   A. When excess glucose is present, the liver removes it from the blood and converts it to glycogen for storage.
   B. As needed, glycogen is degraded, and glucose is returned to the blood.
   C. When glycogen stores are depleted, liver cells convert amino acids and fat into glucose.
VII. Most lipids are ingested as fats. Meat and other animal foods are rich in saturated fats and cholesterol.
   A. Lipids are used as fuel, as components of cell membranes, and to make steroid hormones and other substances.
   B. Fat is stored in adipose tissue. When blood-glucose levels fall, fat is mobilized for use as fuel.
VIII. Proteins are degraded to amino acids during digestion. Amino acids are utilized primarily in anabolic metabolism.
   A. Amino acids are used to make structural proteins, enzymes, and functional proteins such as hemoglobin, actin, and myosin.

B. Excess amino acids are deaminated in the liver and the remaining part of the amino acid is converted to carbohydrate fuel or to lipid for storage as fat.

C. When the amount of nitrogen entering the body daily equals that excreted from amino acid deamination, the body is in nitrogen balance.

IX. Body weight remains constant when energy input equals energy output.

A. When energy input exceeds output, the excess nutrients are stored as fat and body weight increases.

B. When energy input is less than energy output, the body draws on its fuel reserves (fat) and body weight decreases.

X. Obesity is a serious form of malnutrition; the best reducing diets are well-balanced diets with normal proportions of carbohydrates, fats, and proteins.

## POST TEST

1. Synthesizing proteins is an example of the phase of metabolism called _____.

2. Oxidizing glucose is an example of the phase of metabolism called _____.

*Select the most appropriate answer choice from Column B for each item in Column A. You may use an answer once, more than once, or not at all.*

| Column A | Column B |
|---|---|
| 3. _____ Needed for hemoglobin synthesis | a. vitamin A |
| 4. _____ Mineral needed for blood clotting and bone | b. vitamin D |
|  | c. vitamin K |
| 5. _____ Makes tooth enamel resistant to decay | d. calcium |
| 6. _____ Deficiency results in rickets | e. fluorine |
|  | f. iron |
| 7. _____ One of the B complex vitamins | g. niacin |
| 8. _____ Vitamin essential for blood clotting | h. vitamin C |
| 9. _____ Deficiency may cause blindness | |
| 10. _____ Needed for collagen synthesis; deficiency causes scurvy | |

11. Inorganic nutrients ingested in the form of salts dissolved in food or water are called _____.

12. Organic compounds that usually function as coenzymes are called _____.

13. Most digestible carbohydrates are ingested in the form of _____.

14. Most lipids in the diet are ingested in the form of _____.

15. High-quality proteins contain a nutritional balance of essential _____ _____.

16. In the liver excess _____ _____ are deaminated.

17. When the body excretes more nitrogen than it takes in, it is in a state of _____ nitrogen balance.

18. When energy input is greater than energy output _____.

## REVIEW QUESTIONS

1. List the general classes of nutrients and tell why each is required.
2. Would you classify each of the following as anabolism or catabolism: (a) hemoglobin synthesis (b) cellular respiration (c) deamination of amino acids?
3. What are the consequences of deficiencies of each of the following: (a) iron (b) vitamin A (c) vitamin D (d) essential amino acids?
4. Draw a diagram to summarize the fate of carbohydrates in the body. Do the same for amino acids and for lipids.
5. What happens to excess glucose? excess amino acids?
6. Distinguish between basal metabolic rate and total metabolic rate.
7. What happens when energy input is greater than energy output? when energy input equals energy output?
8. Why is it more difficult to obtain adequate amounts of amino acids in a vegetarian diet? How can a nutritious vegetarian diet be planned?

# VI

# REGULATION OF FLUIDS AND ELECTROLYTES

# The Urinary System

LEARNING OBJECTIVES

**After you study this chapter you should be able to**
1. Identify the principal metabolic waste products and the organs that excrete them.
2. Label a diagram of the structures of the urinary system and give the function of each.
3. Describe the structures of a nephron and give the functions of the following structures: Bowman's capsule, glomerulus, renal tubule, collecting duct, afferent arteriole, efferent arteriole. (Be able to label a diagram of a nephron.)
4. Trace a drop of filtrate from glomerulus to urethra, listing in sequence each structure through which it passes.
5. Describe the process of urine formation and give the composition of urine.
6. Summarize the regulation of urine volume, including the role of ADH.
7. Summarize the functions of the kidney in maintaining homeostasis.
8. Describe the process of urination.

As cells carry on metabolic activities, they produce waste products. If permitted to accumulate, metabolic wastes would eventually reach toxic concentrations and threaten homeostasis. To prevent this threat metabolic wastes must be excreted. The term **excretion** refers to the removal of metabolic wastes, whereas **elimination** refers to discharging undigested or unabsorbed food from the digestive tract.

## METABOLIC WASTES AND THEIR EXCRETION

The principal metabolic waste products are water, carbon dioxide, and nitrogenous (nitrogen-containing) wastes (including urea, uric acid, and creatinine). Recall that amino acids and nucleic acids contain nitrogen. During the breakdown of excess amino acids in the liver, the nitrogen-containing amino group is removed, a process known as **deamination**. The amino group is converted to ammonia, which is then chemically converted to **urea**. Somewhat similarly, **uric acid** is formed from the breakdown of nucleic acids. Urea and uric acid are transported from the liver to the kidneys by the circulatory system. **Creatinine** is a nitrogenous waste produced from phosphocreatine in the muscles.

Although metabolic wastes are excreted mainly by the urinary system, the skin, lungs, and digestive system also have waste disposal functions (Fig. 18–1). Sweat glands in the skin excrete 5 to 10% of all metabolic wastes. Sweat contains the same substances—water, salts, and nitrogenous wastes—as urine but is much more dilute.

The lungs excrete carbon dioxide and water (in the form of water vapor). The liver excretes bilirubin and other pigments, which are breakdown products of hemoglobin. These pigments pass into the intestine as part of the bile and then leave the body with the feces.

## ORGANS OF THE URINARY SYSTEM

The principal organs of the urinary system are the paired **kidneys**, which remove wastes from the blood and produce the urine (Fig. 18–2). From the kidneys urine is conducted to the urinary bladder by the paired **ureters.** The single urinary bladder collects and stores urine, which is eventually discharged from the body through the single urethra.

## THE KIDNEYS

The urinary system is located behind the peritoneum lining the abdominal cavity and so is described as **retroperitoneal** (re″-trow-per″-i-tow-

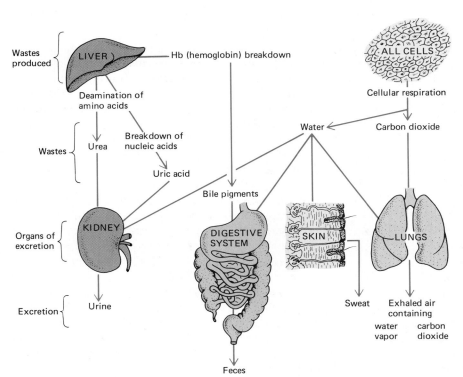

***Figure 18–1.*** *The kidneys, lungs, skin, and digestive system all participate in the disposal of metabolic wastes. Nitrogenous wastes are produced by the liver and transported to the kidneys. The kidneys excrete these wastes in the urine. All cells produce carbon dioxide and some water during cellular respiration.*

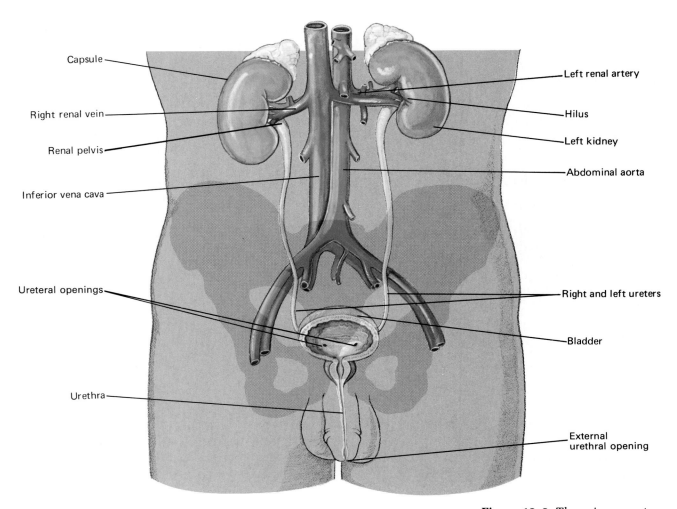

*Figure 18–2.* The urinary system.

nee'-al). The **kidneys** are located near the posterior body wall just below the diaphragm. They are protected by the lower ribs. Each kidney receives blood from a renal artery and is drained by a renal vein.

Each kidney looks something like a large, dark-red lima bean about the size of a fist. The ureters and blood vessels connect with the kidney at its **hilus** (**hi'**-lus), the indentation on its medial border. Covering the kidney is a strong capsule of connective tissue, the **renal capsule**.

The kidney consists of an outer **renal cortex** and an inner **renal medulla** (Fig. 18–3). Urine flows into a hollow structure, the **renal pelvis**, which is continuous with the ureter. The renal pelvis branches into four to eight funnel-shaped cups, the **major calyces** (**kay'**-li-seez). Each major calyx receives urine from two or more smaller **minor calyces**. The minor calyces, in turn, drain collecting ducts.

The renal medulla is composed of several cone-shaped regions known as **pyramids**. The tip of each pyramid, called a **papilla** (pa-**pill'**-ah), is surrounded by a minor calyx. Each papilla has several pores, the openings of the collecting ducts, through which urine passes into the minor calyx.

## The Nephron

Each kidney contains more than a million microscopic units called **nephrons** (**nef'**-rons). A nephron consists of two main structures: a **renal corpuscle** and a **renal tubule**. The nephrons filter the blood and produce urine. Basically, blood is filtered in the renal corpuscle. Then, the filtered fluid, or **filtrate**, passes through the renal tubule. As the filtrate moves through the long tubule, substances needed by the body are returned to the blood. Waste products, excess water, and other substances not needed by the body pass into the collecting ducts as urine.

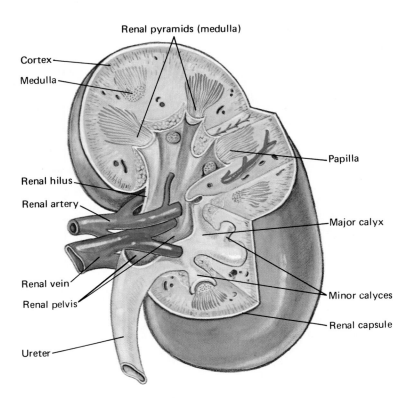

Renal pyramids (medulla)

Cortex

Medulla

Papilla

Renal hilus

Renal artery

Major calyx

Renal vein

Renal pelvis

Minor calyces

Renal capsule

Ureter

*Figure 18–3. Structure of the kidney.*

The renal corpuscle consists of a network of capillaries, the **glomerulus**, which is surrounded by a cuplike structure known as **Bowman's capsule** (Fig. 18–4). Blood flows into the glomerulus through a small **afferent arteriole** and leaves the glomerulus through an **efferent arteriole**. This arteriole conducts blood to a second set of capillaries, the **peritubular capillaries**, which surround the renal tubule.

Bowman's capsule has an opening in its bottom through which filtrate passes into the renal tubule. The first part of the renal tubule is the coiled **proximal convoluted tubule**. After passing through the proximal convoluted tubule filtrate flows into the **loop of Henle (hen′-lee)** and then into the **distal convoluted tubule**. Urine from the distal convoluted tubules of several nephrons drains into a collecting duct. A portion of the distal convoluted tubule curves upward and contacts the afferent and efferent arterioles (Fig. 18–5). Some cells of the distal convoluted tubule and some cells of the afferent arteriole become modified to form the **juxtaglomerular (juks″-tuh-glom-err′-yoo-lar) apparatus**, a structure that helps regulate blood pressure in the kidney.

The renal corpuscle, the proximal convoluted tubule, and the distal convoluted tubule of each nephron are located within the renal cortex. Loops of Henle dip down into the medulla.

## Urine Formation

Urine formation involves three processes: (1) glomerular filtration, (2) tubular reabsorption, and (3) tubular secretion.

### Glomerular Filtration

The first step is **glomerular filtration**. The afferent arteriole is larger in diameter than the efferent arteriole so blood enters the glomerulus more rapidly than it can leave. This causes the blood pressure to be higher in the glomerular capillaries than in other capillaries. As a result plasma and substances dissolved in the plasma are forced out of the capillaries of the glomerulus and into Bowman's capsule. Thus, the filtrate consists of blood plasma containing glucose, salts, and other small, dissolved molecules. Blood cells and proteins are too large to pass through the capillary and capsule membranes. When these do appear in the urine, it is a symptom of a problem with glomerular filtration.

Almost 25% of the cardiac output is delivered to the kidneys each minute, so every 4 minutes the kidneys receive a volume of blood equal to the total volume of blood in the body. Every 24 hours about 180 l (about 45 gallons) of filtrate are produced. Common sense suggests that we could not

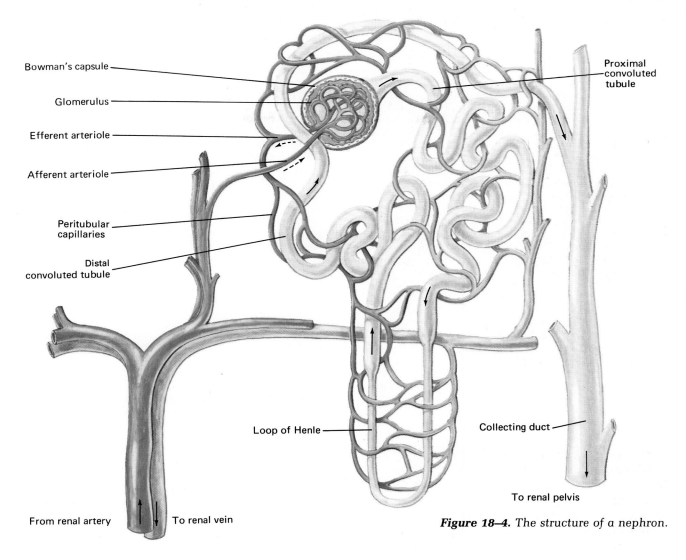

Bowman's capsule

Glomerulus

Efferent arteriole

Afferent arteriole

Peritubular capillaries

Distal convoluted tubule

Proximal convoluted tubule

Loop of Henle

Collecting duct

To renal pelvis

From renal artery    To renal vein

**Figure 18–4.** The structure of a nephron.

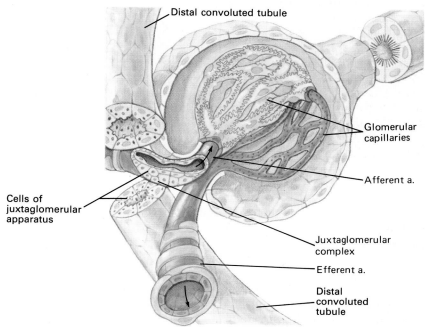

Distal convoluted tubule

Glomerular capillaries

Afferent a.

Juxtaglomerular complex

Efferent a.

Distal convoluted tubule

Cells of juxtaglomerular apparatus

**Figure 18–5.** Close-up view of the glomerulus and Bowman's capsule.

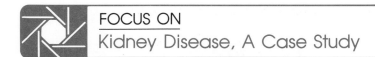

## FOCUS ON
## Kidney Disease, A Case Study

"How could this be happening to me? I'm only 52." Etta sat stunned as her physician informed her that laboratory tests confirmed his diagnosis of glomerular disease. Dr. Nef explained that she was in **renal failure**. Because her kidneys were not functioning effectively, she was losing large amounts of protein in her urine. She had developed edema due to retention of water, and the concentration of hydrogen ions was elevated, causing acidosis. Nitrogenous wastes were accumulating in her blood and tissues, producing **uremia**. Dr. Nef gently explained that, if untreated, the acidosis and uremia could cause coma and eventually death. He recommended kidney dialysis and, perhaps, eventual kidney transplant.

Later, Etta read in the pamphlet Dr. Nef had given her that kidney disease ranks fourth among major diseases in the United States. Kidney function can be impaired by infections, certain drugs, kidney stone formation, poisoning caused by substances such as mercury or carbon tetrachloride, neoplasms, or certain circulatory diseases. Etta knew that her disease, a type of *glomerulonephritis* (glow-mer″-u-low-nef-**rie**′-tis), was linked with a malfunction of her immune system.

The next day a tube was surgically inserted into both an artery and a vein in Etta's arm. During dialysis, these tubes were connected to a dialysis machine through a circuit of plastic tubing. Etta's blood flowed slowly through the tubing, which was immersed in a solution containing normal blood plasma components. Etta was told that the wastes from her blood would dialyze through minute pores in the cellophane tubing and pass into the surrounding solution. The wall of the tubing was a semipermeable membrane. As the blood flowed repeatedly through the tubing in the machine, dialysis continued. After 4 hours of dialysis treatment most of Etta's blood chemistry values had been adjusted to more normal ranges. Kidney dialysis would be repeated three times each week.

Some weeks later Dr. Nef spoke to Etta about a kidney transplant. He explained that a functioning kidney would be far more effective than the dialysis machine. With a successful kidney transplant Etta would be able to live a more normal life with less long-term expense. At present more than two-thirds of kidney transplants are successful for several years. Etta agreed to tissue typing and is waiting for a matched kidney to become available.

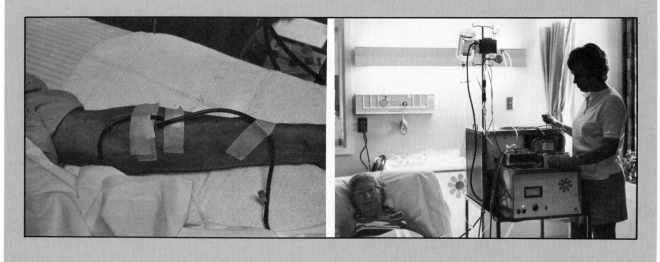

excrete urine at the rate of 180 l/day. At that rate of fluid loss dehydration would become a life-threatening problem within a few moments.

### Tubular Reabsorption and Secretion

Dehydration does not normally occur because about 99% of the filtrate is returned to the blood, leaving only about 1.5 l to be excreted as urine during a 24-hour period. **Tubular reabsorption** is the job of the renal tubules and collecting ducts.

Glomerular filtration is not a selective process. Useful substances such as glucose, amino acids, and salts are present in the filtrate. Tubular reabsorption, however, is highly selective. Wastes, surplus salts, and excess water are retained as part of the filtrate, whereas glucose, amino acids, and other needed substances are reabsorbed into the blood.

A few substances are actively secreted from the blood into the renal tubules. **Tubular secretion** is important in regulating the potassium and hydrogen ion concentrations in the blood. Some toxic substances and certain drugs, such as penicillin, are removed from the body by tubular secretion.

### Composition of Urine

By the time the filtrate reaches the ureter, its composition has been precisely adjusted. Useful materials have been returned to the blood while wastes and excess materials have been cleaned, or cleared, from the blood. The adjusted filtrate, called **urine**, is composed of about 96% water, 2.5% nitrogenous wastes (mainly urea), 1.5% salts, and traces of other substances. Healthy urine is sterile; however, urine rapidly decomposes when exposed to bacterial action, forming ammonia and other products. It is the ammonia that causes diaper rash in infants.

### Regulation of Urine Volume

When you drink a large amount of water, a larger volume of urine is produced. Excess water absorbed from the digestive tract into the blood is removed by the kidneys. When you drink too little water, only a small volume of urine is produced. By regulating urine volume, the body maintains a steady volume and composition of blood.

The kidney receives information regarding the state of the blood by a somewhat indirect route (Fig. 18–6). When fluid intake is low, the body begins to dehydrate. When the volume of the blood decreases, the concentration of dissolved salts is greater, causing an increase in the osmotic pressure of the blood. Specialized receptors in the brain and in certain large blood vessels are sensitive to such change. The posterior lobe of the pituitary gland responds by releasing **antidiuretic hormone (ADH)**. This hormone serves as a chemical messenger carrying information from the brain to the distal convoluted tubules and collecting ducts of the kidneys. There it causes the walls of these ducts to become more permeable to water so that

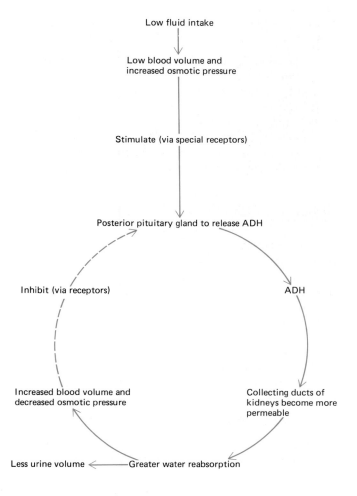

*Figure 18–6. Regulation of urine volume reflects the blood volume and osmotic pressure.*

much more water is reabsorbed into the blood. Blood volume increases and homeostasis of fluid volume is restored. Only a small amount of concentrated urine is produced.

On the other hand, when a great deal of fluid is consumed, the blood becomes diluted and its osmotic pressure falls. Release of ADH by the pituitary gland decreases, reducing the amount of water reabsorbed from the distal tubules and collecting ducts. This results in production of a large volume of dilute urine.

ADH regulates the excretion of water by the kidneys. Salt excretion is regulated by hormones, mainly aldosterone, secreted by the adrenal glands.

Certain chemicals, called **diuretics**, increase urine volume by inhibiting reabsorption of water. Coffee, tea, and alcoholic beverages all contain diuretics. Some diuretics inhibit secretion of ADH, whereas others act directly on the tubules in the kidneys.

## Overview of Kidney Function

The kidneys are vital in maintaining homeostasis. Their functions include the following:

1. Excretion of metabolic wastes such as water, urea, and uric acid.
2. Disposal of excess water and salts.
3. Regulation of pH of blood and body fluids. Acids and bases that are not needed are not reabsorbed and so become part of the urine. The tubules also secrete hydrogen ions when necessary to maintain an appropriate pH.

## URINE TRANSPORT AND STORAGE

Urine passes from the kidneys through the paired **ureters** (u-**ree**'-ters), ducts about 25 cm (10 inches) long, which conduct it to the urinary bladder. Urine is forced along through the ureter by peristaltic contractions.

The **urinary bladder** is a temporary storage sac for urine. Smooth muscle in its wall and a specialized epithelial lining permits the bladder to stretch so that it can hold up to 800 ml (about 1.5 pints) of urine.

When urine leaves the bladder, it flows through the **urethra**, a duct leading to the outside of the body. In the male the urethra is lengthy and passes through the prostate gland and the penis. Semen, as well as urine, is transported through the male urethra. In the female the urethra is short and transports only urine. Its opening to the outside is just above the opening into the vagina. Bladder infections are more common in females than in males because the length of the male urethra discourages bacterial invasion.

## URINATION

The process of emptying the bladder and expelling urine is referred to as **urination**, or **micturition** (mik-too-**rish**'-un). When the volume of urine in the bladder reaches about 300 ml, special nerve endings, called stretch receptors, in the bladder wall are stimulated. These receptors send neural messages to the spinal cord initiating a micturition reflex. This reflex contracts the bladder wall and also relaxes the internal urethral sphincter, a ring of smooth muscle at the upper end of the urethra. These actions stimulate a conscious desire to urinate. If the time and place are appropriate, the external urethral sphincter, located a short distance below the internal sphincter, is voluntarily relaxed, allowing urination to occur. Voluntary control of urination cannot be exerted by an immature nervous system, so most babies under the age of 2 automatically urinate every time the bladder fills.

## SUMMARY

I. The principal waste products are water, carbon dioxide, and nitrogenous wastes (urea, uric acid, creatinine).
II. The kidneys produce urine, which passes through the ureters to the urinary bladder for storage. During urination urine is discharged through the urethra to the outside of the body.
III. Each kidney consists of an outer renal cortex and an inner renal medulla.
   A. The renal medulla consists of pyramids. Collecting ducts open through the papilla of each pyramid and empty their contents into a minor calyx.
   B. The minor calyx opens into a major calyx, which empties into the renal pelvis.
IV. Each nephron consists of a renal corpuscle and a renal tubule.
   A. The renal corpuscle is composed of a glomerulus, which fits into a Bowman's capsule.
   B. The renal tubule consists of a proximal convoluted tubule, a loop of Henle, and a distal convoluted tubule.

V. Urine formation is accomplished by glomerular filtration, tubular reabsorption, and tubular secretion.
- A. Blood delivered to the glomerular capillaries by the afferent arteriole is under high pressure; some plasma containing dissolved substances is filtered out of the capillaries and into Bowman's capsule.
  1. A large volume of filtrate is produced.
  2. Glomerular filtration is not a selective process so useful materials, as well as wastes, become part of the filtrate.
- B. About 99% of the filtrate is returned to the blood by tubular reabsorption.
  1. Tubular reabsorption is accomplished by the renal tubules and collecting ducts.
  2. Tubular reabsorption is highly selective; wastes, excess water, and surplus salts are retained in the filtrate, whereas glucose, amino acids, and other needed substances are reabsorbed into the blood.
- C. Tubular secretion is important in regulating potassium and hydrogen ion concentration in the blood.

VI. The adjusted filtrate is called urine; it consists of water, nitrogenous wastes, salts, and traces of other substances.

VII. Urine volume is regulated by the hormone ADH released by the posterior lobe of the pituitary gland. ADH makes the distal convoluted tubules and collecting ducts more permeable to water.

VIII. The kidneys help maintain homeostasis by excreting metabolic wastes, ridding the body of excess water and salts, and helping to regulate pH.

IX. The micturition reflex occurs when the volume of urine in the bladder reaches about 300 ml; if the external urethral sphincter is relaxed, urination occurs.

## POST TEST

1. The process of disposing of metabolic wastes is called _____.
2. Urea is produced mainly in the _____, then transported to the _____ by the circulatory system.
3. Urine is conducted from the renal pelvis to the urinary bladder by the _____.
4. Urine in the major calyces next passes into the _____ _____.
5. A nephron consists of two main structures: the _____ _____ and the _____ _____.
6. The outer portion of the kidney is the _____ _____; the inner portion is the _____ _____.
7. The renal corpuscle consists of a tuft of capillaries, the _____, surrounded by _____ _____.
8. Blood flows into the glomerulus through an _____ arteriole.
9. From the proximal convoluted tubule filtrate flows into the _____ _____ _____.
10. In glomerular _____ plasma leaves the glomerular capillaries and passes into _____ _____.
11. The process of returning most of the filtrate to the blood is known as _____ _____.
12. The adjusted filtrate is called _____.
13. _____ hormone causes the walls of the collecting ducts to be more permeable.
14. The urinary _____ is a temporary storage sac for urine.
15. During micturition, urine is discharged through the _____.
16. Label the diagram on the following page.

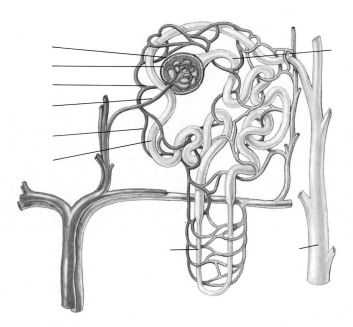

## REVIEW QUESTIONS

1. What is the difference between excretion and elimination? Give specific examples.
2. What are the principal metabolic waste products? What organs excrete them?
3. In what ways do the kidneys help maintain homeostasis?
4. Trace a drop of filtrate from the glomerular capillaries to the renal pelvis.
5. Trace a drop of urine from the renal pelvis to the urethra.
6. What are the main steps in urine production? Where does each occur?
7. If a large amount of protein is found in the urine what type of malfunction might you suspect?
8. The micturition reflex can be consciously facilitated or inhibited. What does this mean?

# 19

# Fluid and Electrolyte Balance

LEARNING OBJECTIVES

**After you study this chapter you should be able to**
1. Identify the fluid compartments of the body.
2. Summarize the principal routes for fluid input and fluid output.
3. Describe how fluid output is regulated.
4. Describe the mechanisms responsible for sodium and potassium homeostasis.
5. Describe dehydration, water intoxication, and edema and relate to fluid and electrolyte imbalance.

Whether you drink 1 l or 4 l water, whether you are on a salt-restricted diet or eat a bag of potato chips, the fluid and salt content of your body is maintained within homeostatic limits. To keep the quantities of these substances stable, the body has mechanisms that ensure that water and salt losses will be replaced and that excesses will be excreted. Normal body function, and even survival, depend on homeostasis of body fluids.

The term **body fluid** refers to the water in the body and the substances dissolved in it. Among the most important components of body fluid are **electrolytes** (e-**lek**′-troe-lites), compounds such as salts that form ions (electrically charged particles) in solution. Most organic compounds dissolved in the body fluid are nonelectrolytes, compounds that do not form ions. Examples of nonelectrolytes in the body fluid are glucose and urea.

## FLUID COMPARTMENTS

The human body is about 60% water by weight. Water and electrolytes are distributed in certain regions, or **compartments**. The two principal compartments are the **intracellular compartment** and the **extracellular compartment**.

About two-thirds of the body fluid is found in the intracellular compartment, that is, within cells (Fig. 19–1). This fluid is referred to as *intracellular fluid*. The remaining third, the *extracellular fluid*, is located outside the cells in the extracellular compartment. The extracellular fluid includes the **interstitial** (in″-tur-**stish**′-ul) **fluid**, also called **tissue fluid**, found in the tissue spaces between cells; the plasma and lymph; the cerebrospinal fluid; and other fluids in the body.

Fluid constantly moves from one compartment to another. However, in a healthy person the volume of fluid in each compartment remains about the same. The movement of fluid from one compartment to another depends on blood pressure and osmotic concentration. Recall that fluid leaves the plasma at the arteriole ends of capillaries and enters the tissues because of blood pressure. Excess tissue fluid returns to the blood at the venous ends of capillaries because of osmotic pressure. (Plasma proteins in the plasma exert a pulling force on fluid.) Excess tissue fluid is also returned to the blood by way of the lymphatic system. Fluid movement between the intracellular and extracellular compartments occurs mainly as a result of changes in osmotic pressure.

There are important differences in composition between the intracellular fluid and the extracellular fluid. For example, sodium ion concentration is much higher in the extracellular fluid than in the intracellular fluid. In contrast, potassium ion concentration is much higher within cells than in the extracellular fluid. To maintain these differences in ion distribution, cells must pump specific kinds of ions into or out of the cell. This is a form of cellular work known as *active transport*.

## FLUID INTAKE AND OUTPUT

Normally, fluid input equals fluid output so that the total amount of fluid in the body remains constant (Fig. 19–2). Fluid is ingested in the foods we eat and liquids we drink. Normally we ingest about 2500 ml each day. Fluid is absorbed from the digestive tract into the blood. Water is also produced during catabolic processes.

Most fluid (about 1500 ml/day) is discharged by the kidneys. Fluid is also lost through the skin, the lungs, and the digestive tract.

### Regulation of Fluid Intake

Fluid intake is regulated by the thirst mechanism (Fig. 19–3). Dehydration raises the osmotic

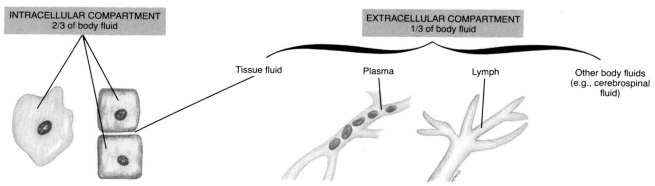

*Figure 19–1. Fluid compartments.*

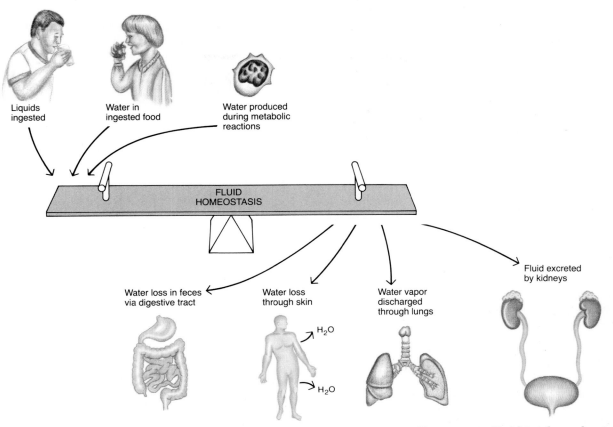

**Figure 19–2.** Fluid intake and output.

pressure of the blood (when there is less fluid, the blood is saltier). The increased osmotic pressure stimulates receptors in the thirst center of the hypothalamus. This results in the sensation of thirst and the desire to drink fluids. Dehydration also leads to a decrease in saliva secretion, which results in dryness in the mouth and throat. This dryness also signals thirst. The thirst mechanism is activated when total body fluid is decreased more than 1 to 2%.

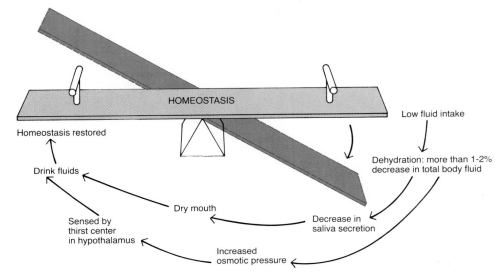

**Figure 19–3.** Regulation of fluid intake.

## Regulation of Fluid Output

The kidneys are primarily responsible for fluid output. This output is regulated by antidiuretic hormone (ADH). Recall from Chapter 18 that ADH, secreted by the posterior lobe of the pituitary gland, regulates the volume of urine. This hormone controls the permeability of the distal convoluted tubules and collecting ducts to water. When the body begins to get dehydrated, ADH secretion increases (Fig. 19–4). This occurs because, when the osmotic pressure of the plasma increases (plasma becomes saltier owing to fluid loss), special receptors in the hypothalamus signal the posterior pituitary to release more ADH. The ADH causes the distal tubules and collecting ducts to become more permeable to water. More water is reabsorbed into the blood and only a small volume of concentrated urine is excreted.

When blood volume increases, less ADH is secreted. Less water is reabsorbed, so that a large volume of dilute urine is excreted. In this way fluid homeostasis is restored.

## ELECTROLYTE BALANCE

Normally, a person obtains adequate amounts of electrolytes in the food and fluid ingested. When the amounts of the various electrolytes taken into the body equal the amounts lost, the body is in **electrolyte balance**. Because electrolytes are dissolved in the body fluid, electrolyte balance and fluid balance are interdependent. When the fluid content changes, the electrolytes become more concentrated or more diluted.

Electrolytes produce positively and negatively charged ions. Positively charged ions are referred to as **cations**; negatively charged ions are **anions**. Among the important cations in the body fluid are sodium, potassium, calcium, hydrogen, magnesium, and iron. Important anions include chloride and phosphate.

## Sodium

About 90% of the extracellular cations are sodium ions. Sodium is needed for the transmission of impulses in nervous and muscle tissue. A low sodium concentration can cause headache, mental confusion, rapid heart rate, low blood pressure, and even circulatory shock. Severe sodium depletion can result in coma.

Sodium concentration is controlled mainly by regulating the amount of water in the body (Fig. 19–5). When the sodium concentration is too high, the person feels thirsty and drinks water. In addition, secretion of ADH increases, causing increased reabsorption of water in the kidneys. The increased water dilutes the sodium in the extracellular fluid so that its concentration returns to normal. However, now blood volume has also increased.

When blood volume increases above normal, ar-

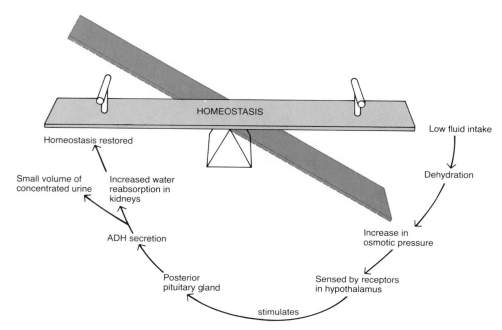

***Figure 19–4.*** *Regulation of fluid output.*

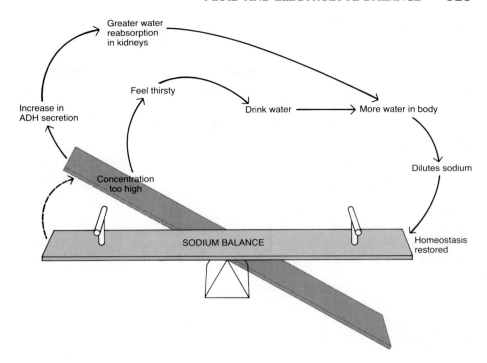

*Figure 19–5.* Sodium balance.

terial blood pressure begins to rise. This causes an increase in the rate of glomerular filtration and more fluid is excreted in the urine. The blood volume returns to normal.

Sodium concentration is also regulated to some extent by the hormone aldosterone secreted by the adrenal cortex. Aldosterone stimulates the distal convoluted tubules and collecting ducts to increase their reabsorption of sodium.

## Potassium

Most intracellular cations are potassium ions. These cations are important in nervous and muscle tissue function. Potassium ions are also important in maintaining the fluid volume within cells and they help to regulate pH. An abnormally low level of potassium may cause mental confusion, fatigue, and cramps and may affect the heart.

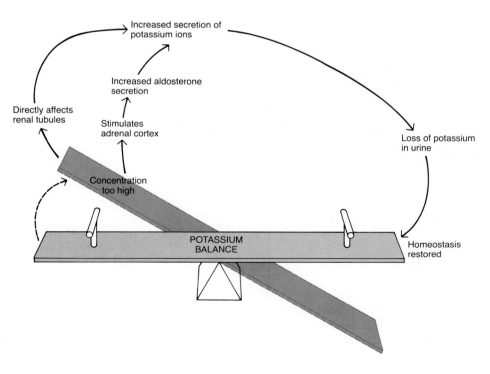

*Figure 19–6.* Potassium balance.

When the potassium concentration is too high nerve impulses are not effectively transmitted and the strength of muscle contraction decreases. In fact, a high potassium concentration can weaken the heart and lead to death from heart failure.

When the concentration of potassium ions is too high, potassium ions are secreted from the blood into the renal tubules, and the ions are excreted in the urine. This is due to a direct effect of the potassium ions on the tubules (Fig. 19–6). A high potassium ion concentration also stimulates the adrenal cortex to increase its output of aldosterone. The aldosterone further stimulates secretion of potassium. Loss of large numbers of potassium ions in the urine brings the potassium concentration in the body back to homeostatic levels. When the potassium concentration becomes too low, aldosterone secretion decreases and potassium secretion decreases almost to zero.

## FLUID AND ELECTROLYTE IMBALANCE

Deficiencies, excesses, or imbalance of fluids and electrolytes can cause serious health problems and even lead to coma and death.

**Dehydration** occurs when fluid output is greater than fluid input. Although dehydration can result from water deprivation or profuse sweating, it generally occurs as a complication of some disease state. Prolonged vomiting or diarrhea cause serious fluid loss. Dehydration can lead to fever, mental confusion, coma, and death. Infants and elderly adults are especially vulnerable to dehydration. This condition is treated by replacing needed water and electrolytes.

**Water intoxication** can occur when a person drinks fluids more rapidly than the kidneys can excrete the excess. It can also occur when a large amount of pure water (without electrolytes) is given to a dehydrated patient. The imbalance that results can lead to convulsions, coma, and death.

**Edema** (e-**dee′**-muh) is the accumulation of excessive tissue fluid. It can be caused by a decrease in concentration of plasma proteins, which lowers the osmotic pressure of the blood. Decreased plasma protein concentration can result from liver or kidney disease or from severe protein malnutrition. Edema can also be due to blockage in lymphatic vessels, increased capillary permeability, or increased venous pressure.

## SUMMARY

I. Body fluid is the water in the body and the substances dissolved in it.
II. Body fluid is distributed in the intracellular and extracellular compartments.

A. About two-thirds of body fluid is located in the intracellular compartment.
B. The remaining third is located in the extracellular compartment; this includes the tissue fluid, the plasma and lymph, and the cerebrospinal fluid.
C. Fluid continuously moves from one compartment to another but the volume in each compartment remains fairly constant.
D. There are differences in composition between the intracellular fluid and the extracellular fluid.
III. Normally, fluid input equals fluid output. We ingest about 2500 ml each day so about 2500 ml must be discharged from the body. Most fluid is excreted by the kidneys.
IV. When total body fluid is decreased by 1 to 2% the thirst mechanism is activated.
V. The kidneys are the organs mainly responsible for fluid output.
A. When the body begins to get dehydrated, the posterior pituitary increases its secretion of ADH. This hormone stimulates the distal tubules and collecting ducts in the kidneys to reabsorb more water; fluid is conserved for the body.
B. When excess fluid is present, ADH secretion decreases and less water is reabsorbed; a large volume of dilute urine is excreted.
VI. When the amounts of the various electrolytes taken into the body equal the amounts lost, the body is in electrolyte balance.
A. Sodium ions account for about 90% of the extracellular cations.
1. Sodium concentration is regulated mainly by adjusting the amount of water in the body.
2. Sodium concentration is regulated to some extent by aldosterone, which stimulates reabsorption of sodium.
B. Potassium ions account for most intracellular cations.
1. When the concentration of potassium ions rises above normal, potassium ions are secreted into the renal tubules and excreted in the urine.
2. A high potassium ion concentration also stimulates aldosterone secretion; aldosterone stimulates potassium secretion.
3. When the potassium concentration becomes too low, aldosterone secretion decreases and potassium is conserved.
VII. Dehydration, water intoxication, and edema are common fluid imbalances.

## POST TEST

1. Compounds such as salts that form ions in solution are called _____.
2. Most of the body fluid is located in the _____ compartment.
3. The movement of fluid from one compartment to another depends on blood _____ and _____ concentration.
4. Sodium ion concentration is much higher in the _____ fluid.
5. Fluid output is mainly the job of the _____.
6. When total body fluid is decreased more than 2% the _____ mechanism is activated.
7. Excretion of water by the kidneys is regulated by the hormone _____.
8. ADH causes the distal tubules and collecting ducts to reabsorb _____ (more, less) water; a _____ (small, large) volume of urine is excreted.
9. Aldosterone results in _____ (greater, less) reabsorption of sodium.
10. Aldosterone results in _____ (greater, less) reabsorption of potassium.
11. When fluid output is greater than fluid input _____ occurs.
12. The accumulation of excessive tissue fluid is called _____.

## REVIEW QUESTIONS

1. What is body fluid? What are electrolytes?
2. What are the main compartments in the body where fluid is located? Describe each.
3. What is meant by fluid balance? How are fluid and electrolyte balance related?
4. What are some differences in composition between intracellular and extracellular fluid? How are these differences maintained?
5. How is fluid intake regulated?
6. What is the role of ADH in regulating fluid output? Explain.
7. How is sodium concentration regulated?
8. How is potassium concentration regulated?
9. What are some of the causes of dehydration? What is water intoxication? What is edema?

# VII

## PERPETUATING THE SPECIES

# Reproduction

LEARNING OBJECTIVES

**After you study this chapter you should be able to**
1. Label a diagram of the male reproductive system and describe the functions of each structure.
2. Trace the passage of sperm from the seminiferous tubules through the conducting tubes, describing changes that may occur along the way.
3. Describe the composition of semen and give reasons for male sterility.
4. Describe the physiological bases for erection and ejaculation.
5. Describe the actions of the male gonadotropic hormones and of testosterone.
6. Label diagrams of internal and external female reproductive organs and describe their structures and functions.
7. Trace the development of an ovum and its passage through the female reproductive system.
8. Describe the principal events of the menstrual cycle and summarize the interactions of hormones that regulate the cycle.
9. Describe the physiological changes taking place during sexual response; compare male and female responses.
10. Describe the process of fertilization and identify the time of the menstrual cycle at which

sexual intercourse is most likely to result in pregnancy.

11. Describe the common methods of birth control and give advantages and disadvantages of each.

12. Describe methods of inducing abortion and discuss the safety of abortion.

---

Reproductive processes include formation of **gametes** (eggs and sperm), physiological preparation for pregnancy, sexual intercourse, **fertilization** (union of sperm and egg), pregnancy, and **lactation** (producing milk for nourishment of the infant). These events are exquisitely orchestrated by the interaction of hormones secreted by the anterior pituitary gland and the **gonads** (sex glands).

## THE MALE

The reproductive responsibility of the male is to produce sperm cells and to deliver them into the female reproductive tract. A sperm contributes half the genetic endowment of the offspring and determines its sex. Male reproductive structures include the testes and scrotum, conducting tubes that lead from the testes to the outside of the body, accessory glands, and the penis (Fig. 20–1).

## The Testes—Production of Sperm

In the adult male millions of sperm cells are manufactured each day within the paired male gonads, the **testes** (tes'-teez). Each **testis** (tes'-tis) is a small oval organ about 4 to 5 cm (1.6 to 2 inches) long and 2.5 cm (about 1 inch) wide and thick. Each testis is filled with about 1000 threadlike, coiled **seminiferous** (sem"-i-**nif**'-ur-us) **tubules**, the sperm cell factories (Fig. 20–2). In an adult male these structures produce millions of sperm cells each day.

Perhaps the smallest cell in the body, the mature sperm is highly specialized. The sperm is an elongated cell with a tail that propels it and enables it to move toward an egg.

The testes develop in the abdominal cavity of the male embryo, but about 2 months before birth they descend into the **scrotum** (skrow'-tum), a skin-covered bag suspended from the groin. As the

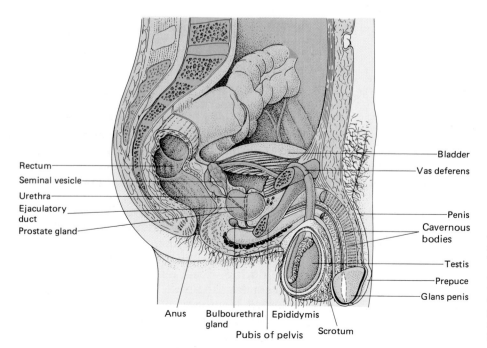

*Figure 20–1.* Anatomy of the human male reproductive system. The scrotum, penis, and pelvic region have been cut sagittally to show their internal structures. Identify the accessory glands and try to trace the conducting tubes from the testis to the urethra.

Labels on figure:
Rectum
Seminal vesicle
Urethra
Ejaculatory duct
Prostate gland
Bladder
Vas deferens
Penis
Cavernous bodies
Testis
Prepuce
Glans penis
Anus
Bulbourethral gland
Pubis of pelvis
Epididymis
Scrotum

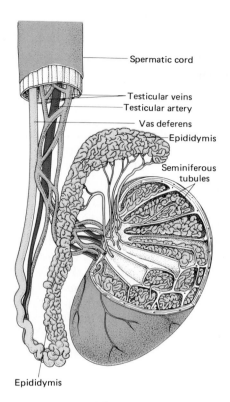

Spermatic cord

Testicular veins
Testicular artery
Vas deferens
Epididymis
Seminiferous tubules

Epididymis

**Figure 20–2.** *Structure of the testis and epididymis. The testis is shown in sagittal section to illustrate the arrangement of the seminiferous tubules.*

testes descend, they move through the **inguinal canals**, the passageways connecting the scrotal and abdominal cavities. The testes pull their arteries, veins, nerves, and conducting tubes after them. These structures, surrounded by the cremaster muscle and by layers of connective tissue make up the **spermatic cord**.

> The inguinal region remains a weak place in the abdominal wall and therefore a common site of hernia in the male. Straining the abdominal muscles by lifting a heavy object may result in a tear through which a loop of intestine can bulge into the scrotum; this is called an **inguinal hernia**.

Sperm cells are not able to develop at body temperature and the scrotum serves as a cooling unit, maintaining them at about 2°C below body temperature. An abundance of both sweat glands and blood vessels in the wall of the scrotum promotes heat loss and so helps maintain the cool temperature. In hot weather involuntary muscles in the scrotal wall relax, positioning the testes away from the body so that the sperm remain cool. In cold weather these muscles contract, drawing the testes up close to the abdominal wall, where they are kept warm.

> If the testes fail to descend into the scrotum, viable sperm cells are not produced. This condition termed **cryptorchidism** (krip-**tor**′-ki-dizm), meaning "hidden testes," can be corrected by hormone therapy, which stimulates descent, or by surgery before age 5. If cryptorchidism is not treated, the seminiferous tubules eventually degenerate and the male becomes **sterile**, that is, unable to father offspring. Masculinity is not affected, however, because secretion of male hormone is not affected by body temperature.

## The Conducting Tubes— Sperm Transport

From the seminiferous tubules sperm pass through a network of small tubules and into a large tube, the epididymis (Fig. 20–2). The **epididymis** (ep″-ih-**did**′-ih-mis) of each testis is a highly coiled tube in which sperm complete their maturation and are stored. The epididymis empties into a straight tube, the **vas deferens**, or sperm duct. The vas deferens passes from the scrotum through the inguinal canal as part of the spermatic cord. After entering the pelvic cavity, the vas deferens loops over the side and then down the posterior surface of the urinary bladder.

The vas deferens is joined by the duct from the seminal vesicles (see below) to become the **ejaculatory duct**. This short duct passes through the prostate gland (see below) and then opens into the urethra. The single **urethra** (which conducts both urine and semen) passes through the penis to the outside of the body.

## The Accessory Glands— Semen Production

**Semen** (**see**′-mun) is a thick, whitish fluid consisting of sperm cells suspended in secretions of the accessory glands. The paired **seminal vesicles** are saclike glands. A seminal vesicle empties into each vas deferens. The mucuslike fluid secreted by the seminal vesicles contains the sugar fructose plus other nutrients that nourish and provide fuel for the sperm cells. Secretions of the seminal vesicles account for about 60% of the semen volume.

The single **prostate** (**pros**′-tate) **gland** surrounds the urethra as the urethra emerges from the bladder. It contributes about 20% of the semen volume, producing a thick, milky, alkaline secretion that is important in neutralizing the mild acidity of the other fluids contributed to the semen. This change in pH activates the sperm cells.

In older men the prostate gland often enlarges and exerts pressure on the urethra, making urination difficult. When necessary, a portion or all of the prostate can be removed surgically, often with no adverse effect on sexual performance. Cancer of the prostate is a common disorder in men over 50.

The **bulbourethral** (bul″-bow-yoo-**ree′**-thrul) **glands** (also called **Cowper's glands**) are about the size and shape of two peas, one on each side of the urethra, into which they secrete. With sexual arousal they release a few drops of clear, alkaline fluid, which neutralizes the acidity of the urethra in preparation for ejaculation and also lubricates the urethra and penis.

About 3 ml of semen, on the average, is ejaculated during sexual orgasm. Semen consists of about 300 million sperm cells (about 100 million per ml) suspended in the secretions of the accessory glands. Sperm cells are so tiny that they account for little (less than 1%) of the semen volume.

Men with fewer than 20 million sperm per milliliter of semen usually are sterile. When a couple's attempts to produce a child are unsuccessful, sperm counts and analyses may be undertaken in clinical laboratories. Sometimes semen is found to contain large numbers of abnormal sperm or, occasionally, no sperm at all. Fever or infection of the testes may cause temporary sterility. In about one-fourth of mumps cases in adult males the testes become inflamed and in some of these cases the immature sperm deteriorate, resulting in sterility.

## The Penis

The **penis** is an erectile copulatory organ designed to deliver sperm into the female reproductive tract during sexual intercourse. It consists of a long **shaft** that enlarges to form an expanded tip, the **glans** (Fig. 20–1). Part of the loose-fitting skin of the penis folds down and covers the proximal portion of the glans, forming a cuff called the **prepuce** (**pree′**-pyous), or **foreskin**. This cuff of skin is removed during **circumcision**.

Under the skin the penis consists of three cylinders of erectile tissue known as the cavernous bodies (corpora cavernosa). One of these columns of erectile tissue surrounds the portion of the urethra that passes through the penis. The erectile tissue of these cylinders consists of large blood vessels called venous sinusoids.

When the male is sexually stimulated, nerve impulses signal the arteries of the penis to dilate. Blood rushes into the sinusoids of the erectile tissue. As this tissue fills with blood, it swells, com-

pressing veins that conduct blood away from the penis. As a result more blood enters the penis than can leave and the erectile tissue becomes engorged with blood. The penis becomes **erect**, that is, longer, larger in circumference, and firm. The average penis is about 9 cm long when flaccid (relaxed) and 16 to 19 cm when erect.

When the level of sexual excitement reaches a peak, ejaculation occurs. *Ejaculation* is the discharge of semen from the penis. Like erection, ejaculation is a reflex action.

## Male Hormones

Between the seminiferous tubules in the testes are small islands of **interstitial cells**, which produce the male hormone **testosterone** (tes-**tos′**-tur-own). Before birth testosterone stimulates the development of the male genital structures. **Puberty** (**pew′**-bur-tee), the period of sexual maturation, begins at about age 12 or 13 years in the male. At puberty the hypothalamus begins to secrete releasing hormones that stimulate the anterior lobe of the pituitary gland to secrete gonadotropic hormones. These hormones are follicle-stimulating hormone (FSH) and luteinizing hormone (LH). FSH stimulates development of the testes and promotes sperm production. LH stimulates the interstitial cells in the testes to secrete testosterone.

An important action of testosterone is to promote body growth. When large quantities of this hormone circulate in the blood during puberty, the adolescent growth spurt occurs. Testosterone is responsible for the development of both primary and secondary sexual characteristics in the male. Primary characteristics include the growth of the penis and scrotum and the growth and activity of internal reproductive structures. Secondary characteristics include deepening of the voice, muscle development, and growth of pubic, facial, and underarm hair. Testosterone also stimulates the oil glands in the skin, predisposing the adolescent to acne.

What if testosterone is absent? When a male is **castrated** (that is, his testes are removed) before puberty, he becomes a **eunuch**. His sex organs remain childlike and he does not develop secondary sexual characteristics. If castration occurs after puberty, increased secretion of male hormone by the adrenal cortex helps to maintain masculinity.

## THE FEMALE

The female reproductive system is designed to produce **ova** (eggs), to receive the penis and the sperm released from it during sexual intercourse, to house and nourish the embryo during its prenatal development, and to nourish the infant. Because it must perform all these diverse functions, the physiology of the female reproductive system is more complex than that of the male. Much of its activity centers about the **menstrual cycle**, the monthly preparation for possible pregnancy.

Principal organs of the female reproductive system (Figs. 20–3 and 20–4) are the ovaries (which produce ova and female hormones), the uterine tubes (where fertilization takes place), the uterus (incubator for the developing child), the vagina (which receives the penis and serves as a birth canal), the vulva (external genital structures), and the breasts.

## The Ovaries—Production of Ova and Hormones

The paired **ovaries**, the female gonads, produce ova and the female sex hormones, **estrogen** (**es'**-trow-jin) and **progesterone** (pro-**jes'**-ter-own). About the size and shape of large almonds, the ovaries are located close to the lateral walls of the pelvic cavity (Fig. 20–3). The ovaries are held in position by several connective tissue ligaments. The **ovarian ligament**, for example, anchors the medial end of the ovary to the uterus.

Each ovary is covered with a single layer of epithelium. Internally it consists mainly of connective tissue, called stroma, through which ova (eggs) in various stages of maturation are scattered. Together the ovum and the cluster of cells that surrounds it make up a **follicle**.

With the onset of puberty a few follicles develop each month in response to FSH secreted by the anterior lobe of the pituitary gland. Cells of the follicle secrete estrogen. As a follicle matures it moves close to the wall of the ovary and looks like a fluid-filled blister on the ovarian surface. Mature follicles are called **graafian follicles**. Normally, only one follicle matures each month. Several others may develop for about a week and then deteriorate.

In response to FSH and LH from the anterior pituitary gland, the mature follicle ruptures after about 2 weeks of development. During this process, called **ovulation**, the ovum is ejected through the wall of the ovary and into the pelvic cavity. The part of the follicle that remains behind in the ovary develops into an important endocrine structure, the **corpus luteum** ("yellow body"). LH stimulates the development of the corpus luteum. This temporary endocrine structure secretes progesterone and estrogen, female hormones needed to stimulate the uterus to prepare for possible pregnancy.

## The Uterine Tubes—Ovum Transport

At ovulation the mature ovum is released into the pelvic cavity. The free end of the **uterine tube** (also called the **fallopian tube**) is strategically located and designed so that the ovum enters it almost immediately (Fig. 20–4).

Each uterine tube is about 12 cm long. Its free end is shaped like a funnel and has long, fingerlike projections called **fimbriae**. Movements of the

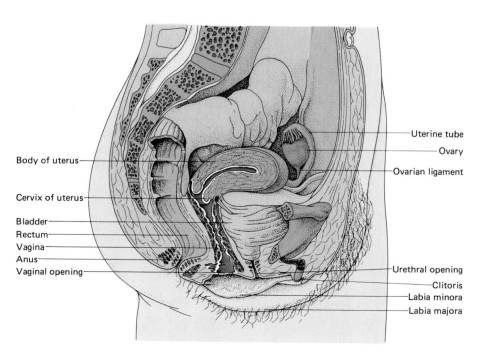

*Figure 20–3. Midsagittal section of female pelvis showing reproductive organs. Note the position of the uterus relative to the vagina.*

Body of uterus

Cervix of uterus

Bladder
Rectum
Vagina
Anus
Vaginal opening

Uterine tube
Ovary
Ovarian ligament

Urethral opening
Clitoris
Labia minora
Labia majora

fimbriae and the current created by the beating of cilia in the lining of the tube help to draw the ovum into the uterine tube. Peristaltic contractions of the muscular wall, as well as the action of the cilia, help to move the ovum toward the uterus. The ovum is not capable of independent locomotion.

Fertilization takes place in the upper third of the uterine tube and the **zygote** (**zye'**-goat) (fertilized egg) begins its development as it is moved toward the uterus. If fertilization does not occur, the ovum degenerates in the uterine tube.

Because the uterine tubes open into the peritoneal cavity, microorganisms that enter through the vagina can cause serious clinical problems. This route of infection has led to many deaths from abortions performed under nonsterile conditions and may also be involved in the spread of some sexually transmitted infections, especially gonorrhea.

Inflammation of the uterine tubes (**salpingitis**) is often caused by gonorrheal infection. Scarring that sometimes occurs may partially constrict the tube, resulting in sterility because passage of the ovum is blocked. Sometimes partial tubal constriction results in **tubal pregnancy**, in which the embryo begins to develop in the wall of the uterine tube because it cannot pass through to the uterus. Such pregnancies must be diagnosed early so that the tube can be surgically removed before it ruptures, endangering the life of the mother. Uterine tubes are not adapted to bear the burden of a developing embryo. Tubal pregnancies are the most common type of **ectopic pregnancy**, a pregnancy in which the embryo begins to develop outside the uterus.

## The Uterus—Incubating the Embryo

Each month during a woman's reproductive life, the **uterus**, or womb, prepares for possible pregnancy. Should pregnancy occur, the uterus serves as the incubator for the developing embryo. The tiny embryo actually implants itself in the wall of the uterus and develops there as a parasite until it is able to live independently. When that time comes, the uterine wall contracts powerfully and rhythmically (the process of **labor**), expelling the new baby from the mother's body. Each month, if pregnancy does not occur, the inner lining of the uterus sloughs off and is discarded. This process is called **menstruation** (men"-stroo-**ay'**-shun).

The uterus is a single hollow organ shaped somewhat like a pear. In the nonpregnant condition it is about the size of a small fist—about 7.5 cm (3 inches) in length and 5 cm (2 inches) in width at its widest region. The uterus lies in the

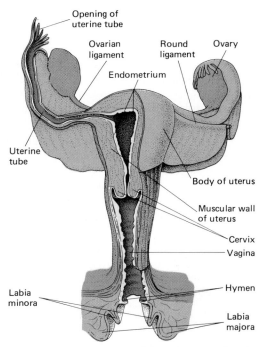

**Figure 20—4.** *Anterior view of female reproductive system. Some organs have been cut open to expose the internal structure. The ligaments are solid cords of tissue that help to hold the reproductive organs in place.*

bottom of the pelvic cavity, anterior to the rectum and posterior to the urinary bladder.

The main portion of the uterus is its **corpus**, or **body**. Above the level of the entrance of the uterine tubes, the rounded portion of the uterus is the **fundus**. The lower narrow portion is the **cervix** (**sur'**-viks). Part of the cervix projects into the vagina.

Lining the uterus is a mucous membrane, the **endometrium** (en-doe-**mee'**-tree-um). Just as the ovary develops a new ovum each month, the uterus is also cyclic in its activity. Each month, in response to estrogen and progesterone from the ovary, the endometrium prepares for possible pregnancy. Its functional layer becomes thick and vascular and develops glands that secrete a nutritive fluid. If pregnancy does not occur, part of the endometrium sloughs off during menstruation. Beneath the endometrium the wall of the uterus consists of a thick layer of muscle.

*Cancer of the cervix* is one of the most common types of cancer in women, accounting for about 13,000 deaths per year in the United States alone. About 50% of cases of cervical cancer are now detected at early stages when cures are most likely. Detection is aided by the routine Papanicolaou test (Pap smear), in which a few cells are scraped from the cervix during a routine gynecological examination and studied microscopically.

## The Vagina

The **vagina** (va-**jie'**-nuh) functions as the sexual organ that receives the penis during sexual intercourse. It also serves as an exit through which the discarded endometrium is discharged during menstruation and as the lower part of the birth canal.

Located anterior to the rectum and posterior to the urethra and urinary bladder, the vagina is an elastic, muscular tube capable of considerable distension. It extends from the cervix to its orifice (opening) to the outside of the body. The vagina surrounds the end of the cervix; the recesses formed between the vaginal wall and cervix are called **fornices** (**for'**-ne-seez).

The vagina is normally collapsed so that its walls touch each other, and the lumen appears in cross section as no more than a slit. Two longitudinal ridges run along anterior and posterior walls and there are numerous **rugae** (folds). During intercourse when the penis is inserted into the vagina or during childbirth when the baby's head emerges into the vagina, the rugae straighten out, greatly enlarging the vagina.

A thin ring of mucous membrane, the **hymen**, partially blocks the entrance to the vagina. Through the ages the hymen has been heralded as the symbol of virginity because it is often ruptured during the woman's first coitus (sexual intercourse). All the attention focused on the hymen is not merited, however, because it is not necessarily a reliable indicator of virginity. In some women the hymen is elastic and may persist despite coitus. And in many cases it ruptures during strenuous physical exercise in childhood or as a result of inserting tampons to absorb the menstrual flow.

## The Vulva—External Genital Structures

The term **vulva** (**vul'**-vah), refers to the external female genital structures. They include the mons pubis, labia majora, labia minora, clitoris, and vestibule of the vagina (Fig. 20–5). The **mons pubis** is a mound of fatty tissue that covers the pubic symphysis. At puberty it becomes covered by coarse pubic hair.

The paired **labia** (**lay'**-be-ah) **majora** (meaning "large lips") are folds of skin that pass from the mons pubis to the region behind the vaginal opening. Normally the labia majora meet in the midline, providing protection for the genital structures beneath. After puberty the outer epidermis of the lips is pigmented and covered with coarse hair. Sensory receptors are abundant. Two thin folds of

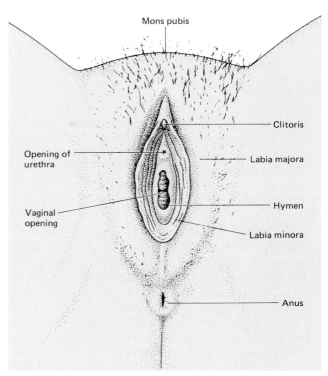

***Figure 20–5.*** *The vulva, the external female genital structures.*

skin, the **labia minora** (meaning "small lips"), are located just within the labia majora. Anteriorly they merge to form the prepuce of the clitoris.

The **clitoris** (**klit'**-o-ris) is a small body of erectile tissue, which corresponds to the male glans penis. It projects from the anterior end of the vulva at the anterior junction of the labia minora. Although it is about 2 cm long and 0.5 cm in diameter, most of the clitoris is not visible because it is embedded in the tissues of the vulva. The clitoris is a main focus of sexual sensation in the female.

The space enclosed by the labia minora is the **vestibule**. Two openings are apparent in the vestibule, the opening of the urethra anteriorly and the opening of the vagina posteriorly.

Two small **Bartholin's glands** (**greater vestibular glands**), which secrete mucus, open on each side of the vaginal orifice. A group of smaller glands (lesser vestibular) open into the vestibule near the urethral orifice and also secrete mucus. The vestibular glands help to lubricate the tissues during sexual intercourse. These glands are vulnerable to infection, especially from the bacteria that cause gonorrhea.

Two elongated masses of erectile tissue, the **bulbs of the vestibule**, are located beneath the surface on each side of the vaginal opening. In both male and female the diamond-shaped region between the pubic arch and the anus is the **peri-**

**neum**. In the female the region between the vagina and anus is referred to as the **clinical perineum**.

## The Breasts

The breasts, containing the **mammary glands**, overlie the pectoral muscles and are attached to them by connective tissue. Fibrous bands of tissue called **ligaments of Cooper** firmly connect the breasts to the skin. The function of the breasts is **lactation**, production of milk for the nourishment of the young.

Each breast is composed of 15 to 20 lobes of glandular tissue. A duct drains milk from each lobe and opens onto the surface of the nipple. Thus, there are 15 to 20 openings on the surface of each nipple (Fig. 20–6). (Some types of baby bottle nipples emulate this natural arrangement by having many small openings in the nipple rather than a single one, as in old-fashioned bottle nipples.)

The amount of adipose tissue around the lobes of the glandular tissue determines the size of the breasts and accounts for their soft consistency. The size of the breasts does not affect their capacity to produce milk.

The nipple consists of smooth muscle that can contract to make the nipple erect in response to sexual or certain other stimuli. In the pinkish **areola** surrounding the nipple several rudimentary milk glands (the areolar glands) may be found.

In childhood the breasts contain only rudimentary glands. At puberty, estrogen and progesterone (in the presence of growth hormone and prolactin) stimulate development of the glands and ducts and the deposition of fatty tissue characteristic of the adult breast.

### Lactation

During pregnancy high concentrations of estrogen and progesterone produced by the corpus luteum and by the placenta (the organ of exchange between mother and developing baby) stimulate the glands and ducts to develop, resulting in increased breast size. For the first few days after childbirth the mammary glands produce a fluid called **colostrum**, which contains protein and lactose but little fat. After birth, prolactin secreted by the anterior pituitary stimulates milk production, and by the third day after delivery, milk itself is produced.

When the infant suckles at the breast, a reflex action results in release of prolactin and oxytocin from the pituitary gland. Oxytocin permits actual release of milk from the glands and from the breasts.

> Breast-feeding a baby offers many advantages, including promoting a close bond between the mother and child. Breast milk is tailored to the nutritional needs of a human infant, whereas cow's milk is more likely to produce allergies to dairy products. Furthermore, breast-fed babies receive antibodies from the colostrum and from breast milk that are thought to play a protective role, resulting in a lower incidence of infantile diarrhea and of respiratory infection during the second 6 months of life. Breast-feeding also helps the uterus to recover from childbirth because oxytocin stimulates it to contract to nonpregnant size.

### Breast Cancer

The breasts are the most common site of cancer in women. Incidence has increased in recent years and **breast cancer** now strikes 1 in every 13 women and is the leading cause of cancer deaths in women.

About 50% of breast cancers begin in the upper outer quadrant of the breast. As a malignant tumor grows it may adhere to the deep connective tissue of the chest wall. Sometimes it extends to the skin, causing dimpling. Eventually the cancer spreads to the lymphatic system, often to the axillary nodes or the nodes along the internal mammary artery. About two-thirds of breast cancers have metastasized (that is, spread) to the lymph nodes by the time the cancer is first diagnosed.

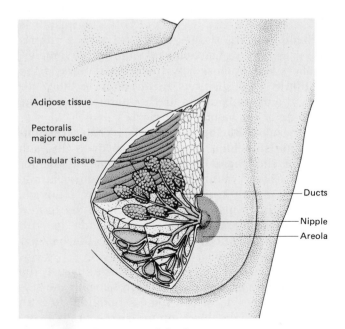

**Figure 20–6.** *Structure of the breast.*

Mastectomy (surgical removal of the breast) and radiation treatment are the most common methods of treating breast cancer. When diagnosis and treatment begin early, 80% of patients survive for 5 years and 62% for 10 years or longer. Untreated patients have only a 20% 5-year survival rate.

Because early detection of these cancers greatly increases the chances of cure and survival, campaigns have been launched to educate women on the importance of self-examination. **Xeromammography**, a soft-tissue radiological study of the breast, is a technique helpful in detecting small lesions that might not be identified by palpation (Fig. 20–7).

## Actions of Estrogen and Progesterone

Like testosterone in the male, **estrogen** (es'-tro-jen) is responsible for the growth of sex organs at puberty and for the development of secondary sex characteristics—initiation of breast development, broadening of the pelvis, and characteristic distribution of fat and muscle. During the menstrual cycle estrogen enhances the growth of follicles, stimulates growth of the endometrium, increases peristaltic movements of the uterine tubes, and makes the cervical mucus thinner and more alkaline, changes that are more favorable to sperm survival.

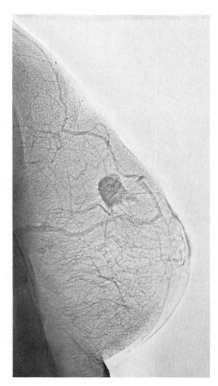

**Figure 20–7.** Xeromammogram showing cancer of the breast.

**Progesterone** (pro-jes'-ter-own) is a steroid secreted by the corpus luteum and by the placenta during pregnancy. One of its most important actions is to stimulate the endometrium to complete its preparation for pregnancy. Under its influence, glands of the endometrium secrete glycogen, which serves as nourishment for the early embryo.

## The Menstrual Cycle

As a female approaches puberty the anterior pituitary gland secretes the gonadotropic hormones FSH and LH, which signal the ovaries to begin functioning. Interaction of FSH and LH with estrogen and progesterone from the ovaries regulates the menstrual cycle, which runs its course every month from puberty until menopause, the end of a woman's reproductive life. The menstrual cycle stimulates production of an ovum each month and prepares the uterus for pregnancy.

Although there is wide variation, a "typical" menstrual cycle is 28 days long. The first day of menstruation marks the first day of the cycle. Ovulation occurs about 14 days before the next cycle begins; in a 28-day cycle this would correspond to about the fourteenth day (Fig. 20–8).

During menstruation, which lasts for about the first 5 days of the menstrual cycle, the thickened endometrium of the uterus sloughs off. Total blood loss is about 35 ml (1 fluid ounce), but an additional 35 ml of fluids from the uterine glands is also discharged. During this phase of the menstrual cycle FSH is the principal hormone released by the pituitary gland. It stimulates a group of follicles to develop in the ovary.

During the **preovulatory phase** of the menstrual cycle, estrogen released from the theca of the developing follicles in the ovary stimulates the growth of the endometrium once again. Its blood vessels and glands begin to develop anew. At midcycle an increase in estrogen secretion from the follicles is followed by release of LH from the anterior pituitary. LH is necessary for final maturation of the follicle, for ovulation, and later for development of the corpus luteum.

After ovulation the **postovulatory phase** begins. The corpus luteum releases progesterone, as well as estrogen, and these hormones stimulate continued thickening of the endometrium. Progesterone especially affects the small glands in the endometrium, stimulating them to secrete a fluid rich in nutrients. Should fertilization occur, this nutritive fluid nourishes the early embryo when it arrives in the uterus on about the fourth day of development.

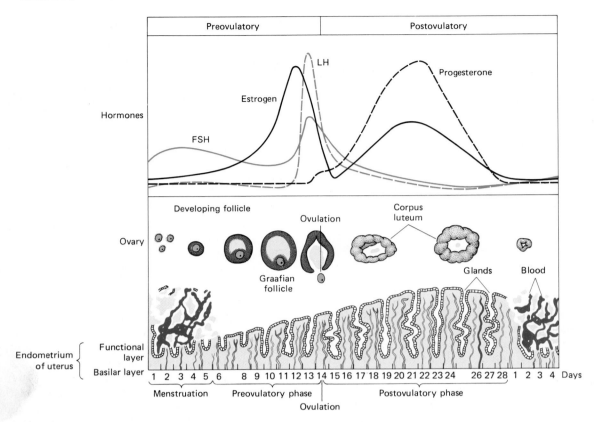

**Figure 20—8.** *The menstrual cycle. The events that take place within the pituitary, ovary, and uterus are precisely synchronized. When fertilization does not occur, the cycle repeats itself about every 28 days.*

On about the seventh day after fertilization the embryo begins to implant itself in the thick endometrium of the uterus. The placenta begins to develop and secretes a hormone called **human chorionic gonadotropin (HCG)**, which signals the corpus luteum to continue to function.

If pregnancy does not occur, the corpus luteum begins to degenerate and progesterone and estrogen levels in the blood fall markedly. Spiral arteries in the uterine wall constrict and the part of the endometrium they supply becomes ischemic (oxygen-deprived). Menstruation begins once again as cells begin to die and damaged arteries rupture and bleed.

## Menopause

At about age 48 to 52 years **menopause** begins. The ovaries become less responsive to gonadotropic hormones and the amount of estrogen and progesterone secreted diminishes. Perhaps there are not enough follicles left to develop and secrete hormones. The ovaries then begin to degenerate and the menstrual cycle becomes irregular and eventually halts. A sensation of heat ("hot flashes") sometimes occurs, probably because of the effect of decreased estrogen on the temperature-regulating center in the hypothalamus. Estrogen deficiency may also contribute to headaches and to feelings of depression experienced by some women. The vaginal lining thins and the breasts and vulva begin to atrophy.

Despite these physical changes, menopause does not usually affect a woman's interest in sex or her sexual performance. Although replacing missing hormones has been used to alleviate many of the symptoms of menopause, this is no longer widely practiced, as continued use of estrogen has been linked to increased risk of cancer.

## PHYSIOLOGY OF SEXUAL RESPONSE

Two basic physiological responses to sexual stimulation are **vasocongestion** and **myotonia** (increase in muscle tension). Vasocongestion occurs as blood flow is increased to the genital structures and to certain other tissues such as the breasts, skin, and earlobes. These structures become engorged with blood and the penis and clitoris become erect.

In describing physiological changes, it is helpful to divide sexual response into four phases—excitement, plateau, orgasm, and resolution. To function in sexual intercourse, or **coitus**, the penis must be erect. During the **excitement phase** physiological or physical stimulation, usually both, provides the needed arousal. In the female, vaginal lubrication is the first response to effective sexual stimulation. The wall of the vagina lacks glands; the fluid produced is a product of the vasocongestion that occurs in the vaginal walls. During the excitement phase the vagina lengthens and expands in preparation for receiving the penis. The clitoris and breasts become vasocongested, and the nipples become erect. In both sexes the heart rate increases and blood pressure is elevated.

If the erotic stimuli continue, sexual excitement heightens to the **plateau phase**. During this phase excitement intensifies and sexual climax is approached. During coitus the penis is moved back and forth in the vagina by movements known as pelvic thrusts. Physical and psychological sensations resulting from this friction and from the intimacy experienced lead to **orgasm**, the climax of sexual excitement.

Though lasting only a few seconds, orgasm is the achievement of maximum sexual tension and its release. In the male, orgasm is marked by ejaculation of the semen. Contraction of the vas deferens propels sperm into the ejaculatory duct, while the accessory glands contract, adding their secretions. Contractions of the ejaculatory ducts, muscles in the pelvic floor, and urethra eject the semen from the penis. After ejaculation the urethra, ducts, accessory glands, and muscles surrounding the root of the penis continue to contract at 0.8-second intervals. After the first several contractions their intensity decreases and they become less regular and less frequent. In both sexes heart rate and respiration more than double and blood pressure rises to a peak.

Stimulation of the clitoris is important in heightening the sexual excitement that leads to orgasm in the female. Orgasm is marked by rhythmical contractions of the pelvic muscles and vagina starting at 0.8-second intervals and recurring 5 to 12 times. (One of the muscles involved is the pubococcygeus muscle, which controls flow of urine as well as constriction of the vagina.) After the first three to six contractions the intensity of the contractions decreases and the time interval between them increases. Orgasm in the female is not accompanied by fluid ejaculation. In the **resolution phase**, the body is restored to its normal state.

Erection of the penis is necessary for effective coitus. Chronic inability to sustain an erection is referred to as **erectile dysfunction**. Although almost all men experience erectile dysfunction, when chronic this condition is often associated with psychological issues. Erectile dysfunction should not be confused with sterility, although both may result in failure to produce offspring.

## FERTILIZATION

During coitus sperm are released in the vicinity of the cervix, but during most of the menstrual cycle the female reproductive tract is a hostile environment for sperm. The acidic nature of the vagina is **spermicidal** (meaning that it kills sperm) and a thick plug of mucus blocks the cervix. As the time of ovulation approaches, however, this situation begins to change. The vagina becomes slightly alkaline and the cervical mucus thins, permitting sperm to pass into the uterus.

Only one sperm **fertilizes** the ovum, yet millions are required. Apparently many die or lose their way, because only about 2000 succeed in reaching the "correct" upper uterine tube; many probably traverse the "wrong" tube. (Remember that only one ovum is released each month, and it moves into the uterine tube nearest the ovary that produced it.) It is thought that large numbers of sperm are also necessary to penetrate the follicle cells surrounding the ovum. As soon as one sperm penetrates the ovum, no other sperm is able to get through.

After ejaculation sperm remain viable for about 48 hours. The ovum remains fertile for about 24 hours after ovulation. Thus there are only about 3 days each menstrual cycle (perhaps days 12 to 15 in a regular cycle) when sexual intercourse is likely to result in fertilization.

## BIRTH CONTROL

Any method for deliberately separating sexual intercourse from the production of a baby may be considered a form of **birth control**. **Contraception** (literally "against conception") is specifically the prevention of conception. When a sexually active woman uses no form of birth control, her chances of becoming pregnant during the course of a year are about 90%. Highly effective contraceptive methods are now available (Table 20–1) but all have side effects, inconveniences, or other disadvantages. A completely ideal contraceptive has not yet been developed.

Table 20–1
**Contraceptive Methods**

| Method | Failure Rate[1] (%) | Mode of Action | Advantages | Disadvantages |
|---|---|---|---|---|
| Oral contraceptives | 0.3; 5 | Prevent ovulation; may also affect endometrium and cervical mucus and prevent implantation | Highly effective; sexual freedom; regular menstrual cycle | Minor discomfort in some women; possible thromboembolism; hypertension, heart disease in some users |
| Intrauterine device (IUD) | 1; 5 | Unknown; probably sets up minor inflammation, which leads to destruction of sperm and/or prevention of implantation | Provides continuous protection; highly effective | Cramps; increased menstrual flow; spontaneous expulsion; pelvic inflammatory disease and possible resultant infertility; because of these possible side effects IUDs are being prescribed less frequently |
| Spermicides (foams, jellies, creams, sponges) | 3; 22 | Chemically kill sperm | No known side effects; vaginal sponges are effective in vagina for up to 24 hours after insertion | Unreliable; recent epidemiological evidence suggests that when used at or around the time of conception, spermicides may cause birth defects (e.g., Down's syndrome and limb malformations) or miscarriages |
| Contraceptive diaphragm (with jelly)[2] | 3; 13 | Diaphragm mechanically blocks entrance to cervix; jelly is spermicidal | No side effects | Must be prescribed (and fitted) by physician; must be inserted prior to coitus |
| Condom | 2.6; 10 | Mechanical; prevents sperm from entering vagina | No side effects; some protection against STD | Interruption of foreplay to fit; slightly decreased sensation for male |
| Rhythm[3] | 35, but varies greatly | Abstinence during fertile period | No side effects | Not reliable |
| Douche | 40 | Flushes semen from vagina | No side effects | Unreliable; sperm beyond reach of douche within seconds |
| Withdrawal (coitus interruptus) | 20? | Male withdraws penis from vagina prior to ejaculation | No side effects | Unreliable; contrary to powerful drives present as orgasm is approached; sperm present in fluid secreted before ejaculation may be sufficient for conception |
| Sterilization | | | | |
| Tubal ligation | 0.04 | Prevents ovum from leaving uterine tube | Most reliable method | Usually not reversible |
| Vasectomy | 0.15 | Prevents sperm from leaving scrotum | Most reliable method | Usually not reversible |
| Chance (no contraception) | About 90 | | | |

[1]The first figure is the failure of the method; the second figure includes method failure plus failure of the user to utilize the method correctly. Both are based on number of failures per 100 women who use the method per year in the United States.

[2]Failure rate is lower when used together with spermicidal foam.

[3]There are several variations of the rhythm method. For those who use the calendar method alone, the failure rate is about 35%. However, if a woman takes her temperature daily and keeps careful records (because temperature rises after ovulation), the failure rate can be reduced. Also, by keeping a daily record of the type of vaginal secretions, she can note changes in cervical mucus and use them to determine time of ovulation. This type of rhythm contraception is also slightly more effective. When women use the temperature or mucus method and wait more than 48 hours after ovulation to have intercourse, the failure rate can be reduced to about 7%.

Short of total abstinence, the only foolproof method of contraception is **sterilization**. An estimated 1 million **vasectomies** are performed each year in the United States. In this procedure a small incision is made on each side of the scrotum. Then, each vas deferens is cut and its ends are tied or clipped so that they cannot grow back together (Fig. 20–9). Vasectomies can be performed in a physician's office using only a local anesthetic. Because testosterone secretion and transport are not affected, a vasectomy in no way affects masculinity. Sperm continue to be produced, though at a much slower rate, and are destroyed by macrophages in the testes. No change in the amount of semen ejaculated is noticed because sperm account for little of the semen volume.

Surgeons have been able to reverse sterilization in about 30% of attempts made by reuniting the

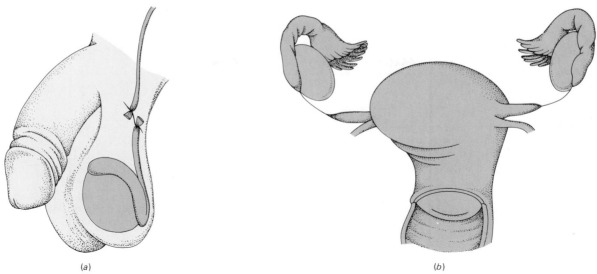

(a)                                                                                          (b)

**Figure 20–9.** *Sterilization. (a) In vasectomy the vas deferens (sperm duct) on each side is cut and tied. (b) In tubal ligation each uterine tube is cut and tied so that ovum and sperm can no longer meet.*

ends of the vasa deferentia. The success rate is low, partly because some sterilized men eventually develop antibodies against their own sperm, making the sperm nonviable.

Several techniques are in current use for preventing transport of ova. Most of them involve **tubal ligation**, cutting and tying the uterine tubes (Fig. 20–9). Although this can be done through the vagina, it is usually performed through an abdominal incision and requires general anesthesia. Female sterilization carries with it an estimated risk of 25 deaths per 100,000 procedures performed, whereas there is almost no risk of death in vasectomy. New techniques are being developed that would make tubal ligation a simpler, safer procedure and also improve chances of reversing it. As in the male, hormone balance and sexual performance are not affected.

## ABORTION

More than 1 million abortions are performed each year in the United States, and an estimated 40 million worldwide. There are three kinds of abortion. **Spontaneous abortions** (popularly known as miscarriages) occur without intervention and often are nature's way of destroying a defective embryo. **Therapeutic abortions** are performed to preserve the health of the mother or when there is reason to believe that the embryo is grossly abnormal. The third type of abortion—the kind performed as a means of birth control—is the most controversial. All societies use abortion to prevent unwanted births and abortion is thought to be the

most widely used method of birth control in the world.

Most first-trimester abortions (those done in the first 3 months of pregnancy) and some later ones are performed using a suction method. After the cervix is dilated, a suction aspirator is inserted into the uterus and the fetus and other products of conception are quickly evacuated.

Later in pregnancy abortions are performed using saline injections. Amniotic fluid surrounding the embryo is removed with a needle and replaced with a salt solution. The fetus dies within 1 or 2 hours and labor begins several hours later. Prostaglandins are being used experimentally to induce abortions during both first and second trimesters. They appear to be a safe, nonsurgical method of chemically terminating pregnancy.

What about the safety of abortions? When performed during the first trimester by skilled medical personnel, the maternal mortality rate is about 1.9 per 100,000 abortions performed. After the first trimester this rate rises to 12.5 per 100,000. The death rate from illegal abortions performed by medically untrained individuals is about 100 per 100,000.

## SEXUALLY TRANSMITTED DISEASES

**Sexually transmitted diseases** (also called venereal diseases) are, next to the common cold, the most common communicable diseases in the world. The World Health Organization estimates that more than 250 million people are infected

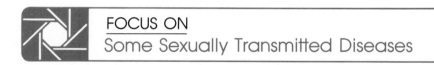

## FOCUS ON
## Some Sexually Transmitted Diseases

| Disease and Causative Organism | Course of Disease | Treatment |
|---|---|---|
| Gonorrhea (*Gonococcus* bacterium) | Infection by sexual contact; bacterial toxin may produce redness and swelling at infection site; symptoms in males: painful urination and discharge of pus from penis; in about 60% of infected women no symptoms occur in initial stages; can spread to epididymis (in males) or uterine tubes and ovaries (in females), causing sterility; can cause widespread pelvic or other infection, plus damage to heart valves, meninges (outer coverings of brain and spinal cord), and joints | Penicillin, or other antibiotic if penicillin-resistant strain involved. |
| Syphilis (*Treponema pallidum*, a spirochete bacterium) | Bacteria enter body through defect in skin near site of infection; spread throughout body by lymphatic and circulatory routes; primary chancre (small, painless ulcer) forms at site of initial infection and heals in about a month, highly infectious at this stage; secondary stage follows, in which widespread rash and influenzalike symptoms may occur, scaly lesions may occur that teem with bacteria and are highly infectious; latent stage that follows can last 20 years, eventually, lesions called gummae may occur, consuming parts of the body surface or damaging liver, bone, or spleen; serious brain damage may occur; death results in 5 to 10% of cases | Penicillin; sensitive blood tests can detect antibodies and hence infection; about one-third of cases recover spontaneously |
| Genital herpes (herpes simplex type 2 virus) | Tiny, painful blisters appear on genitals, may develop into ulcers; influenzalike symptoms may occur; recurs periodically; threat to fetus or newborn infant; may predispose to cervical cancer in females | No effective cure; some drugs may shorten outbreaks or reduce severity of symptoms |
| Pelvic inflammatory disease (PID) (usually chlamydial bacteria) | Generalized infection of reproductive organs and pelvic cavity, usually chronic and difficult to treat; may lead to sterility (more than 15% of cases); PID now most common STD in the U.S. | Antibiotics, surgical removal of affected organs |
| Trichomoniasis (a protozoan) | Symptoms include itching, discharge, soreness; can be contracted from dirty toilet seats and towels | Drugs |
| Yeast infections (genital candidiasis) (yeasts) | Irritation, soreness, discharge; especially common in females | Drugs |

Note: AIDS is discussed in Chapter 14.

each year with gonorrhea and more than 50 million with syphilis. (See Focus on Some Sexually Transmitted Diseases.)

## SUMMARY

I. The reproductive function of the male is to produce sperm cells and to deliver them into the female reproductive tract.
   A. Sperm are produced in the seminiferous tubules of the testes.
   B. From the seminiferous tubules in the testes sperm pass into an epididymis, where they complete maturation and may be stored. From the epididymis they enter the vas deferens for further storage. During ejaculation, sperm pass into the ejaculatory duct and then into the urethra, which extends through the penis.
   C. Most of the volume of the semen is produced by the seminal vesicles and the prostate gland. The bulbourethral glands produce a few drops of alkaline fluid prior to ejaculation.
   D. The penis consists of three columns of erectile tissue. When the large venous sinusoids of this tissue become engorged with blood, the penis becomes erect.
   E. The anterior lobe of the pituitary gland releases the gonadotropic hormones FSH and LH.
      1. FSH stimulates development of the seminiferous tubules and promotes sperm production.
      2. LH stimulates the interstitial cells to release testosterone.
   F. Testosterone is responsible for the development of reproductive structures and the development and maintenance of secondary sex characteristics.
II. The reproductive role of the female includes production of ova, reception of sperm, incubation and nourishment of the developing embryo, and lactation.
   A. Ova develop in the ovaries as part of follicles.
      1. After puberty a few follicles begin to develop each month when stimulated by FSH.
      2. At ovulation the ovum is ejected into the pelvic cavity. It then passes into the uterine tube, where it is either fertilized or deteriorates.
   B. If fertilized, the ovum begins to develop, and the tiny embryo passes into the uterus, which serves as its incubator.
   C. The vagina is the lower part of the birth canal. It also receives the penis during sexual intercourse and serves as an outlet for menstrual discharge.
   D. The term vulva refers to the external female genital structures.
   E. The mammary glands within the breasts function in lactation.
   F. The first day of menstrual bleeding marks the first day of the menstrual cycle.
      1. In a "typical" 28-day cycle ovulation occurs on about the fourteenth day.
      2. Events of the menstrual cycle are coordinated by the interaction of gonadotropic and ovarian hormones.
         a. FSH stimulates follicle growth during the preovulatory phase of the cycle.
         b. Estrogen released from the developing follicles stimulates the endometrium to thicken.
         c. LH released from the pituitary stimulates ovulation and the development of the corpus luteum.
         d. The corpus luteum secretes progesterone during the postovulatory phase of the cycle. Progesterone stimulates the glands in the endometrium to secrete a nutritive fluid.
         e. If fertilization does not occur, the corpus luteum begins to degenerate.
         f. With the degeneration of the corpus luteum, estrogen and progesterone levels fall and the endometrium begins to slough off again (menstruation).
   G. Estrogen is responsible for the development and maintenance of secondary sex characteristics; with progesterone it prepares the endometrium each month for possible pregnancy.
III. The cycle of sexual response includes the excitement phase, plateau phase, orgasm, and resolution. Vasocongestion and increased muscle tension are the two basic physiological responses to sexual stimulation.
IV. Millions of sperm are required for fertilization even though only one sperm actually fertilizes the ovum.
V. Although an ideal contraceptive has not yet been developed, effective methods of birth control, such as oral contraceptives, are available. Sterilization is accomplished by vasectomy in the male and by tubal ligation in the female.
VI. Gonorrhea, syphilis, and genital herpes are three serious and common varieties of sexually transmitted disease.

## POST TEST

1. Sperm cells are produced in the _____ tubules of the _____.

2. From the epididymis sperm pass into the _____ _____.

3. Most of the semen is produced by the _____ _____.

4. The interstitial cells of the testes produce _____.
5. The term castration refers to the removal of the _____.
6. The two ovarian hormones are _____ and _____.

*Select the most appropriate answer from Column B for each item in Column A. You may use an answer once, more than once, or not at all.*

|  | **Column A** | **Column B** |
|---|---|---|
| 7. _____ | Place where ova are produced. | a. vulva |
| 8. _____ | Site of fertilization | b. uterine tube |
| 9. _____ | Part of uterus that projects into vagina | c. ovary |
| 10. _____ | Embryo implants here | d. uterus |
| 11. _____ | External female genital structures | e. cervix |

12. Ejection of the ovum from the follicle is called _____.
13. In the female FSH is released by the _____ _____ of the _____ gland and stimulates development of _____.
14. The number of sperm that fertilizes an ovum is _____.
15. Sterilization is commonly accomplished surgically by _____ in the male and by _____ _____ in the female.
16. Label the diagram below.

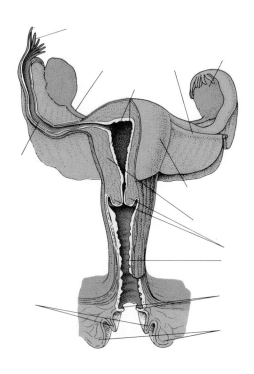

## REVIEW QUESTIONS

1. The testes are located in the scrotum outside of the pelvic cavity. Why?
2. What are the actions of testosterone?
3. Trace the path traveled by a sperm cell from the tubules of the testes until it is discharged from the body.
4. What is erectile dysfunction? What is sterility? What is castration?
5. What is the function of the corpus luteum? What hormone is necessary for its development?
6. In a typical 28-day menstrual cycle, when does ovulation occur? When does menstruation occur? When is a woman most likely to become pregnant?
7. What is puberty? What is menopause?
8. Is masculinity affected by vasectomy? Why or why not?

# Development

LEARNING OBJECTIVES

**After you study this chapter you should be able to**
1. Trace the development of the embryo from conception until it becomes a fetus.
2. Give the functions of the amnion and placenta.
3. Describe the general course of development from the third month until birth.
4. Describe the birth process, distinguishing among the three stages of labor.
5. Distinguish between fraternal and identical twins, describing how each develops.
6. Describe how the embryo can be affected by nutrients, drugs, oxygen deprivation, pathogens, and ionizing radiation.
7. Trace the stages of the human life cycle.
8. Summarize changes that occur with aging.

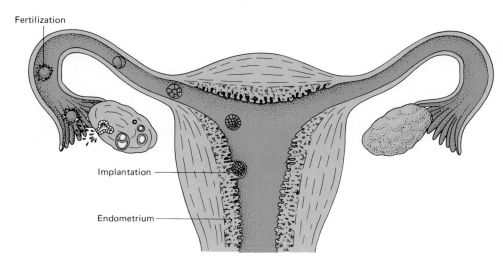

Fertilization

Implantation

Endometrium

*Figure 21–1. Cell division takes place as the embryo is moved through the uterine tube to the uterus.*

How does the microscopic **zygote** (fertilized egg) develop into a fully formed and functioning baby? The single-celled zygote divides to form a two-cell **embryo**. Then each of these cells divides to form four cells. As these first cell divisions take place, the embryo is pushed along the uterine tube (Fig. 21–1). By the time the embryo reaches the uterus on the fifth day of development, it is a tiny cluster of 16 cells.

## EARLY DEVELOPMENT

On about the seventh day of development the embryo begins to implant itself in the wall of the uterus. Cells of the embryo secrete enzymes that erode away an area of the uterine wall just large enough to enable it to work its way down into the underlying connective tissues. This process is called **implantation**. All further **prenatal development** (development before birth) takes place within the wall of the uterus.

## The Amnion and Placenta

Several fetal membranes develop around the embryo. These help protect, nourish, and support the developing embryo and are discarded at birth. The **amnion**, a sac that surrounds the embryo, is filled with a clear fluid that keeps the embryo moist (Fig. 21–2). The *amniotic fluid* also serves as an effective shock absorber so that when the pregnant woman bumps her abdomen the embryo is protected from mechanical injury.

The **placenta** is the organ of exchange between the blood of the mother and that of the embryo. It provides nutrients and oxygen for the embryo and

removes wastes from the embryo, which are then excreted by the mother's kidneys. The placenta also produces a hormone called **human chorionic gonadotropin (HCG)**, which signals the corpus luteum that pregnancy is in process. In response, the corpus luteum increases in size and releases large amounts of estrogen and progesterone, which stimulate the continued development of the endometrium and placenta. Without HCG the corpus luteum degenerates and the embryo is aborted. Af-

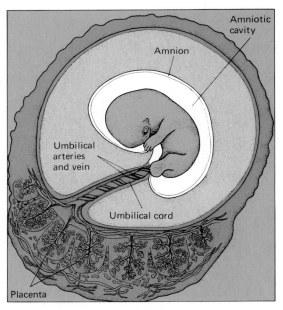

Amniotic cavity

Amnion

Umbilical arteries and vein

Umbilical cord

Placenta

*Figure 21–2. At about 45 days the embryo and its membranes together are about the size of a Ping-Pong ball and the mother still may be unaware of her pregnancy. The amnion filled with amniotic fluid surrounds and cushions the embryo. Blood circulation has been established between the embryo and the maternal circulation by blood vessels that run through the umbilical cord to the placenta.*

ter about the eleventh week of pregnancy the placenta itself produces enough estrogen and progesterone to maintain pregnancy.

The placenta brings maternal blood close to the blood of the embryo but the two circulatory systems are completely separate. The blood does not normally mix. Oxygen and nutrients diffuse out of the maternal blood through the placental tissue and into the embryo's blood.

An **umbilical cord** develops, connecting the embryo with the placenta. Two umbilical arteries deliver blood from the embryo to the placenta and an umbilical vein returns blood to the embryo.

## Development of Organs

Development proceeds in an orderly, predictable sequence. By 4 weeks the embryo has developed the rudiments of many of its organs (Fig. 21–3). The brain and spinal cord are among the first organs to develop, and by 4 weeks the eye and ear are visible. A simple, but functional circulatory system is also working by this time. At this stage the heart is an S-shaped tube that beats about 60 times each minute. Limb buds appear by the end of the first month and slowly lengthen and differentiate to form the limbs.

## LATER DEVELOPMENT

After the second month the embryo is referred to as a **fetus**. During the third month the fetus be-

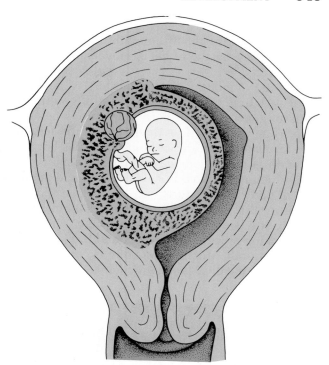

*Figure 21–4.* Human embryo at 10 weeks, 6 cm (2.4 inches) long.

comes recognizably human (Fig. 21–4). By 3 months the external genital structures differentiate so that the sex of the fetus can be determined by inspection. By the end of the third month the fetus is almost 56 mm (2.2 inches) in length and weighs about 14 g (0.5 ounce) (Fig. 21–5). By 5 months of

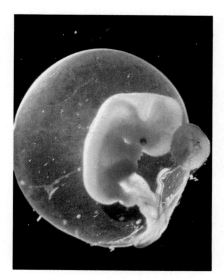

*Figure 21–3.* Photograph of human embryo at 5½ weeks, about 1 cm (0.4 inch) long. Note the developing limb buds. (Guigoz, Petit Format, Photo Researchers, Inc.)

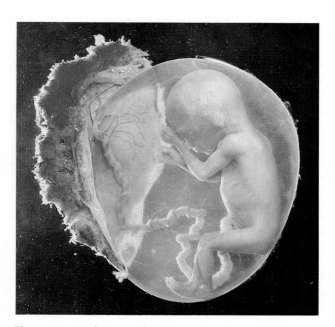

*Figure 21–5.* Photograph of human embryo at 16 weeks, about 16 cm (6.4 inches) long. (From Nilsson, L.: A Child Is Born. New York, Dell Publishing Co., Inc., 1977.)

---

development the fetus moves about in the amniotic cavity. During the fifth month the mother usually becomes aware of fetal movements (quickening).

The last 3 months (last trimester) of development are a time of rapid growth and differentiation of tissues and organs. If born prematurely before 7 months or weighing less than 1000 g, the fetus is able to move about and cry but often dies because its brain is not developed enough to sustain such vital functions as rhythmical breathing and regulation of body temperature.

During the seventh month the cerebrum grows rapidly and becomes highly convoluted. The grasp and sucking reflexes are present and the fetus may suck its thumb. Much of the body is covered with a downy hair called **lanugo**, which is usually shed

before birth. At birth the full-term baby weighs about 3000 g (7 pounds) and measures about 52 cm (20 inches) in length.

## BIRTH

From the time of conception about 266 days are required for the baby to complete its prenatal development. Late in pregnancy the placenta begins to degenerate. The uterus is distended to its fullest capacity. Several days before birth the fetus usually assumes an upside-down position preparing it to enter the birth canal head first. The factors that actually initiate the birth process are not well understood.

Childbirth, or **parturition**, begins with a long se-

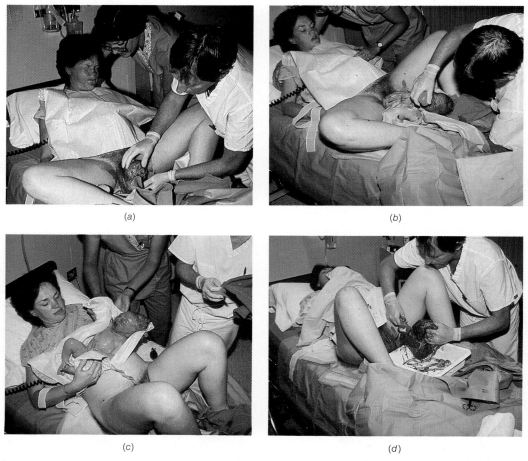

(a)  (b)  (c)  (d)

***Figure 21–6.*** *Birth of a baby. In about 95% of all human births the baby descends through the cervix and vagina in the head-down position. (a) The mother bears down hard with her abdominal muscles, helping to push the baby out. When the head fully appears, the physician or midwife can gently grasp it and guide the baby's emergence into the outside world. (b) Once the head has emerged, the rest of the body usually follows readily. The physician gently aspirates the mouth and pharynx to clear the upper airway of any amniotic fluid, mucus, or blood. At this time the neonate usually takes its first breath. (c) The baby, still attached to the placenta by its umbilical cord, is presented to its mother. (d) During the third stage of labor the placenta is delivered. (Courtesy of Dan Atchison.)*

ries of involuntary contractions of the uterus, referred to as labor contractions. *Labor* may be divided into three stages.

During the **first stage** regular uterine contractions occur. At first they may occur at about 30-minute intervals, but then they become more intense, rhythmical, and frequent, occurring as often as every minute (or even less) later in labor. As this stage progresses, the cervix becomes dilated to about 10 cm (4 inches) and effaced (that is, continuous with the uterine wall, so it cannot be distinguished from the adjoining portion of the uterus), allowing passage of the fetal head. Rupture of the amnion with release of the amniotic fluid through the vagina may occur during this stage. The first stage of labor is the longest, often lasting 8 to 24 hours in a first pregnancy.

The **second stage** begins when the cervix is fully dilated and ends with the delivery of the baby (Fig. 21–6). By contracting her abdominal muscles the mother can help push the baby along through the vagina. Just before birth the physician usually makes a surgical incision called an *episiotomy*, extending from the vagina toward the anus. This facilitates delivery of the baby and prevents tearing of the vagina. After the delivery the incision is sutured and usually heals within a few weeks. When the **neonate** (newborn) emerges it is still connected to the placenta by the umbilical cord. Most physicians clamp and cut the cord immediately after the infant has been delivered.

During the **third stage** of labor the placenta separates from the uterus and is expelled. Generally this occurs within 10 to 20 minutes after the birth of the baby. Now referred to as the afterbirth, the placenta is inspected for abnormalities and later discarded.

## MULTIPLE BIRTHS

In the United States twins are born once in about 88 births, triplets once in 88 squared (7744), and quadruplets once in 88 cubed births. Twins (or other multiple births) can be either fraternal or identical. **Fraternal twins** develop when a woman ovulates two eggs and each is fertilized by a different sperm. Each fertilized egg has its own unique genetic endowment and the twins that develop are no more alike than any two siblings. Identical twins develop when the tiny mass of cells that makes up the early embryo subdivides to form two independent groups of cells, and each develops into a baby. Because the cells of each twin have developed from one fertilized egg, they have identical genes and are indeed **identical twins**. Rarely,

the two masses of cells do not separate completely and develop into **conjoined** (Siamese) **twins**.

## ENVIRONMENTAL INFLUENCES ON THE EMBRYO

About 7% of all babies born alive in the United States, or 175,000 babies per year, arrive with a birth defect of clinical significance. Such birth defects account for about 10% of deaths among newborn babies. Birth defects result from environmental or genetic factors, or from a combination of the two.

Prenatal development is affected by maternal nutrition, the air the mother breathes, disease organisms, chemicals, drugs, and radiation. Because most organs form during the first three months of embryonic life, the developing baby is most susceptible to environmental conditions during this early period. Table 21–1 describes some of the environmental factors that can affect development.

Physicians can now diagnose some birth defects during early development. In **amniocentesis** a sample of amniotic fluid is withdrawn through the abdominal wall and used in diagnosing certain genetic disorders. Figure 21–7 shows two **sonograms**, photographs taken of the embryo using ultrasound. Such previews are helpful in diagnosing defects and also in determining the position of the fetus and whether a multiple birth is pending.

## THE HUMAN LIFE CYCLE

Development begins at conception and continues through the stages of the human life cycle until death (Table 21–2). In this chapter we have briefly examined the development of the **embryo** and **fetus**. The **neonatal period** extends from birth to the end of the first month of postnatal life. **Infancy** follows the neonatal period and lasts until age 2 years; some consider infancy to end when the infant can assume an erect posture and walk, usually between the ages of 10 and 14 months. **Childhood**, also a period of rapid growth and development, continues from infancy until adolescence.

**Adolescence** is the time of development between puberty and adulthood. During adolescence a young person experiences the physical and physiological changes that result in physical and reproductive maturity. This is also a time when young people make the psychological adjustments that prepare them to assume the responsibility of

Table 21–1
**Environmental Influences on the Embryo**

| Factor | Example and Effect | Comment |
|---|---|---|
| Nutrition | Severe protein malnutrition doubles number of defects; fewer brain cells are produced, and learning ability may be permanently affected | Growth rate mainly determined by rate of net protein synthesis by embryo's cells |
| Excessive amounts of vitamins | Vitamin D essential, but excessive amounts may result in form of mental retardation; too much vitamins A and K may also be harmful | Vitamin supplements are normally prescribed for pregnant women, but some women mistakenly reason that if one vitamin pill is beneficial, four or five might be even better |
| Drugs | Many drugs affect development of fetus: even aspirin has been shown to inhibit growth of human fetal cells (especially kidney cells) cultured in laboratory; it may also inhibit prostaglandins, which are concentrated in growing tissue | Common prescription drugs are generally taken in amounts based on body weight of mother, which may be hundreds or thousands of times too much for tiny embryo |
| Alcohol | When woman drinks heavily during pregnancy, baby may be born with fetal alcohol syndrome, that is, deformed and mentally and physically retarded; low birth weight and structural abnormalities have been associated with as little as two drinks a day; some cases of hyperactivity and learning disabilities may be caused by alcohol intake of pregnant mother | Fetal alcohol syndrome thought to be an important cause of mental retardation in United States |
| Heroin | Heroin results in high mortality rate and high prematurity rate | Infants that survive are born addicted and must be treated for weeks or months |
| Methadone | Methadone results in fetal addiction | |
| Thalidomide | Thalidomide, marketed as mild sedative, was responsible for more than 7000 grossly deformed babies born in the late 1950s in 20 countries; principal defect was **phocomelia**, condition in which babies are born with extremely short limbs, often with no fingers or toes | This drug interferes with cellular metabolism; most hazardous when taken during fourth to sixth weeks, when limbs are developing |
| Cigarette smoking | Cigarette smoking reduces amount of oxygen available to fetus because some of maternal hemoglobin is combined with carbon monoxide; may slow growth and can cause subtle forms of damage; in extreme form carbon monoxide poisoning causes such gross defects as hydrocephaly | Mothers who smoke deliver babies with lower-than-average birth weights and have higher incidence of spontaneous abortions, stillbirths, and neonatal deaths; studies also indicate possible link between maternal smoking and slower intellectual development in offspring |
| Rubella | Rubella (German measles) virus crosses placenta and infects embryo; interferes with normal metabolism and cell movements; causes syndrome that involves blinding cataracts, deafness, heart malformations, and mental retardation; risk is greatest (about 50%) when rubella is contracted during first month of pregnancy; risk declines with each succeeding month | Rubella epidemic in the United States in 1963–1965 resulted in about 20,000 fetal deaths and 30,000 infants born with gross defects |
| Syphilis | Syphilis is transmitted to fetus in about 40% of infected women; fetus may die or be born with defects and congenital syphilis | Pregnant woman are routinely tested for syphilis during prenatal examinations |
| Ionizing radiation | When mother is subjected to x-rays or other forms of radiation during pregnancy, infant has higher risk of birth defects and leukemia | Radiation was one of earliest teratogens to be recognized |

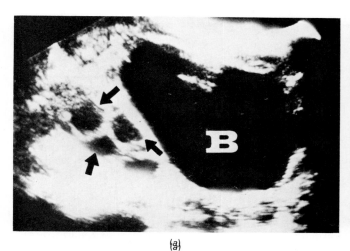

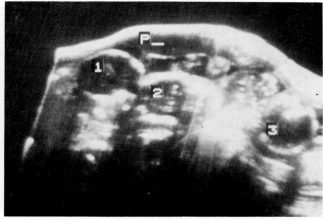

**Figure 21–7.** *Ultrasonic techniques can be used to monitor follicle maturation and ovulation, as well as to give the physician information about the fetus. (a) Sonogram showing three follicles of equal maturity in the left ovary of a woman. (b) Triplets (1, 2, 3) in the same patient at 16 weeks of pregnancy. P, Placenta. Such previews are valuable to the physician in diagnosing defects and predicting multiple births. (Courtesy of Biserka Funduk-Kurjuk and Asim Kurjak, from Acta Obstetrica et Gynecologica Scandinavica, 61, 1982.)*

Table 21–2
**Stages in the Human Life Cycle**

| Stage | Time Period | Characteristics |
|---|---|---|
| Embryo | Conception to end of eighth week of prenatal development | Development proceeds from single-celled zygote to embryo that is about 30 mm long, weighs 1 g, and has rudiments of all its organs |
| Fetus | Beginning of ninth week of prenatal development to birth | Period of rapid growth, morphogenesis, and cellular differentiation, changing tiny parasite to physiologically independent organism |
| Neonate | Birth to 4 weeks of age | Neonate must make vital physiological adjustments to independent life: it must now process its own food, excrete its wastes, obtain oxygen, and make appropriate circulatory changes |
| Infant | End of fourth week to 2 years of age (sometimes, ability to walk is considered end of infancy) | Rapid growth; deciduous teeth begin to erupt; nervous system develops (myelinization), making coordinated activities possible; language skills begin to develop |
| Child | Two years to puberty | Rapid growth; deciduous teeth erupt, are slowly shed and replaced by permanent teeth; development of muscular coordination; development of language skills and other intellectual abilities |
| Adolescent | Puberty (approximately ages 11–14) to adult | Growth spurt; primary and secondary sexual characteristics develop; development of motor skills; development of intellectual abilities; psychological changes as adolescent approaches adulthood |
| Young adult | End of adolescence (approximately age 20) to about age 40 | Peak of physical development reached; individual assumes adult reponsibilities that may include marriage, fulfilling reproductive potential, and establishing career; after age 30, physiological changes associated with aging begin |
| Middle-aged adult | Age 40 to about age 65 | Physiological aging continues, leading to menopause in women and physical changes associated with aging in both sexes (e.g., graying hair, decline in athletic abilities, wrinkling skin); this is period of adjustment for many as they begin to face their own mortality |
| Old adult | Age 65 to death | Period of senescence (growing old); physiological aging continues; maintaining homeostasis more difficult when body is challenged by stress; death often results from failure of cardiovascular or immune system |

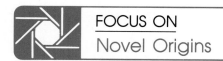

## FOCUS ON
## Novel Origins

About 10,000 children born each year are products of **artificial insemination**. Usually this procedure is sought when the male partner of a couple desiring a child is sterile or carries a genetic defect. Although the sperm donor remains anonymous to the couple involved, his genetic qualifications are screened by physicians.

**In vitro fertilization** is a technique by which an ovum is removed from a woman's ovary, fertilized in a test tube, and then reimplanted in her uterus. Such a procedure may be attempted if a woman's uterine (fallopian) tubes are blocked or if they have been surgically removed. With the help of this technique a healthy baby was born in England in 1978 to a couple who had tried unsuccessfully for several years to have a child. Since that time, many other children have been conceived within laboratory glassware.

Another novel procedure is **host mothering**. In this procedure, a tiny embryo is removed from its natural mother and implanted into a female substitute. The foster mother can support the developing embryo either until birth or temporarily until it is implanted again into the original mother or into an-

other host. This technique has already proved useful to animal breeders. For example, embryos from prize sheep can be temporarily implanted into rabbits for easy shipping by air and then reimplanted into a foster mother sheep, perhaps of inferior quality. Host mothering also has the advantage of allowing an animal of superior quality to produce more offspring than would be naturally possible. In one recent series of experiments mouse embryos were frozen for up to 8 days and then successfully transplanted into host mothers. Host mothering may someday be popular with women who can produce embryos but are unable to carry them to term.

Someday society may have to deal with **cloning** (not yet a reality in humans). In this process the nucleus would be removed from an ovum and replaced with the nucleus of a cell from a person who wished to produce a human copy of himself. Theoretically, any cell nucleus could be used, even a white blood cell nucleus. The fertilized ovum would then be placed into a human uterus for incubation; the resulting baby would be an identical, though younger, twin to the individual whose nucleus was used.

---

adulthood. **Young adulthood** extends from adolescence until about age 40. **Middle age** is usually considered to be the period between ages 40 and 65. **Old age** begins after age 65.

## THE AGING PROCESS

Development includes those biological changes that result in the decreased functional capacities of the mature organism, changes we refer to as **aging**. Various systems of the body become less functional at different times and at different rates. A 75-year-old man has lost about 64% of his taste buds, 44% of his renal glomeruli, and 37% of the axons in his spinal nerves that he had at age 30. His nerve impulses are transmitted 10% more slowly, the blood supply to his brain is about 20% less, and the vital capacity of his lungs is 44% less. The aging process in also marked by a progressive decrease in the body's homeostatic ability to respond to stress.

Several theories have been proposed to explain the aging process—hormonal changes; changes with time in the structure of macromolecules such as collagen; a decrease in the elastic properties of connective tissues owing to an accumulation of calcium, which results in stiffening of the joints and hardening of the arteries; destruction of cells by enzymes released by leaky or broken lysosomes; accumulation of specific waste products within cells; and the development of autoimmune reactions, resulting in destruction of body structures by the body's own antibodies. Other current theories suggest that aging involves the accumulation of mutations caused by continued exposure to cosmic radiation and x-radiation, mutations that decrease the ability of the cell to carry out its normal functions at the normal rate. Aging processes are likely part of the program of timed development built into the genes.

Like other developmental processes, aging may be accelerated by certain environmental influences and may occur at varying rates in different individuals because of inherited differences. For example, there is some experimental evidence that aging, at least in rats, can be delayed by dietary means (by caloric restriction); thin rats generally live longer than fat rats. Genetic predisposition may, however, be the best guarantee of a long life.

## SUMMARY

I. The series of cell divisions that divide the zygote into a mass of cells takes place as the embryo is moved through the uterine tube to the uterus.

II. Fetal membranes protect and nourish the embryo.

  A. The amnion contains fluid that keeps the embryo moist and protects it from mechanical shock.

  B. The placenta is the organ of exchange between mother and embryo and also secretes hormones.

III. By 4 weeks the embryo has developed the rudiments of many of its organs.

IV. After the second month the embryo is referred to as a fetus; during the third month it becomes recognizably human.

V. Labor can be divided into three stages with the actual delivery of the baby occurring during the second stage and the delivery of the placenta occurring during the third stage.

VI. Fraternal twins develop from different zygotes; identical twins develop from the same zygote and therefore have identical genes.

VII. Environmental factors such as nutrition, pathogens, drug intake, chemical and radiation exposure, and cigarette smoking can affect the development of the embryo.

VIII. The human life cycle can be divided into the following stages: embryo, fetus, neonate, infant, child, adolescent, young adult, middle-aged adult, and old adult.

## POST TEST

1. The fertilized egg is called a _____.
2. The embryo develops in a fluid-filled sac called the _____.
3. The _____ is the organ of exchange between mother and embryo.
4. The hormone human chorionic gonadotropin (HCG) signals the _____ _____ that pregnancy has occurred.
5. The _____ _____ connects the embryo with the placenta.
6. After the second month the embryo is called a _____.
7. The baby is delivered during the _____ stage of labor.
8. The newborn infant is referred to as a _____.
9. _____ twins develop from a single zygote.
10. The stage in the human life cycle between puberty and adulthood is _____.

## REVIEW QUESTIONS

1. What is implantation? Describe the process.
2. What are the functions of the amnion? The placenta?
3. What generally prevents survival of a baby born prematurely before 7 months?
4. When during development do most of the organs begin to form?
5. What happens during each stage of labor?
6. Why are fraternal twins no more alike than two nontwin brothers or sisters?
7. What are some specific things a pregnant woman can do (or not do) to promote the well-being of her developing child?
8. Why is the embryo most susceptible to environmental damage during the first three months of development?
9. List the stages of the human life cycle and identify four theories of aging.

# Genetics

LEARNING OBJECTIVES

**After you study this chaper you should be able to**
1. Summarize the relationship among DNA, genes, and chromosomes and define the term gene.
2. Describe how gender of the offspring is determined.
3. Define basic terms related to inheritance, such as dominant gene, recessive gene, genotype, phenotype, homozygous, and heterozygous.
4. Give the chromosomal basis for Down's syndrome.
5. Define mutation and describe its causes and effects.

Identical twins look the same because they have inherited identical genes from their parents. Members of the same family often have many traits in common and are said to exhibit a family resemblance. They have inherited many of the same genes. The transfer of biological information from parent to offspring is called **heredity**. The branch of biology that is concerned with heredity is **genetics**.

## GENES AND CHROMOSOMES

**Chromosomes** are tiny packages in which genetic information is stored. Each chromosome contains thousands of **genes** and each gene contains the information for a specific trait. That information is in the form of a chemical code. The chemical compound that codes genetic information is **deoxyribonucleic acid (DNA)** (Fig. 22–1). In fact, a gene may be defined as a sequence of DNA that codes for a specific protein. The proteins specified by the genes determine what a person looks like (including height, body build and shape, color of skin, hair, and eyes), body chemistry (including blood type and metabolic function), and at least a framework for intelligence and many aspects of behavior. More than 150 human disorders are inherited and genes are thought to determine susceptibility to many diseases.

Every human cell (except the sex cells) contains 23 pairs of chromosomes, or a total of 46 chromosomes. One of each pair is inherited from the father and the other from the mother. Thus, every sperm cell contains 23 chromosomes and every egg cell contains 23 chromosomes. When sperm and egg unite in fertilization they form a single cell, the zygote, which then contains 46 chromosomes.

Before the zygote divides to form the first two cells of the embryo, the complete set of chromosomes is duplicated and then during **mitosis** (my-**tow'**-sis) a complete set of chromosomes is distributed to each end of the cell. When cell division occurs each new cell has an identical set of 46 chromosomes. This process is repeated over and over so that each of the billions of cells of the completed human being contains an identical set of 46 chromosomes.

Only the gametes (the sex cells) are different. Gametes are formed by a special type of cell division known as **meiosis** (my-**oh'**-sis) (Fig. 22–2). During meiosis the members of each pair of chromosomes are separated and distributed to different cells. Each gamete contains only one of each pair of chromosomes, or a total of 23 chromosomes.

During the process of meiosis the chromosomes are thoroughly shuffled so that no two gametes are likely to contain the same chromosomes.

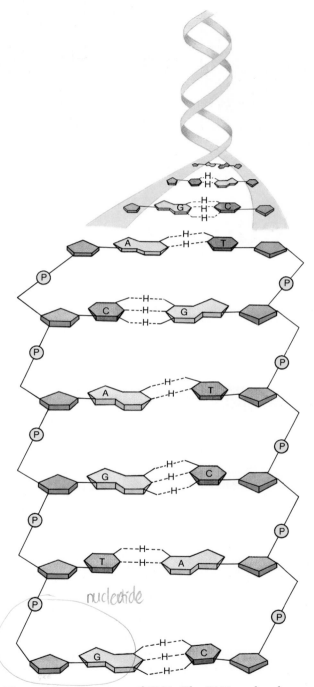

***Figure 22–1.*** *Structure of DNA. The DNA molecule consists of subunits called nucleotides. In turn, each nucleotide is made up of a phosphate group (labeled P), a sugar (shown in green), and a nitrogen base (shown in red or blue). The four types of bases found in DNA are adenine (A), thymine (T), cytosine (C), and guanine (G). The sequence of these bases spells out the genetic code. A sequence of several hundred nucleotides makes up a gene and codes for a specific protein.*

*Figure 22–2.* Meiosis compared with mitosis. (a) Mitosis. Note that each daughter cell has an identical set of four chromosomes (two paris). (b) Meiosis. Two divisions take place, giving rise to four daughter cells. Each daughter cell has only two chromosomes, one of each pair. The chromosomes shown in blue originally came from one parent; those shown in pink came from the other parent.

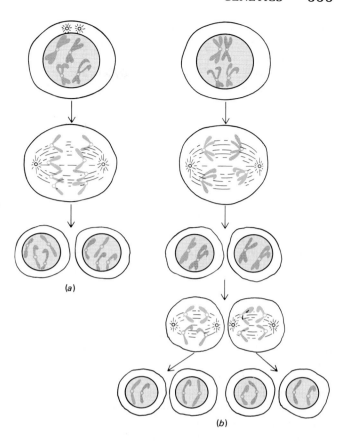

## MALE OR FEMALE? HOW GENDER IS DETERMINED

Of the 23 pairs of chromosomes, 22 pairs appear matched. For example, the two chromosomes of pair 1 look similar to one another (Fig. 22–3). One pair of chromosomes, the sex chromosomes, are alike in females but different in males. Every normal female has two X chromosomes in each of her body cells, whereas every normal male cell contains one X chromosome and one smaller Y chromosome. As a result every egg cell contains an X chromosome and every sperm cell contains *either* an X chromosome *or* a Y chromosome. (Recall that during meiosis one of each pair of chromosomes is distributed to each new cell.)

Gender of the offspring is determined by the sperm cell at the moment of fertilization (Fig. 22–4). If the egg cell is fertilized by a sperm cell containing an X chromosome, the baby that develops will be a female. If the egg is fertilized by a Y-bearing sperm cell, the baby will be male.

## HOW GENES FUNCTION

The gene for any particular trait occupies a specific location on a specific chromosome. Members of a pair of chromosomes have genes for similar traits arranged in similar order. For example, persons with albinism are unable to make the pigment melanin, which is responsible for most of the color of skin, hair, and eyes. Let us say that the recipe for producing melanin is encoded in a gene that we will specify as *A*. We can symbolize the abnormal (mutated) version of this gene as *a*. In a normal person with no history of albinism both members of the pair of chromosomes that code for melanin production will contain a normal gene (*A*). In a person who is a genetic carrier for albinism, one chromosome will carry a normal gene (*A*) and the other chromosome will carry the abnormal gene (*a*). An albino will have two defective genes (*aa*). Thus, every individual will have one of the following genetic makeups, or **genotypes** (**jee'**-no-types): *AA*, *Aa*, or *aa*.

When the two genes for the same trait are the same, for example, *AA* or *aa*, the individual is said to have a **homozygous** (ho-mow-**zy'**-gus) **genotype** for the trait. When the two genes for a trait are different, the individual has a **heterozygous** (het-er-oh-**zy'**-gus) **genotype** for that trait.

In albinism (as in most genetic disorders) the normal gene is the **dominant gene**; when present, it dominates over the abnormal gene. The abnor-

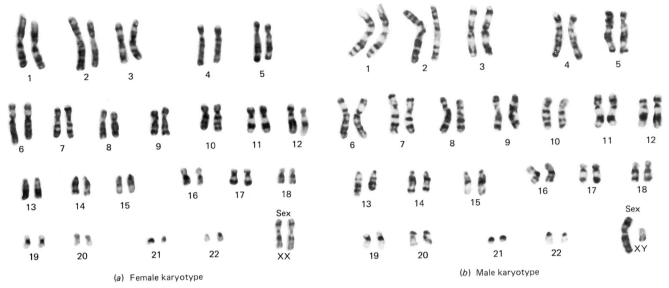

**Figure 22–3.** Human chromosomes. By careful study of such chromosome photographs, known as karyotypes, it is possible to diagnose some hereditary diseases. Such diagnoses can often be made before birth from cells sloughed off into the amniotic fluid surrounding the fetus. The fluid can be sampled by the process known as amniocentesis.

mal gene (a) is a **recessive gene**. It is expressed only in the absence of a normal counterpart. For this reason, a person must have two abnormal genes for melanin production to be an albino (Fig. 22–5). The term **phenotype (fee'-no-type)** refers to how the genes are expressed. A person with two normal genes (AA) for melanin production has a different genotype than a carrier for albinism (Aa) but both have a normal phenotype for pigmentation.

Many genes are not clearly dominant or recessive. They may be codominant, in which case both are fully expressed (this is true in human blood types), or they may be incompletely dominant, in which the trait expressed tends to be a compromise. The expression and interaction of genes can be quite complex. A single gene may have multiple effects, for example.

In analyzing the probable combinations of genes, special charts called **Punnett squares** can be constructed (Fig. 22–5). The types of eggs can be represented across the top and the types of sperm indicated along the left side of the square. The squares are then filled with the resulting zygote

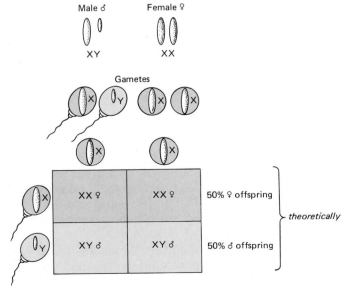

**Figure 22–4.** The inheritance of sex. Sex is determined by the sperm at the moment of fertilization. When the egg is fertilized by an X-bearing sperm, the offspring will be female. When the egg is fertilized by a Y-bearing sperm, the zygote will contain an X and a Y chromosome and the offspring will be male.

*Figure 22–5. Normal skin color is dominant over albinism. (a) The cross between a homozygous normal and an albino parent produces an offspring with a normal phenotype. However, notice that the offspring is a carrier for albinism. (b) The offspring of two heterozygous parents can result in three possible genetic combinations in the offspring. There is a 25% chance that the child will be homozygous normal; a 50% chance that the child will be normal but a carrier for albinism; and a 25% probability that the child will be an albino.*

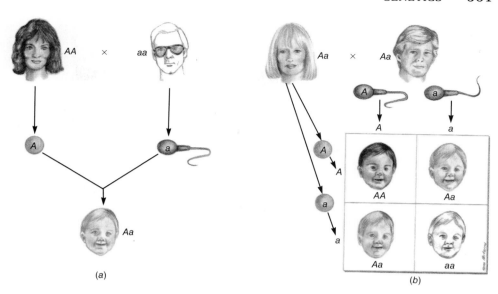

(a)

(b)

combinations so that the letters in each square indicate the genotype of one genetic type of offspring.

## CHROMOSOMES AND DISEASE

Occasionally something goes wrong and a pair of chromosomes fails to separate duing meiosis or sometimes a part of a chromosome may break off and attach to another chromosome. Having three (instead of two) of one kind of chromosome is called a **trisomy**. A trisomy can result in serious imbalance of body chemistry (because the extra genes may be causing production of extra proteins). Trisomies of most chromosome pairs are lethal and result in spontaneous abortion. Trisomy of chromosome 21 results in **Down's syndrome**, a disorder characterized by profound mental retardation, short stature, an epicanthic skin fold, cardiac defects, and other deformities (Fig. 22–6). The frequency of Down's syndrome is about 1 in 700 live births and the disorder is most common in the offspring of older women.

## GENES AND DISEASE

Genetic diseases result from genetic mutations. A **mutation** (mew-**tay′**-shun) is an abrupt, permanent change in a gene that causes it to have a different effect than it originally had. Radiation and exposure to certain chemicals and drugs can cause mutations. However, we do not understand the causes of all mutations. Many mutations occur

when chromosomes are being duplicated. A mistake in the assembly of subunits of DNA can change the code so that it no longer contains the information needed to produce the particular protein. Among the disorders linked to mutations are sickle cell anemia, hemophilia (bleeder's disease), cystic fibrosis, Tay-Sachs disease, and phenylketonuria (PKU).

### Genetic Counseling

Couples who have had one abnormal child or who have a familial history of hereditary disease may seek genetic counseling. Genetic clinics offering such counseling are available in most metropolitan centers. Modern enzyme analysis and other sophisticated chemical techniques can now be used to detect many recessive genetic diseases in the heterozygous state. Carriers of many genetic diseases can be identified by analyzing blood samples. Screening programs have been set up in more than 50 major cities for Tay-Sachs disease, a degenerative neurological disease that causes death in early childhood.

When both parents are known to be carriers for a genetic disease, the fetus can be evaluated early in development. Amniocentesis is used to remove samples of amniotic fluid. Then embryonic cells found in the fluid can be analyzed.

Some genetic diseases are now treatable. In phenylketonuria (PKU) an enzyme needed to metabolize a common amino acid (phenylalanine) is lacking. When untreated, a high percentage of children with PKU become mentally retarded. When treated with a special diet (low in phenylalanine), mental retardation is prevented. In many states all babies are routinely screened during the first days of life for this genetic disease.

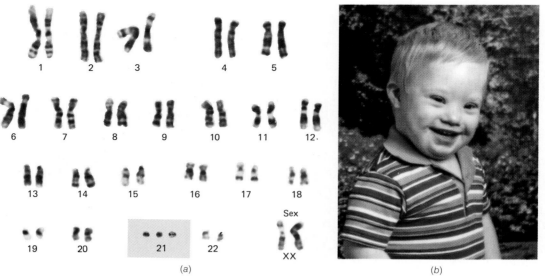

**Figure 22–6.** Downs syndrome, a disease usually associated with trisomy of the 21st chromosome. (a) A karyotype (photomicrograph of the chromosomes) of a child with Downs syndrome. Note the extra chromosome 21. (b) A 2-year-old boy with Downs syndrome. (Courtesy of Mr. and Mrs. Beny Peretz.)

## FOCUS ON
## Some Chromosome Abnormalities

| Aneuploidy | Common Name | Description |
|---|---|---|
| Trisomy 13 | | Multiple defects, with death by 1–3 months |
| Trisomy 15 | | Multiple defects, with death by 1–3 months |
| Trisomy 18 | | Ear deformities, heart defects, spasticity, and other damage; death by 1 year |
| Trisomy 21 | Down's syndrome (mongolism) | Overall frequency is about 1 in 700 live births; true trisomy usually found among children of older (40+) mothers, but translocation resulting in equivalent of trisomy may occur in children of younger women; a 35-year-old mother has 1:200 chance of producing mongoloid child; a 40-year-old mother has 1:50 chance of doing so, and the risk at 44 is 1:20; epicanthic skin fold, though not same as that in Mongolian race, produces superficial resemblance, hence older name "mongolian idiocy"; varying degrees of mental retardation, usually IQ below 70, though more intelligent exceptions are known; Short stature, protruding furrowed tongue, transverse palmar crease, cardiac deformities common; patients usually die by age 30–35, 50% die by age 3 or 4; unusually susceptible to leukemia and respiratory infections; females are fertile if they live to sexual maturity, producing 50% mongoloid offspring |
| Trisomy 22 | | Similar to Down's syndrome but with more skeletal deformities |
| XO | Turner's syndrome | Female with short stature, webbed neck, sometimes slight mental retardation; ovaries degenerate in late embryonic life, leading to rudimentary sexual characteristics; similar disorders occur sometimes in XX individuals, perhaps resulting from abnormalities of X-chromosome inactivation and, very rarely, in XY individuals |
| XXY | Klinefelter's syndrome | Male with slowly degenerating testes, enlarged breasts, and developing eunuchoidism |
| XYY | | Unusually tall male, heavy acne, some tendency to mild mental retardation |
| XXX | | Despite triploid X chromosomes, usually fertile, normal females |
| Short 5 | Cri-du-chat | Microcephaly, severe mental retardation. In infancy, cry resembles that of cat. Defective chromosome is heterozygous. |

## SUMMARY

I. Each chromosome contains thousands of genes; the genes are composed of DNA.
   A. A gene is a sequence of DNA that codes for a specific protein.
   B. Every human cell (except the sex cells) contains 23 pairs of chromosomes.
II. Gender of the offspring is determined by the sperm cell at the moment of fertilization.
   A. If an X-bearing sperm fertilizes the egg the offspring will be female.
   B. If a Y-bearing sperm fertilizes the egg the offspring will be male.
III. A dominant gene dominates over a recessive gene. An individual exhibits the phenotype for the recessive trait only when the genotype is homozygous.
IV. Genetic diseases result from mutations.
   A. Down's syndrome, a trisomy of chromosome 21, is an example of a chromosomal disorder.
   B. A mutation is a permanent change in a gene that causes it to have a different effect than it had before the change.
   C. Mutations may be caused by radiation or by exposure to certain chemicals and drugs.
   D. Diseases caused by mutations include hemophilia, sickle cell anemia, and PKU.

## POST TEST

1. The branch of biology concerned with heredity is _____.
2. Genes are found within _____.
3. A gene is a sequence of _____ that codes for a specific protein.
4. Each human cell contains _____ pairs of chromosomes, or a total of _____ chromosomes.
5. Gametes are formed by a special type of cell division called _____.
6. When a Y-bearing sperm fertilizes an ovum the offspring will be _____.
7. The term _____ refers to an individual's genetic makeup, whereas the term _____ refers to how the genes are expressed.
8. The gene for normal pigmentation is _____ over the gene for albinism.
9. Having three of one type of chromosome is a condition referred to as _____.
10. A _____ is an abrupt, permanent change in a gene.

## REVIEW QUESTIONS

1. What do you think would happen if eggs and sperm cells contained 46 chromosomes like other cells?
2. In former days a king would sometimes dispose of his queen if she did not produce a male heir to the throne for him? Was this genetically justified? Why or why not?
3. How could two people with normal skin pigmentation have an albino child? Explain.
4. Use a Punnett square to show the probability that a homozygous man and a woman who is a carrier for PKU could have a baby with PKU.
5. In what ways is genetic counseling useful?

# Appendices

# Dissecting Terms
## Common Prefixes, Suffixes, and Word Roots

*Your task of mastering new terms will be greatly simplified if you learn to dissect each new word. Many terms can be divided into a prefix (the part of the word that precedes the main root), the word root itself, and often a suffix (a word ending that may add to or modify the meaning of the root). As you progress in your study of anatomy and physiology, you will learn to recognize the more common prefixes, word roots, and suffixes. Such recognition will help you analyze new terms so that you can determine their meaning and will also help you remember them.*

## PREFIXES

**a-, ab-** from, away, apart (*ab*duct, lead away, move away from the midline of the body)

**a-, an-** un-, -less, lack, not (*a*symmetrical, not symmetrical)

**ad-** (also **af-, ag-, an-, ap-**) to, toward (*ad*duct, move toward the midline of the body)

**ambi-** both sides (*ambi*dextrous, able to use either hand)

**ante-** forward, before (*ante*flexion, bending forward)

**anti-** against (*anti*coagulant, a substance that prevents coagulation of blood)

**bi-** two (*bi*ceps, a muscle with two heads of origin)

**bio-** life (*bio*logy, the study of life)

**brady-** slow (*brady*cardia, abnormally slow heart beat)

**circum-, circ-** around (*circum*cision, a cutting around)

**co-, con-** with, together (*con*genital, existing with or before birth)

**contra-** against (*contra*ception, against conception)

**crypt-** hidden (*crypt*orchidism, undescended or hidden testes)

**cyt-** cell (*cyt*ology, the study of cells)

**di-** two (*di*saccharide, a compound made of two sugar molecules chemically combined)

**dis-** (also **di-** or **dif-**) apart, un-, not (*dis*sect, cut apart)

**dys-** painful, difficult (*dys*pnea, difficult breathing)

**end-, endo-** within, inner (*endo*plasmic reticulum, a network of membranes found within the cytoplasm)

**epi-** on, upon (*epi*dermis, upon the dermis)

**eu-** good, well (*eu*phoria, a sense of well-being)

**ex-, e-, ef-** out from, out of (*ex*tension, a straightening out)

**extra-** outside, beyond (*extra*embryonic membrane, a membrane such as the amnion that protects the embryo)

**hemi-** half (cerebral *hemi*sphere, lateral half of the cerebrum)

**hetero-** other, different (*hetero*geneous, made of different substances)

**homo-, hom-** same (*homo*logous, corresponding in structure)

**hyper-** excessive, above normal (*hyper*secretion, excessive secretion)

**hypo-** under, below, deficient (*hypo*dermic, below the skin; *hypo*thyroidism, insufficiency of thyroid hormones)

**in-, im-** not (*im*balance, condition in which there is no balance)

**inter-** between, among (*inter*stitial, situated between parts)

**intra-** within (*intra*cellular, within the cell)

**iso-** equal, like (*iso*tonic, equal strength)

**mal-** bad, abnormal (*mal*nutrition, poor nutrition)

**mega-** large, great (*mega*karyocyte, giant cell of bone marrow)

**meta-** after, beyond (*meta*phase, the stage of mitosis after prophase)

**neo-** (*neo*natal, newborn during the first 4 weeks after birth)

**oo-** egg (*oo*cyte, developing egg cell)

**oligo-** small, deficient (*oligo*uria, abnormally small volume of urine)

**para-** near, beside, beyond (*para*central, near the center)

**peri-** around (*peri*cardial membrane, membrane that surrounds the heart)
**poly-** multiple, complex (*poly*saccharide, a carbohydrate composed of many simple sugars)
**post-** after, behind (*post*natal, after birth)
**pre-** before (*pre*natal, before birth)

**retro-** backward (*retro*peritoneal, located behind the peritoneum)

**semi-** half (*semi*lunar, half-moon)
**sub-** under (*sub*cutaneous tissue, tissue immediately under the skin)
**super-, supra-** above (*supra*renal, above the kidney)
**syn-** with, together (*syn*drome, a group of symptoms that occur together and characterize a disease)

**trans-** across, beyond (*trans*port, carry across)

## SUFFIXES

**-able, -ible** able (vi*able*, able to live)
**-ac** pertaining to (cardi*ac*, pertaining to the heart)
**-ad** used in anatomy to form adverbs of direction (cephal*ad*, toward the head)
**-asis, -asia, -esis** condition or state of (hemost*asis*, stopping of bleeding)

**-cide** kill, destroy (bio*cide*, substance that kills living things)

**-ectomy** surgical removal (append*ectomy*, surgical removal of the appendix)
**-emia** condition of blood (an*emia*, without enough blood)

**-gen** something produced or generated or something that produces or generates (patho*gen*, something that can cause disease)
**-gram** record, write (electrocardio*gram*, a record of the electrical activity of the heart)
**-graph** record, write (electrocardio*graph*, an instrument for recording the electrical activity of the heart)

**-itis** inflammation of (appendic*itis*, inflammation of the appendix)

**-logy** study or science of (physio*logy*, study of the function of the body)

**-oid** like, in the form of (thyr*oid*, in the form of a shield)
**-oma** tumor (carcin*oma*, a malignant tumor)
**-osis** indicates disease (psych*osis*, a mental disease)
**-ous, -ose** full of (poison*ous*, full of poison)

**-scope** instrument for viewing or observing (micro*scope*, instrument for viewing small objects)
**-stomy** refers to a surgical procedure in which an artifical opening is made (colo*stomy*, surgical formation of an artificial anus)

**-tomy** cutting or section (append*ectomy*, cutting out the appendix)

**-uria** refers to urine (poly*uria*, excessive production of urine)

## SOME COMMON WORD ROOTS

**aden** gland, glandular (*aden*osis, a glandular disease)
**alg** pain (neur*alg*ia, nerve pain)
**arthr** joint (*arthr*itis, inflammation of the joints)

**bi, bio** life (*bio*logy, study of life)
**blast** a formative cell, germ layer (osteo*blast*, cell that gives rise to bone cells)
**brachi** arm (*brachi*al artery, blood vessel that supplies the arm)
**bronch** branch of the trachea (*bronch*itis, inflammation of the bronchi)
**bry** grow, swell (em*bry*o, an organism in the early stages of development)

**carcin** cancer (*carcin*ogenic, cancer-producing)
**cardi** heart (*cardi*ac, pertaining to the heart)
**cephal** head (*cephal*ad, toward the head)
**cerebr** brain (*cerebr*al, pertaining to the brain)
**cervic, cervix** neck (*cervic*al, pertaining to the neck)
**chol** bile (*chol*ecystogram, an x-ray of the gallbladder)
**chondr** cartilage (*chondr*ocyte, a cartilage cell)
**chrom** color (*chrom*osome, deeply staining body in nucleus)
**cran** skull (*cran*ial, pertaining to the skull)
**cyt** cell (*cyt*ology, study of the cells)

**derm** skin (*derm*atology, study of the skin)
**duct, duc** lead (*duct*, passageway)

**ecol** dwelling, house (*ecol*ogy, the study of organisms in relation to their environment)
**enter** intestine (*enter*itis, inflammation of the intestine)
**evol** to unroll (*evol*ution, descent of complex organisms from simpler ancestors)

**gastr** stomach (*gastr*itis, inflammation of the stomach)
**gen** generate, produce (*gen*e, a hereditary factor)
**glyc, glyco** sweet, sugar (*glyc*ogen, storage form of glucose)
**gon** semen, seed (*gon*ad, an organ producing gametes)

**hem, em** blood (*hem*atology, the study of blood)
**hepat, hepar** liver (*hepat*itis, inflammation of the liver)
**hist** tissue (*hist*ology, study of tissues)
**hom, homeo** same, unchanging, steady (*homeo*stasis, reaching a steady state)
**hydr** water (*hydr*olysis, a breakdown reaction involving water)

**leuk** white (*leuk*ocyte, white blood cell)

**macro** large (*macro*phage, large janitor cell)

**mamm** breast (*mamm*ary glands, the glands that produce milk to nourish the young)

**micro** small (*micro*scope, instrument for viewing small objects)

**morph** form (*morph*ogenesis, development of body form)

**my, mys** muscle (*my*ocardium, muscle layer of the heart)

**nephr** kidney (*nephr*on, microscopic unit of the kidney)

**neur, nerv** nerve (*neur*algia, pain associated with nerve)

**neutr** neither one nor the other (*neutr*on, a subatomic particle that is neither positively nor negatively charged)

**occiput** back part of the head (*occip*ital, back region of the head)

**ost, oss** bone (*ost*eology, study of bones)

**path** disease (*path*ologist, one who studies disease processes)

**ped** child (*ped*iatrics, branch of medicine specializing in children)

**ped, pod** foot (bi*ped*, organism with two feet)

**phag** eat (*phag*ocytosis, process by which certain cells ingest particles and foreign matter)

**phil** love (hydro*phil*ic, a substance that attracts water)

**proct** anus (*proct*oscope, instrument for examining rectum and anal canal)

**psych** mind (*psych*ology, study of the mind)

**scler** hard (athero*scler*osis, hardening of the arterial wall)

**som** body (chromo*som*e, deeply staining body in the nucleus)

**stas, stat** stand (*stas*is, condition in which blood stands, as opposed to flowing)

**thromb** clot (*thromb*us, a clot within the body)

**ur** urea, urine (*ur*ologist, a physician specializing in the urinary tract)

**visc** pertaining to an internal organ or body cavity (*visc*era, internal organs)

# APPENDIX B
# The Metric System

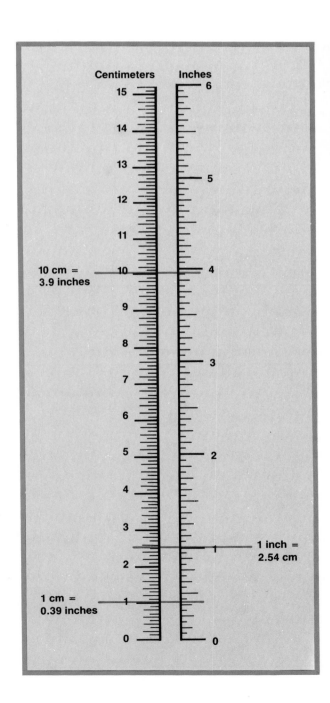

## Think Metric!

A 154-lb person weighs 70 kilograms (kg).

A 5′ 6″ person is 165 cm long.

You are driving down the highway at 85.8 km per hour. That is the same speed as 55 mph.

A 70-kg human male has 5.6 liters of blood. That is about 6 quarts.

## APOTHECARY SYSTEM OF WEIGHT AND VOLUME*

| Metric weight | | Apothecary weight | Metric volume | | Apothecary volume |
|---|---|---|---|---|---|
| 30 g | = | 1 ounce | 1,000 ml | = | 1 quart |
| 15 g | = | 4 drams | 500 ml | = | 1 pint |
| 10 g | = | 2.5 drams | 250 ml | = | 8 fl ounces |
| 4 g | = | 60 grains | 90 ml | = | 3 fl ounces |
| | | (= 1 dram) | 30 ml | = | 1 fl ounce |
| 2 g | = | 30 grains | | | |
| 1 g | = | 15 grains | | | |

*Used by pharmacists in preparing medications.

**Temperature conversions**

$$°C = \frac{(°F - 32) \times 5}{9}$$

$$°F = \frac{°C \times 9}{5} + 32$$

**Some equivalents**

1°C = 1.8°F

10°C = 18°F

16°C = 61°F

# Think Celsius!

**When room temperature is 20°C, you should not feel cold. That is the same as 68°F.**

**When the temperature reaches 100°C, water boils.**

**At 0°C, water freezes.**

**Normal human body temperature is about 37°C.**

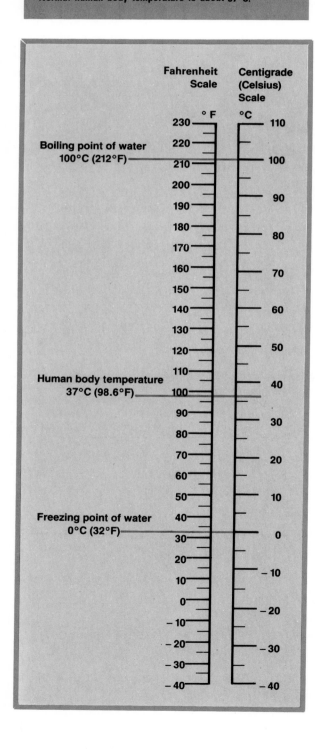

**Fahrenheit Scale** / **Centigrade (Celsius) Scale**

Boiling point of water 100°C (212°F)

Human body temperature 37°C (98.6°F)

Freezing point of water 0°C (32°F)

## SOME COMMON UNITS OF VOLUME

| Unit | Abbreviation | Equivalent |
|---|---|---|
| liter | l | approximately 1.06 qt |
| milliliter | ml | $10^{-3}$ l (1 ml = 1 cm$^3$ = 1 cc) |
| microliter | $\mu$l | $10^{-6}$ l |

**Volume conversions**

| | | | |
|---|---|---|---|
| 1 tsp = 5 ml | | 1 ml = 0.03 fl oz | |
| 1 tbsp = 15 ml | | 1 l = 2.1 pt | |
| 1 fl oz = 30 ml | | 1 l = 1.06 qt | |
| 1 cup = 0.241 l | | 1 l = 0.26 gal | |
| 1 pt = 0.47 l | | | |
| 1 qt = 9.95 l | | | |
| 1 gal = 3.8 l | | | |

| *To convert* | *Multiply by* | *To obtain* |
|---|---|---|
| fluid ounces | 30 | milliliters |
| quart | 0.95 | liters |
| milliliters | 0.03 | fluid ounces |
| liters | 1.06 | quarts |

## SOME COMMON UNITS OF WEIGHT

| Unit | Abbreviation | Equivalent |
|---|---|---|
| kilogram | kg | $10^3$ g (approximately 2.2 lb) |
| gram | g | approximately 0.035 oz |
| milligram | mg | $10^{-3}$ g |
| microgram | $\mu$g | $10^{-6}$ g |
| nanogram | ng | $10^{-9}$ g |
| picogram | pg | $10^{-12}$ g |

**Weight conversions**

| | | |
|---|---|---|
| 1 oz = 28.3 g | 1 g = 0.035 oz | |
| 1 lb = 453.6 g | 1 kg = 2.2 lb | |
| 1 lb = 0.45 kg | | |

| *To convert* | *Multiply by* | *To obtain* |
|---|---|---|
| cunces | 28.3 | grams |
| pounds | 453.6 | grams |
| pounds | 0.45 | kilograms |
| grams | 0.035 | ounces |
| kilograms | 2.2 | pounds |

# APPENDIX C
# Post Test Answers

## CHAPTER 1

1. anatomy; physiology
2. molecules
3. cells
4. organs
5. endocrine
6. homeostasis
7. d
8. b
9. f
10. c
11. e
12. a
13. b
14. f
15. e
16. a
17. g
18. sagittal
19. transverse (cross)
20. axial; appendicular
21. viscera
22. b
23. c
24. d
25. e
26. a
27. f
28. diaphragm

## CHAPTER 2

1. electrons
2. $CaCl_2$
3. ionic
4. cations
5. right
6. electrons
7. acid
8. alkaline (basic); acidic
9. pH
10. carbon
11. b
12. e
13. c
14. d
15. a

## CHAPTER 3

1. d
2. b
3. c
4. f
5. e
6. h
7. g
8. a
9. cell; surrounding solution
10. phagocytosis
11. energy
12. mitosis
13. d
14. a
15. c
16. c
17. b
18. ducts
19. connective
20. hormones

## CHAPTER 4

1. integumentary
2. epidermis; dermis
3. basale
4. keratin
5. corneum
6. subcutaneous tissue
7. follicle
8. Sebaceous; sebum
9. water; salts
10. keratin
11. pigment cells
12. inflammation
13. swelling; redness; heat; pain
14. first
15. nines
16. basal cell carcinoma

## CHAPTER 5

1. marrow
2. periosteum
3. diaphysis
4. osteons
5. lacunae
6. break down bone
7. axial
8. cranial; facial
9. Sinuses
10. spinal cord
11. pectoral girdle
12. thoracic
13. centrum
14. synarthroses
15. Synovial
16. flexion; abduction
17. hinge
18. b
19. d
20. e
21. a
22. c
23. h
24. g
25. f

## CHAPTER 6

1. fibers
2. endomysium
3. myosin; actin
4. motor neuron
5. calcium ions
6. ATP
7. energy
8. muscle tone
9. antagonist
10. synergists
11. d
12. b
13. e
14. a
15. c
16. g
17. f.
18. see Figure 6—7

## CHAPTER 7

1. brain; spinal cord
2. peripheral
3. afferent
4. glial
5. neurons
6. cell body
7. axon
8. neurotransmitter
9. ganglion; nucleus
10. reception
11. synapse
12. sensory; association; motor
13. sodium
14. refractory period
15. sodium pumps
16. dura mater
17. cerebrospinal fluid
18. ventricles
19. brain stem
20. d
21. c
22. b
23. a
24. f
25. b
26. c
27. a
28. see Figure 7—8

## CHAPTER 8

1. somatic
2. optic; vagus
3. VII; facial
4. olfactory; olfactory bulbs of cerebrum
5. cochlea; organs of equilibrium in inner ear
6. 8; 12
7. sensory fibers
8. plexus
9. dermatome
10. autonomic
11. sympathetic
12. acetylcholine
13. norepinephrine
14. sympathetic
15. parasympathetic.
16. see Figure 8—3

## CHAPTER 9

1. h
2. d
3. a
4. e
5. i
6. b
7. f
8. g
9. g
10. d
11. e
12. a
13. f
14. b
15. c
16. h
17. see Figures 9—1 and 9—3

# CHAPTER 10

1. ducts; hormones
2. chemical messenger
3. cyclic AMP
4. hypothalamus
5. oxytocin
6. prolactin
7. anterior lobe of the pituitary gland
8. hypothalamus
9. posterior lobe of the pituitary gland
10. pituitary dwarf
11. metabolism
12. raise blood sugar level
13. insulin
14. diabetes mellitus
15. cortisol
16. calcium
17. pituitary gland; adrenal gland

# CHAPTER 11

1. oxygen
2. plasma
3. antibodies
4. clotting
5. bone marrow
6. anemia
7. defend against disease organisms
8. white blood cell
9. bone marrow
10. fibrin; thrombin
11. thrombus
12. B; A
13. Rh; Rh negative; Rh positive

# CHAPTER 12

1. pericardium
2. outer
3. myocardium
4. interventricular septum
5. mitral
6. semilunar
7. papillary
8. sinoatrial (SA) node
9. Purkinje fibers
10. intercalated discs
11. systole; diastole
12. stroke volume
13. cardiac output
14. parasympathetic (vagus); sympathetic (accelerator)
15. venous return
16. all the blood delivered to it
17. P; atria
18. see Figure 12–4

# CHAPTER 13

1. arteries
2. capillaries
3. blood; pressure
4. systemic
5. pulmonary trunk (artery)
6. oxygen-rich
7. aorta
8. common iliac
9. superior vena cava
10. aorta; common; subclavian
11. coronary; right atrium
12. circle of Willis
13. internal carotid; vertebral
14. hepatic portal; liver
15. renal; inferior vena cava
16. pulse
17. blood pressure
18. blood pressure
19. returns interstitial fluid to blood; defends body against disease by producing lymphocytes; absorbs lipids from intestine
20. lymph tissue
21. filter lymph; produce lymphocytes
22. lymphatics
23. blood
24. thymus
25. lymph
26. see Figure 13–5

# CHAPTER 14

1. pathogens
2. redness; heat; swelling (edema); pain
3. phagocytes
4. phagocytosis
5. interferon
6. antigens
7. antibodies
8. antibody
9. cell
10. memory cells
11. antigens
12. complement
13. passive
14. immunization
15. graft rejection
16. allergens; IgE antibody; mast

# CHAPTER 15

1. larynx; trachea
2. alveoli
3. diaphragm
4. epiglottis
5. cough reflex
6. visceral pleura
7. alveoli
8. breathing
9. inspiration; expiration
10. hemoglobin
11. phrenic
12. constriction
13. see Figure 15–1

# CHAPTER 16

1. ingestion
2. Digestion
3. mucosa
4. visceral peritoneum
5. peristalsis
6. greater omentum
7. 32
8. crown; root
9. dentin; enamel
10. parotids
11. polysaccharides (starch); maltose; small polysaccharides
12. rugae
13. enzymes (pepsin); hydrochloric acid
14. duodenum; jejunum; ileum
15. villi, microvilli
16. gallbladder
17. stomach mucosa; gastric glands
18. amino acids
19. villi
20. descending colon
21. see Figure 16–1

# CHAPTER 17

1. anabolism
2. catabolism
3. f
4. d
5. e
6. b
7. g
8. c
9. a
10. h
11. minerals
12. vitamins
13. starch
14. fats
15. amino acids
16. amino acids
17. negative
18. weight is gained

# CHAPTER 18

1. excretion
2. liver; kidneys
3. ureter
4. renal pelvis
5. renal corpuscle; renal tubule
6. renal cortex; renal medulla
7. glomerulus; Bowman's capsule
8. afferent
9. loop of Henle
10. filtration; Bowman's capsule
11. tubular reabsorption
12. urine
13. Antidiuretic (ADH)
14. bladder
15. urethra
16. see Figure 18–4

# CHAPTER 19

1. electrolytes
2. intracellular
3. pressure; osmotic
4. extracellular
5. kidneys
6. thirst
7. ADH
8. more; small
9. greater
10. less
11. dehydration
12. edema

# CHAPTER 20

1. seminiferous; testes
2. vas deferens
3. seminal vesicles
4. testosterone
5. testes
6. estrogen; progesterone
7. c
8. b
9. e
10. d
11. a
12. ovulation
13. anterior lobe; pituitary; follicles
14. one
15. vasectomy; tubal ligation
16. see Figure 20–4

## CHAPTER 21

1. zygote
2. amnion
3. placenta
4. corpus luteum

5. umbilical cord
6. fetus
7. second

8. neonate
9. Identical
10. adolescence

## CHAPTER 22

1. genetics
2. chromosomes
3. DNA
4. 23; 46

5. meiosis
6. male
7. genotype; phenotype

8. dominant
9. trisomy
10. mutation

# Glossary/Index

Note: Page numbers in *italics* refer to illustrations; those followed by t refer to tables; **boldface** page numbers indicate pages on which index term is defined; page numbers followed by f refer to focus boxes.

377

Embolus (**em**-buh-lus) A circulating fragment of foreign matter in the blood, such as a blood clot, foreign object, cancer cells, air, or tissue.

Embryo (**em**-bree-oh) The developing human organism until the end of the second month, after which it is referred to as a fetus, **334**, *348, 349*

Embryology, **4**

Emphysema, pulmonary, **269**

Enamel, of tooth, **278**

Endocardium (en-dow-**kar**-dee-um) The inner layer of the heart wall, consisting of an endothelial lining resting upon connective tissue, **211**

Endocrine glands (**en**-doe-krin) Ductless glands that depend upon interstitial fluid and blood for transport of their secretions, which are called hormones, **50**

Endocrine system, 177–191
  disorders of, 180, 183, 185, 187, 190
  glands of, 178–179t
  hormones of, 178–179t
  mechanism of action of, 178–180
  regulation of, 180, *188*

Endogenous (en-**dodj**-e-nus) Produced within the body or due to internal causes.

Endolymph (**en**-doe-limf) The fluid of the membranous labyrinth of the ear, **170**

Endometrium, **334**

Endomysium (en-doe-**mis**-ee-um) The connective tissue between the fibers of a muscle bundle, **103**

Endoplasmic reticulum (**en**-doe-plas-mik ret-**ik**-yoo-lum) Intracellular system of membranes continuous with the cell membrane; functions in intracellular transport of materials, *39*, **40**

Endorphins (en-**dor**-fins) Peptides in the central nervous system that affect pain perception and other aspects of behavior; may function as neurotransmitters, **137**

Endosteum (en-**dos**-tee-um) The thin layer of connective tissue lining the marrow cavity of a bone, **72**

Endothelium (en-doe-**theel**-ee-um) The simple epithelial tissue that lines the cavities of the heart and of the blood and lymph vessels, 211

Energy
  and metabolism, 294, 298, 301
  and valence electrons, 27–29, *28*

Environmental influences on the human embryo, 351, 352t

Enzyme (**en**-zime) An organic protein catalyst that promotes or regulates a biochemical reaction, **32**, 40–41, 280, 285

Eosinophil (e-o-**sin**-o-fil) A type of white blood cell,

Epidermis (ep-i-**dur**-mis) The outermost layer of the skin, including dead cells of the stratum corneum and the living sublayers of cells that give rise to them, **60**–61, *61*

Epididymis (ep-i-**did**-i-mis) pl. epididymides (ep-i-**did**-i-my-deez) A coiled tube that receives sperm from the testes and conveys it to the vas deferens, **331**

Epidural space, **140**

Epiglottis, 263, 281

Epimysium (ep-i-**miz**-ee-um) The sheath of connective tissue surrounding a muscle, **103**

Epinephrine (ep-i-**nef**-rin) The chief hormone of the adrenal medulla; stimulates the sympathetic nervous system, 188–189

Epiphysis (e-**pif**-i-sis) The end of a long bone, usually wider than the shaft and either made entirely of cartilage or separated from the shaft by a disc of cartilage, **72**

Episiotomy, 351

Epithelial tissue (ep-i-**theel**-ee-al) The type of tissue that covers body surfaces, lines body cavities, and forms glands; also called epithelium, **47**–50, 48t, 49t

Equilibrium, **171**

Erectile dysfunction, 339

Erection of penis, 332

Erythroblastosis fetalis, 205

Erythrocytes (e-**rith**-ro-sites) Red blood cells, 198–199

Erythropoietin (e-rith-row-**poy**-e-tin) A hormone that regulates production of red blood cells.

Erythropoiesis (e-rith-row-poy-**ee**-sis) The production of red blood cells.

Esophagus (e-**sof**-ah-gus) The muscular tube extending from the pharynx to the stomach, 280–281, *280*

Essential amino acids, **300**

Estrogens (**es**-tro-jins) Female sex hormones produced mainly by the ovaries, **333**

Ethmoid. See *Bones, individual; by region.*

Eunuch, **332**

Eustachian tube (you-**stay**-shun) A canal connecting the middle ear with the pharynx; also known as the auditory tube, **169**

Excretion (ek-**skree**-shun) The discharge from the body of a waste product of metabolism (not to be confused with the elimination of undigested food materials), 47

Exhalation. See *Expiration.*

Exocrine gland (**ex**-so-krin) A gland that delivers its secretions to an epithelial surface, usually by way of a duct, **50**

Exogenous (ek-**sodj**-e-nus) Due to or produced by an external cause; not arising within the body.

Expiration, **265**

Extension (ex-**sten**-shun) A straightening out, especially the muscular movement by which a flexed part is made straight.

External auditory meatus, **169**

Exteroceptors (ek-stur-o-**sep**-tors) Sense organs that receive sensory stimuli from the outside world, **166**

Extrinsic muscle (ex-**trin**-sik) A muscle that operates a body part but is located outside of the part it operates.

Eye, 166–169, *167*
  disorders of, 168–169f

Fallopian tube (fa-**low**-pee-un) The uterine tube, **333**

Fascicle (**fas**-i-kul) pl. fasciculi A small bundle or cluster, especially of nerve or muscle fibers, **103**

Fat, 286t
  absorption of, 287
  saturated and unsaturated, 298–299

Feces, 288–289

Feedback systems, 180

Femur, **90**, *92*

Fertilization (fur-ti-li-**zay**-shun) Union of male and female gametes, **330**, 339

Fetal membranes, 348

Fetus, **349**–351

Fever, **247**

Fibrillation (fib-ri-**lay**-shun) Rapid uncoordinated contractions of muscle fibers, such as those in the heart, preventing effective action by the organ or muscle, 218–219

Fibrin (**figh**-brin) The fibrous insoluble protein of blood clots that is formed by the action of thrombin on fibrinogen, **203**